– Staff Library (Education Centre)

# Bone Disease in Rheumatology

**EDITORS**

## ■ MICHAEL MARICIC, M.D.

Associate Professor of Clinical Medicine
University of Arizona
Chief, Section of Rheumatology
Southern Arizona Veterans Affairs Health Care System
Tucson, Arizona

## ■ OSCAR S. GLUCK, M.D.

Codirector, The Arizona Rheumatology Center
Phoenix, Arizona
Clinical Professor, Department of Medicine
University of Arizona School of Medicine
Tucson, Arizona

◆ LIPPINCOTT WILLIAMS & WILKINS
A **Wolters Kluwer** Company
Philadelphia • Baltimore • New York • London
Buenos Aires • Hong Kong • Sydney • Tokyo

*Acquisitions Editor:* Danette Somers
*Developmental Editor:* Nicole T. Dernoski
*Production Manager:* Bridgett Dougherty
*Senior Manufacturing Manager:* Benjamin Rivera
*Marketing Manager:* Kathy Neely
*Cover Designer:* Larry Didona
*Production Services:* Nesbitt Graphics, Inc.
*Printer:* Edwards Brothers

© 2005 by LIPPINCOTT WILLIAMS & WILKINS
530 Walnut Street
Philadelphia, PA 19106 USA
LWW.com

All rights reserved. This book is protected by copyright. No part of this book may
be reproduced in any form or by any means, including photocopying, or utilized by
any information storage and retrieval system without written permission from the
copyright owner, except for brief quotations embodied in critical articles and
reviews. Materials appearing in this book prepared by individuals as part of their
official duties as U.S. government employees are not covered by the above-
mentioned copyright.

Printed in the USA

**Library of Congress Cataloging-in-Publication Data**
Bone disease in rheumatology / [edited by] Michael Maricic, Oscar S. Gluck.
   p. ; cm.
  Includes bibliographical references and index.
  ISBN 0-7817-5301-5
  1. Bone—Diseases. 2. Arthritis. 3. Rheumatism. I. Maricic, Michael J. II. Gluck,
Oscar S., 1949-2003.
  [DNLM: 1. Bone Diseases—diagnosis. 2. Bone Diseases—etiology. 3. Bone
Diseases—physiopathology. 4. Rheumatic Diseases—complications. WE 225
B71256 2005]
  RC930.B6626 2005
  616.7′2—dc22

                             2004023009

Care has been taken to confirm the accuracy of the information presented and to
describe generally accepted practices. However, the authors, editors, and publisher
are not responsible for errors or omissions or for any consequences from application of the information in this book and make no warranty, expressed or implied,
with respect to the currency, completeness, or accuracy of the contents of the publication. Application of this information in a particular situation remains the professional responsibility of the practitioner.

The authors, editors, and publisher have exerted every effort to ensure that drug
selection and dosage set forth in this text are in accordance with current recommendations and practice at the time of publication. However, in view of ongoing
research, changes in government regulations, and the constant flow of information
relating to drug therapy and drug reactions, the reader is urged to check the package
insert for each drug for any change in indications and dosage and for added warn-
ings and precautions. This is particularly important when the recommended agent
is a new or infrequently employed drug.

Some drugs and medical devices presented in this publication have Food and Drug
Administration (FDA) clearance for limited use in restricted research settings. It is
the responsibility of the health care provider to ascertain the FDA status of each
drug or device planned for use in their clinical practice.

10 9 8 7 6 5 4 3 2 1

This book is dedicated to our teachers and our families:
Alison Maricic, Rosemary and Natalie Gluck,
and Vanessa, Benjamin, and Isabelle May.

# Contributors

**JONATHAN D. ADACHI, MD, FRCP (C)** Professor, Department of Medicine, McMaster University, Head, Service of Rheumatology, St. Joseph's Hospital, Hamilton, Ontario, Canada

**ROY D. ALTMAN, MD** Professor of Medicine, Departments of Rheumatology and Immunology, David Geffen School of Medicine at UCLA, Los Angeles, California

**SHREYASEE AMIN, MDCM, FRCP (C), MPH** Rheumatology Assistant Professor, Department of Medicine, Division of Rheumatology, Mayo Clinic College of Medicine, Rochester, Minnesota

**REINA ARMAMENTO-VILLAREAL, MD** Assistant Professor of Medicine, Division of Bone and Mineral Diseases, Department of Medicine, Washington University School of Medicine, St. Louis, Missouri

**DAVID J. BAYLINK, MD** Distinguished Professor of Medicine, Department of Medicine, Loma Linda University; Chief, Musculoskeletal Disease Center, Jerry L. Pettis Veterans Affairs Medical Center, Loma Linda, California

**JOHN P. BILEZIKIAN, MD** Professor of Medicine and Pharmacology, Chief, Division of Endocrinology Medicine, College of Physicians and Surgeons, Columbia University; Attending Physician, Department of Medicine, New York Presbyterian Hospital, New York, New York

**TIM A. BONGARTZ, MD** Fellow of Rheumatology, Department of Internal Medicine I, University Hospital Regensburg, Regensburg, Germany

**LENORE M. BUCKLEY, MD, MPH** Professor, Departments of Internal Medicine and Pediatrics, Virginia Commonwealth University, Richmond, Virginia

**ERNESTO CANALIS, MD** Professor, Department of Medicine, University of Connecticut School of Medicine, Farmington, Connecticut; Director, Department of Research, St. Francis Hospital Medical Center, Hartford, Connecticut

**ROBERTO CIVITELLI, MD** Professor of Medicine, Cell Biology and Physiology, Department of Internal Medicine, Division of Bone and Mineral Diseases, Washington University School of Medicine, St. Louis, Missouri

**TANIA N. CROTTI, PHD** Harvard Medical School, Boston, Massachusettes

**JEFFREY R. CURTIS, MD, MPH** Department of Medicine, Division of Immunology and Rheumatology, University of Alabama at Birmingham; Birmingham, Alabama

**CHAD DEAL, MD** Head, Center for Osteoporosis and Metabolic Bone Disease, Cleveland Clinic Foundation, Cleveland, Ohio

**DAVID W. DEMPSTER, PHD** Professor of Clinical Pathology, Columbia University, New York, New York; Director, Regional Bone Center, Helen Hayes Hospital, West Haverstraw, New York

**ATUL A. DEODHAR, MD** Associate Professor of Medicine and Medical Director, Rheumatology Clinic Division of Arthritis and Rheumatic Diseases, Oregon Health and Science University, Portland, Oregon

**ROBIN DORE, MD** Clinical Professor of Medicine, Division of Rheumatology, David Geffen School of Medicine, University of California at Los Angeles, Los Angeles, California

**DANA FLETCHER, DO** Wayne State University, Detroit, Michigan

**ERIC P. GALL, MD** Chairman, Professor, Department of Medicine, Rosalind Franklin University of Medicine and Science, The Chicago Medical School, North Chicago, Illinois

**LORA GIANGREGORIO, B.SC.** PhD Candidate, Kinesiology, McMaster University, Hamilton, Ontario

**OSCAR S. GLUCK, MD** Codirector, The Arizona Rheumatology Center, Phoenix, Arizona; Clinical Professor Department of Medicine, University of Arizona School of Medicine, Tuscon, Arizona

**DEBORAH T. GOLD, PHD** Associate Professor of Medical Sociology, Department of Psychiatry and Behavioral Sciences, Duke University Medical Center, Durham, North Carolina

**STEVEN R. GOLDRING, MD** Beth Israel Deaconess Medical Center, Harvard Medical School, Boston, Massachusetts

**ELLEN M. GRAVALLESE, MD** Associate Professor of Medicine, Havard Medical School, Attending Rheumatologist, Department of Medicine, Beth Israel Deaconess Medical Center; Boston, Massachusetts

**MARC C. HOCHBERG, MD, MPH** Professor of Medicine and Head, Division of Rheumatology and Clinical Immunology, Department of Medicine, University of Maryland School of Medicine; Baltimore, Maryland

**MICHAEL KLEEREKOPER, MD, FACE** Department of Internal Medicine, Wayne State University; Detroit, Michigan

**CHIN LEE, MD** Attending Physician, Division of Rheumatology, Department of Medicine, Northwestern Memorial Hospital, Instructor of Medicine, Northwestern University, The Feinberg School of Medicine, Chicago, Illinois

**JEFFREY R. LISSE, MD** Professor of Medicine, Department of Internal Medicine, University Medical Center, Acting Chief, Section of Rheumatology, University of Arizona, Tucson, Arizona

**SUSAN MANZI, MD, MPH** Associate Professor of Medicine and Epidemiology, Department of Medicine, Division of Rheumatology, University of Pittsburgh, Pittsburgh, Pennsylvania

**MICHAEL MARICIC, MD,** Associate Professor of Clinical Medicine, University of Arizona; Chief, Section of Rheumatology, Southern Arizona Veterans Affairs Health Care System, Tucson, Arizona

**FIONA M.F. MCQUEEN, MBCHB, MD, FRACP** Associate Professor, Department of Molecular Medicine, Faculty of Medicine and Health Sciences, University of Auckland, Consultant Rheumatologist, Department of Rheumatology, Auckland City Hospital, Auckland, New Zealand

**JOAN M. MEYER, PHD** Proctor and Gamble, Inc.

**PAUL D. MILLER, MD** Clinical Professor of Medicine, University of Colorado Health Science Center, Denver, Colorado; Medical Director, Colorado Center for Bone Research, Lakewood, Colorado

**MIHAIL MOROIANU, MD** Wayne State University, Detroit, Michigan

**ANGELIA D. MOSLEY-WILLIAMS, MD, MS** Assistant Professor, Department of Internal Medicine, Wayne State University, Chief of Rheumatology, Department of Internal Medicine, John D. Dingell Veterans Administration Medical Center, Detroit, Michigan

**DOROTHY A. NELSON, PHD** Professor, Department of Internal Medicine, Wayne State University School of Medicine, Detroit, Michigan

**A. PAPAIOANNU, MD** Associate Professor, Department of Medicine, McMaster University; Geriatrician, Department of Medicine, Hamilton Health Sciences, Hamilton, Ontario

**ALLISON R. PETTIT, PHD** C.J. Martin Research Fellow, Institute for Molecular Bioscience, University of Queensland, St. Lucia, Australia

**ROSALIND RAMSEY-GOLDMAN, MD, DRPH** Professor of Medicine, Department of Medicine, Division of Rheumatology, Northwestern University Feinberg School of Medicine; Attending, Department of Medicine, Northwestern Memorial Hospital, Chicago, Illinois

**MISHAELA R. RUBIN, MD** Instructor in Clinical Medicine, Department of Medicine, Columbia University; Assisting Attending, Department of Medicine, The Presbyterian Hospital, New York, New York

**KENNETH G. SAAG, MD, MSC** Associate Professor of Medicine, Division of Clinical Immunology and Rheumatology, University of Alabama at Birmingham, Birmingham, Alabama

**JÜRGEN SCHÖLMERICH, MD** Professor of Medicine, Chief, Department of Internal Medicine I, University Hospital Regensburg, Regensburg, Germany

**SHONNI J. SILVERBERG, MD** Professor, Department of Medicine, Columbia University, College of Physicians & Surgeons, New York, New York

**STUART L. SILVERMAN, MD, FACP, FACR** Clinical Professor, Departments of Medicine and Rheumatology, UCLA, Cedars-Sinai Medical Center, Los Angeles, California

**APURVA K. SRIVASTAVA, PHD** Assistant Resident Professor, Department of Medicine, Loma Linda University; Research Scientist, Musculoskeletal Disease Center, Loma Linda VA Health Care Systems, Loma Linda, California

**VIBEKE STRAND, MD** Adjunct Clinical Professor, Department of Immunology and Rheumatology, Stanford University, Stanford, California

**RAINER H. STRAUB, MD** Associate Professor of Medicine and Chief of Laboratory, Department of Internal Medicine I, University Hospital Regensburg, Regensburg, Germany

**ROBERT L. SWEZEY, MD, FACP, FACR, FAAPMR** Clinical Professor of Medicine, University of California—Los Angeles, Osteoporosis Prevention & Treatment Center, Los Angeles, California

**DÉSIRÉE VAN DER HEIJDE, MD, PHD** Professor of Rheumatology, Department of Rheumatology, CAPHRI Research Institute; Staff member, Department of Rheumatology; University of Maastricht, The Netherlands

**JEAN M. WEIGERT, MD** Assistant Clinical Professor, Diagnostic Radiology, University of Connecticut, Farmington, Connecticut, Director of Women's Imaging, Mandell and Blau MD's PC, New Britain, Connecticut

**DEBORAH WENKERT, MD** Associate Clinical Professor, Department of Pediatrics, St. Louis University; Pediatric Rheumatologist, Center for Metabolic Bone Disease and Molecular Research, Shriners Hospitals for Children, St. Louis, Missouri

**MICHAEL P. WHYTE, MD** Professor of Medicine, Pediatrics and Genetics, Division of Bone and Mineral Diseases, Washington University School of Medicine, St. Louis, Missouri

# Foreword

Welcome to all readers. Here at last is a text targeted primarily to rheumatologists who are charged with understanding, diagnosing, preventing, and treating periarticular and systemic bone loss in a high proportion of their patients. Every day in practice we deal with people who have limited mobility due to rheumatic diseases. We are expected to identify bone loss early enough to make a meaningful intervention that will reduce the risk of fractures. We expect it of ourselves. We are responsible for making a correct diagnosis of why bone is lost in individuals who already have reduced mobility, advancing age, menopause, and perhaps a systemic inflammatory disease. Is it "ordinary" osteoporosis, or in fact are there elements of hyperparathyroidism or osteomalacia? In older patients with low back pain, is there Paget's Disease as well as lumbar spine degenerative disease? If so, what treatments should be tried, in what order, in what doses? Is pain in the knees of that young person with systemic lupus signaling a flare up of disease, or is it ischemic necrosis of bone? How widely and how often should we be measuring biomarkers and densitometry to evaluate bone mass? How useful are the current and emerging imaging techniques to detect early periarticular erosions and cartilage loss? How does that information change what we do? When we must prescribe corticosteroids, how can we protect the patient from bone loss? These are questions we face on a daily basis.

Here in this volume is an in-depth, practical guide to these problems. Drs. Maricic and Gluck have gathered a large number of experts in bone biology, diagnosis, imaging, biomarkers, and treatment. The text is structured for the rheumatologist and other professionals who deal with patients with acute and chronic musculoskeletal disease. The chapters are organized in a logical order and are packed with useful and thought-provoking information.

Whether you the reader are planning to work your way through this interesting text chapter by chapter, or whether you are looking up a particular item to help you understand, diagnose, or manage bone disease, you are in for a treat. This is an outstanding book. The editors and authors have set a high standard, thus committing themselves to updating a stream of later editions. We thank them.

Bevra Hannahs Hahn, MD, FACR
Professor of Medicine
Vice Chair, Department of Medicine
Chief, Division of Rheumatology
David Geffen School of Medicine at University of
California Los Angeles
USA

June 2004

# Preface

Individuals caring for patients with musculoskeletal disorders frequently encounter bone disease either as a primary process or as a complication of systemic inflammation. In addition to recent advances in our understanding of specific joint and bone abnormalities, there is a renewed appreciation of the interaction between the osseous and the immune systems.

Cells and cytokines from the bone marrow mediate physiological and pathological states affecting both bone and inflammation. Thus, the anatomy and physiology of the osseous and immune systems are intertwined, leading to the concept of osteoimmunology (1).

The primary objective of this text is to review current knowledge of skeletal pathology in both autoimmune illness and common metabolic bone disorders. The initial section covers bone anatomy and physiology and the role of cells and cytokines in bone remodeling and erosions. The following section on measurement tools reviews state-of-the-art methods to assess pathologic processes affecting the skeleton. Section III includes the epidemiology and clinical manifestations of skeletal involvement in the major rheumatic diseases. Section IV discusses generalized bone loss due to the use of glucocorticoids and other medications. Next, is a section on exercise, rehabilitation, and pharmacological agents that maintain or increase bone mass with particular emphasis on their use in autoimmune disease. The final portion of the book is devoted to several metabolic bone disorders, not necessarily inflammatory in etiology, frequently seen in clinical practice.

The World Health Organization has recognized the high prevalence of musculoskeletal disease in society by designating the first decade of the 21st century as "The Bone and Joint Decade" (2). Hopefully, this textbook will contribute significantly to the care of patients with bone and joint disorders.

1. Arron, JR, Choi Y. Osteoimmunology: bone versus immune system. *Nature* 2000;408: 535–536.
2. The consensus document. The Bone and Joint Decade 2000-2010. Inaugural Meeting 17 and 18 April 1998,Lund, Sweden. *Acta Orthop Scand* 1998;69(Suppl 281):67–86.

# In Memoriam

## Oscar S. Gluck, M.D.
## 1949–2004

Oscar Gluck suddenly and tragically passed away on July 23, 2004. He completed his medical studies at Universidad del Valle in Cali, Colombia, and his medical residency and rheumatology fellowship at Washington University School of Medicine in St. Louis. There, under the mentorship of Bevra Hahn, M.D., he developed an interest in osteoporosis and metabolic bone disorders as they relate to rheumatic practice. Bone disease became his professional love for the next 25 years in his career as Director of the Arizona Rheumatology Center and Clinical Professor at the University of Arizona. He was widely published on therapeutics for rheumatoid arthritis, lupus, postmenopausal and glucocorticoid-induced osteoporosis, and was a nationally and internationally known speaker in these areas.

Oscar was a man of incredible energy and drive. For the past 10 years, he worked tirelessly through committees of the American College of Rheumatology, the International Society of Clinical Densitometry, and others to foster communication and educational interactions between the "bone" and "joint" worlds. To honor his lifelong commitment, insight and energy toward this goal, the American College of Rheumatology has posthumously elected to establish the annual "Oscar S. Gluck Osteoporosis Lectureship" at the American College of Rheumatology National meeting.

Above all, Oscar was a superb educator. In his book *The Art of Teaching*, Gilbert Highet wrote that teaching has 3 stages: "First, the teacher prepares the subject. Then he communicates it to his pupils, or those parts of it that he has selected. Then he makes sure they have learnt it". This is the way Oscar approached every talk he gave, and how he edited *Bone Disease in Rheumatology* every day for the last 6 months of his life. He worked hard to make sure that the outstanding contributions of each author flowed cohesively to fit the outline and message that he envisioned.

*Bone Disease in Rheumatology* was Oscar's conception, and would not have been possible without his guidance and energy. It is hoped that this book will be an enduring reflection of his distinguished and unique professional career.

Finally, there was no one more loved in the rheumatology and osteoporosis communities by his patients and colleagues than Oscar Gluck. Our loss is superseded only by that of his wife Rosemary, daughters Vanessa and Natalie, and granddaughter Isabelle to whom he dedicated this book before he passed away.

Michael Maricic, M.D.

# Contents

Contributors  iv
Foreword by Bevra Hannahs Hahn, M.D.  vi
Preface  vii

## SECTION I: ANATOMY AND PHYSIOLOGY OF BONE  1

1  Bone Structure and Function  3
   *David W. Dempster*

2  Pathophysiology of Systemic Bone Loss in Rheumatic Disorders: The Role of Inflammatory Cytokines  8
   *Steven R. Goldring and Tania N. Crotti*

3  Pathogenesis of Focal Bone Loss in Inflammatory Arthritis  15
   *Allison R. Petit and Ellen M. Gravallese*

## SECTION II: MEASUREMENT TOOLS IN OSTEOPOROSIS AND ARTHRITIS  23

4  Biochemical Markers of Bone and Cartilage Turnover  25
   *Apurva K. Srivastava and David J. Baylink*

5  Measurement of Bone Mineral Density
   A. DXA and QCT  35
   *Dorothy A. Nelson, Jean M. Weigert, and Angelia D. Mosley-Williams*

   B. Peripheral Densitometry
   *Paul D. Miller*

   C. Densitometry in Glucocorticoid-Induced Osteoporosis  49
   *Oscar S. Gluck and Michael Maricic*

6  Radiological Measurements of Periarticular Bone Loss, Erosions, and Joint Space
   A. X-Ray Measurement of Erosions and Joint Space Narrowing  53
   *Désirée van der Heijde*

   B. The Use of MRI for the Grading of Erosions and Joint Space Narrowing  59
   *Fiona M.F. McQueen*

7  Quality of Life and Its Measurement in Osteoporosis  67
   *Deborah T. Gold*

## SECTION III: BONE LOSS AND FRAGILITY FRACTURES IN THE RHEUMATIC DISEASES  71

8  Bone Loss and Fractures in Rheumatoid Arthritis  73
   *Shreyasee Amin*

9  Bone Loss and Fractures in Systemic Lupus Erythematosus  79
   *Chin Lee, Susan Manzi, and Rosalind Ramsey-Goldman*

10 Bone Disease in Ankylosing Spondylitis and Psoriatic Arthritis  87
   *Atul Deodhar*

11 Osteoarthritis  91
   *Marc C. Hochberg and Joan M. Meyer*

## SECTION IV: BONE LOSS DUE TO MEDICATIONS  97

12 Glucocorticoid-Induced Osteoporosis
   A. Epidemiology  99
   *Lenore M. Buckley*

   B. Pathophysiology  105
   *Ernesto Canalis*

   C. Prevention and Treatment  111
   *Jeffrey R. Curtis and Kenneth G. Saag*

13 Drug-Induced Bone Loss  120
   *Jonathan D. Adachi, A. Papaioannu, and Lora Giangregorio*

## SECTION V: MANAGEMENT OF BONE LOSS IN PATIENTS WITH RHEUMATIC DISEASES 123

14    Disease-Modifying Antirheumatic Drugs and Biological Therapy in Prevention of Bone Erosions 125
*Vibeke Strand*

15    Exercise and Rehabilitation in Patients with Osteoporosis and Arthritis 131
*Robert L. Swezey*

16    Estrogens and Rheumatic Diseases 134
*Jeffrey R. Lisse*

17    Calcitonin in the Treatment of Rheumatic Diseases 138
*Stuart L. Silverman*

18    The Use of Bisphosphonates in Rheumatic Disease and Osteoporosis 141
*Chad Deal*

19    Selective Estrogen Receptor Modulators in the Prevention and Treatment of Osteoporosis 150
*Michael Maricic and Oscar S. Gluck*

20    The Use of Androgens and Dehydroepiandrosterone in Rheumatic Bone Disease 154
*Tim A. Bongartz, Jürgen Schölmerich, and Ranier H. Straub*

21    The Use of Parathyroid Hormone in Patients with Rheumatic Diseases 161
*Robin Dore*

22    Potential New Biological Therapies for Bone Loss 170
*Reina Armamento-Villareal and Roberto Civitelli*

## SECTION VI: OTHER BONE DISORDERS 175

23    Paget's Disease of Bone 177
*Roy D. Altman*

24    Osteomalacia 181
*Mihail Moroianu, Dana Fletcher, and Michael Kleerekoper*

25    Primary Hyperparathyroidism: Rheumatologic Manifesations and Bone Disease 185
*Mishaela R. Rubin, Shonni J. Silverberg, and John P. Bilezikian*

26    Osteonecrosis 191
*Eric P. Gall*

27    Calcinosis and Heterotopic Ossification 197
*Deborah Wenkert and Michael P. Whyte*

Index 203

# Anatomy and Physiology of Bone

# Bone Structure and Function

*David W. Dempster*

Almost 50 years ago A.M. Cooke wrote the following: "The skeleton, out of site and often out of mind, is a formidable mass of tissue occupying about 9% of the body by bulk and no less than 17% by weight. The stability and immutability of dry bones and their persistence for centuries, and even millions of years after the soft tissues have turned to dust, give us a false impression of bone during life. Its fixity after death is in sharp contrast to its ceaseless activity during life" (1).

In the adult skeleton the ceaseless activity largely refers to the process of bone remodeling. This introductory chapter briefly reviews the structure and function of bone and the cellular mechanisms underlying bone remodeling, a process that sustains both structure and function.

## BONE STRUCTURE AND FUNCTION

Bone is a connective tissue consisting of cells and extracellular fibers embedded in an amorphous ground substance containing tissue fluid. Unlike other connective tissues, the extracellular matrix of bone is calcified, making it hard and unyielding. These properties are essential for bones to fulfill their many and varied functions, which include supporting and protecting the internal organs and the bone marrow, enabling locomotion by acting as levers to amplify the power of the muscles, and serving as a large and accessible store of calcium, base, and growth factors. The ground substance of bone consists primarily of glycoproteins and proteoglycans. The fibers of bone are composed of type-I collagen that is impregnated with mineral, primarily in the form of hydroxyapatite $[3Ca_3(PO_4)_2(OH)_2]$ (2).

Bone is, therefore, a composite material, and it is this that endows it with its impressive strength to weight ratio. The mineral component imparts stiffness and rigidity, while the organic component imparts flexibility and resilience. Unlike man-made composite materials, such as fiberglass and reinforced concrete, bone is a living tissue, and the relative proportions of the components of the composite can vary, resulting in dramatic alterations in physical properties. For example, in osteomalacia, or rickets, the mineral component is reduced and the mechanical properties of the collagen are predominant. Consequently, the bones are soft and malleable and they bend under load. They do not usually break, however, because of the intrinsic toughness of collagen. At the other extreme, osteopetrosis is characterized by hypermineralization of the matrix and the physical properties of the mineral component dominate. Despite the fact that these patients display very high bone mineral density, their bones fracture readily because they are brittle and cannot yield to absorb the load (3).

At the organ level, bone can be subdivided into two principal types: cancellous, or spongy, bone, which is found primarily within the vertebral bodies and in the epiphyses and metaphyses of the long bones, and cortical, or compact, bone, which is primarily found in the shafts of the long bones. Approximately 80% of the adult skeleton is composed of cortical bone, and 20% is cancellous, but the relative proportions of the two types of bone vary considerably among different skeletal sites. For example the ratio of cancellous to cortical bone is estimated to be 75:25 in human vertebrae, 50:50 in the femoral head, and 95:5 in the diaphysis of the radius (4).

### Bone Remodeling

Bone remodeling is achieved by the orchestrated action of numerous cell types (5). The two major processes in the remodeling cycle are resorption and formation (Figs. 1.1 and 1.2), and we focus on these consecutively.

## Resorption

Bone resorption is accomplished by highly specialized cells called osteoclasts. They are formed from circulating precursors in the monocyte lineage, which migrate to the bone microenvironment where they fuse to form large, multinucleated cells (Fig. 1.3). Resorption is a complex undertaking requiring dissolution of the bone mineral and degradation of the organic matrix. To accomplish this, osteoclasts first form a tight, annular seal between themselves and the bone matrix. This is achieved by the binding of integrin receptors in the plasma membrane to specific amino acid motifs in the organic matrix (6). In forming the seal, the osteoclast creates the bone-resorbing compartment, a unique microenvironment, between itself and the bone matrix. Specific types of proton pumps and other ion channels in the membrane transfer protons to the resorbing compartment lowering its pH considerably. pH values as low as 4.0 have been detected in this compartment (7). Acidification of the resorbing compartment is accompanied by secretion of a number of lysosomal enzymes, such as tartrate-resistant acid phosphatase and cathepsin K, as well as matrix metalloproteases including MMP-9 (collagenase) and gelatinase (8). The acidic solution containing enzymes that are most active at low pH effectively dissolves and digests the mineral and organic phases of the matrix, creating saucer-shaped resorption cavities on the surface of the cancellous bone and cylindrical tunnels within the cortex (Fig. 1.1).

One of the major accomplishments in the bone field over the last 10 years has been the identification of the key factors involved in the regulation of osteoclast formation and activity. These are members of the tumor necrosis factor ligand family called receptor activator nuclear factor κB ligand

(RANKL) and its two receptors, RANK and osteoprotegerin (OPG) (9,10). RANKL is constitutively expressed on osteoblast cell membranes as well as on those of bone marrow stromal cells, where its expression is regulated by a number of hormones and cytokines. RANK is expressed on the membrane of the osteoclast precursors, and binding of RANKL to RANK stimulates their differentiation to osteoclasts. RANK is also expressed on mature osteoclasts, and, here, binding of RANKL increases their resorptive activity and prolongs their life span. OPG is a secreted, decoy receptor for RANKL, which functions as a negative regulator of bone resorption by mopping up excess RANKL and, thereby, prevents it from interacting with its receptors on osteoclasts and their precursors. RANKL and OPG production are tightly regulated. Agents that stimulate resorption, for example, PTH, do so by upregulating RANKL synthesis and downregulating that of OPG, whereas the opposite is the case for agents that inhibit resorption, such as estrogen (11,12). This provides for exquisite control of one of the most destructive processes in the body with a dual mechanism analogous to regulation of a car's speed being achieved with both an accelerator and a brake. Another key factor in the regulation of osteoclastogenesis is macrophage-colony stimulating factor (M-CSF), which binds to its receptor, c-fms, on osteoclast precursors and triggers their survival and proliferation (13). The importance of RANKL and M-CSF in osteoclastogenesis is shown by the fact that treatment of human peripheral monocytes in vitro with only these two cytokines is sufficient to generate large numbers of functional osteoclasts (Fig. 1.4)

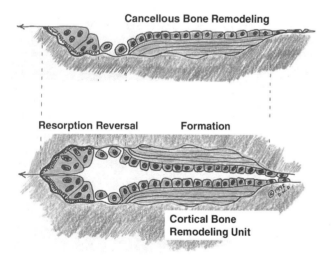

**Figure 1.1** Diagram illustrating the major phase in the bone remodeling cycle in cancellous and cortical bone. The process is similar in each type of bone, but on cancellous bone, the cells work on the surface of the trabeculae, whereas in cortical bone they must penetrate through the tissue.

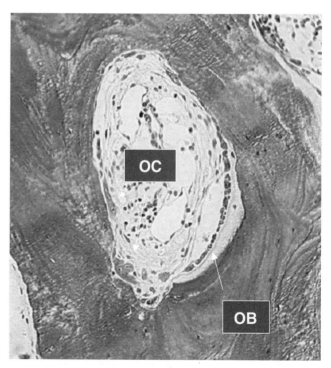

**Figure 1.2** Light micrograph of a bone remodeling unit in human bone. *OC*, osteoclasts; *OB*, osteoblasts.

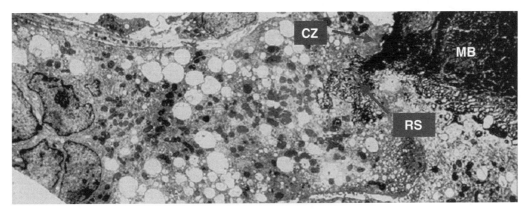

**Figure 1.3** Transmission electron micrograph of a rat osteoclast engaged in bone resorption. The cell is firmly attached to the mineralized bone *(MB)* at the sealing zone (CZ), which surrounds the resorption space *(RS)*. The resorbing osteoclast is highly polarized. Parts of four nuclei are visible at the apical margin. The cell contains numerous mitochondria, indicating that bone resorption requires a substantial amount of energy.

## Formation

Following a brief reversal phase, osteoclastic resorption is followed by osteoblastic new bone formation. In stained bone biopsy sections, the osteoblasts are seen to literally follow the osteoclasts in their sweep across the surface of cancellous bone and through the evolving haversian canal in cortical bone (Fig. 1.2). Osteoblasts arise from mesenchymal stem cells in the bone marrow stroma. The mesenchymal stem cell is in turn derived from pluripotential stem cells, which have the capacity to differentiate into a number of mesenchymal cell types including osteoblasts, chondroblasts, adipocytes, myoblasts, and fibroblasts, depending on the local environmental factors to which they are exposed. This plasticity of the osteoblast precursors is thought to account for the reciprocal relationship that exists between osteoblasts and adipocytes and the long-recognized phenomenon that age-related bone loss is associated with an increase in adipose tissue in bone marrow (14,15).

Mature osteoblasts possess all of the characteristics of a cell engaged in the manufacture and export of proteins, such as abundant rough endoplasmic reticulum, and a well-developed Golgi complex (Fig. 1.5). Once the collagen is secreted, the osteoblasts seed mineralization by releasing small, membrane-bound vesicles, called matrix

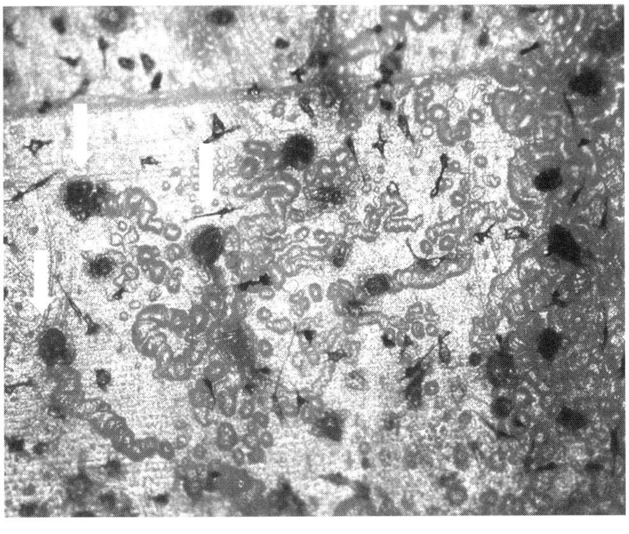

**Figure 1.4** Human osteoclasts *(arrows)* formed in vitro on a thin slice of dentin from monocytes treated with RANKL and M-CSF. Note the extensive resorption "trails" associated with the osteoclasts. (Micrograph courtesy of Dr. Timothy Arnett, University College, London. The osteoclasts were formed from Dr. Arnett's monocytes.)

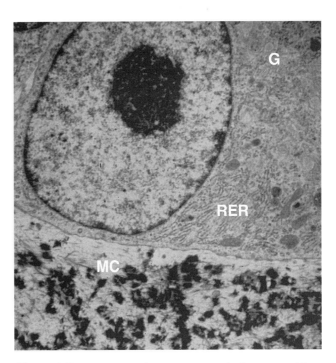

**Figure 1.5** Transmission electron micrograph of a rat osteoblast. The cell contains abundant rough endoplasmic reticulum *(RER)* and a well-developed Golgi complex (G). Clusters of mineral crystals *(MC)* are forming in the organic matrix.

vesicles, which establish suitable conditions for initial mineral deposition by concentrating calcium and phosphate ions and by enzymatically degrading inhibitors of mineralization, such as pyrophosphate and proteoglycans, that are present in the extracellular matrix (16). When the osteoblasts have completed their matrix forming function, they can suffer a number of fates.

Approximately 50% to 70% die by apoptosis, and the remainder are either incorporated into the matrix as osteocytes or remain on the surface as bone lining cells. Recent work indicates new functions for these cells. The bone lining cells were once thought to serve primarily to regulate the flow of ions into and out of the bone extracellular fluid and, in so doing, constitute the anatomical basis of the blood-bone barrier. There is evidence, however, that under special circumstances, the lining cells are capable of reverting to their previous role of bone formation. Such a mechanism has been implicated in the bone formation response to intermittent parathyroid hormone administration and mechanical stimulation (17,18). These two stimuli have synergistic effects on bone formation (19–21).

The function of osteocytes remained elusive until relatively recently. These cells are incarcerated within the mineralized matrix, but they are by no means in solitary confinement. They communicate with each other, as well as with the bone lining cells, via gap junctions between cellular processes that pass through tiny tubular channels in the matrix called canaliculi. There is growing evidence to suggest that such an arrangement permits the osteocytes to sense changes in the mechanical properties of the surrounding matrix. Having detected localized damage to the matrix the osteocytes appear to be capable of initiating targeted remodeling and, thereby, repair of such damage (22,23). The importance of the integrity of the osteocyte network is reinforced by the fact that conditions that are harmful to the skeleton, such as estrogen deficiency and glucocorticoid excess, enhance osteocyte death by apoptosis, whereas pharmaceutical agents that lower fracture risk, including estrogen, bisphosphonates, and teriparatide, all preserve osteocyte viability (24–27).

## Bone Remodeling and Fracture Risk in Osteoporosis

There is a growing appreciation that high remodeling rates confer increased fracture risk in patients with osteoporosis. There are a number of plausible explanations for why this may be the case. High remodeling rates are associated with more rapid bone loss and loss of trabecular microarchitecture (28). Enhanced remodeling also increases the number of osteoclastic resorption cavities that are present on the surface of the trabeculae at any one time concentrating local stress at these sites and, thereby, the probability of mechanical failure (29). Cortical porosity is also increased and the time available for secondary mineralization of the matrix is reduced

(30,31). These observations, coupled with numerous analyses indicating that the degree of fracture risk reduction following treatment with antiresorptive agents is poorly correlated with the change in bone mineral density (32,33), are rapidly changing our concept of the mechanism of action of these drugs (34). The proximate cause of the lowered fracture risk is the rapid reduction in the remodeling rate with the change in bone mineral density and other factors that influence bone strength, such as microarchitecture, stress concentration, and mineralization, being secondary effects.

## REFERENCES

1. Cooke AM. Osteoporosis. *Lancet* 1955; I:878–882.
2. Gokhale JA, Robey PG, Boskey AL. The biochemistry of bone. In: Marcus R, Feldman D, Kelsey A, eds. *Osteoporosis*, vol. 1. San Diego: Academic Press, 2001:107–188.
3. Turner CH. Biomechanics of bone: determinants of skeletal fragility and bone quality. *Osteoporos Int* 2002;13:97–104.
4. Mundy GR, Chen D, Oyajobi BO. Bone remodeling. In: Favus MJ, ed. *Primer on the Metabolic Bone Diseases and Disorders of Mineral Metabolism*. Washington, DC: American Society for Bone and Mineral Research, 2003:46–58.
5. Dempster DW. Bone remodeling. In: Coe FL, Favus MJ, eds. *Disorders of Bone and Mineral Metabolism*, 2nd ed. Philadelphia: Lippincott Williams & Wilkins, 2002:315–343.
6. Duong LT, Lakkakorpi P, Nakamura I, Rodan GA. Integrins and signaling in osteoclast function. *Matrix Biol* 2000;19:97–105.
7. Silver IA, Murrills RJ, Etherington DJ. Microelectrode studies on the acid microenvironment beneath adherent macrophages and osteoclasts. *Exp Cell Res* 1988;175:266–276.
8. Delaisse JM, Andersen TL, Engsig MT, et al. Matrix metalloproteinases (MMP) and cathepsin K contribute differently to osteoclastic activities. *Microsc Res Tech* 2003; 61:504–513.
9. Boyle WJ, Simonet WS, Lacey DL. Osteoclast differentiation and activation. *Nature* 2003;423(6937):337–342.
10. Troen BR. Molecular mechanisms underlying osteoclast formation and activation. *Exp Gerontol* 2003;38:605–614.
11. Huang JC, Sakata T, Pfleger LL, et al. PTH differentially regulates expression of RANKL and OPG. *J Bone Miner* Res 2004; 19(2):235–244.
12. Hofbauer LC, Schoppet M, Schuller P, et al. Effects of oral contraceptives on circulating osteoprotegerin and soluble RANK ligand serum levels in healthy young women. *Clin Endocrinol (Oxf)* 2004;60:214–219.
13. Woo KM, Kim HM, Ko JS. Macrophage colony–stimulating factor promotes the survival of osteoclast precursors by up-regulating Bcl-X(L). *Exp Mol Med* 2002;34:340–346.
14. Akune T, Ohba S, Kamekura S, et al. PPARgamma insufficiency enhances osteogenesis through osteoblast formation from bone marrow progenitors. *J Clin Invest* 2004;113:846–855.
15. Meunier P, Aaron J, Edouard C, Vignon G. Osteoporosis and the replacement of cell populations of the marrow by adipose tissue. A quantitative study of 84 iliac bone biopsies. *Clin Orthop* 1971; 80:147–154.
16. Anderson HC. Matrix vesicles and calcification. *Curr Rheumatol Rep* 2003;5:222–226.
17. Dobnig H, Turner RT. Evidence that intermittent treatment with parathyroid hormone increases bone formation in adult rats by activation of bone lining cells. *Endocrinology* 1995;136:3632–3638.
18. Chow JW, Wilson AJ, Chambers TJ, Fox SW. Mechanical loading stimulates bone formation by reactivation of bone lining cells in 13-week-old rats. *J Bone Miner Res* 1998;13:1760–1767.
19. Li J, Duncan RL, Burr DB, et al. Parathyroid hormone enhances mechanically induced bone formation, possibly involving L-type voltage-sensitive calcium channels. *Endocrinology* 2003;144: 1226–1233.

20. Kim CH, Takai E, Zhou H, et al. Trabecular bone response to mechanical and parathyroid hormone stimulation: the role of mechanical microenvironment. *J Bone Miner Res* 2003;18:2116–2125.

21. Cherian PP, Cheng B, Gu S, et al. Effects of mechanical strain on the function of gap junctions in osteocytes are mediated through the prostaglandin EP2 receptor. *J Biol Chem* 2003;278:43146–43156.

22. Martin RB. Fatigue microdamage as an essential element of bone mechanics and biology. *Calcif Tissue Int* 2003;73:101–107.

23. Noble BS, Reeve J. Osteocyte function, osteocyte death and bone fracture resistance. *Mol Cell Endocrinol* 2000;159:7–13.

24. Tomkinson A, Reeve J, Shaw RW, Noble BS. The death of osteocytes via apoptosis accompanies estrogen withdrawal in human bone. *J Clin Endocrinol Metab* 1997;82:3128–3135.

25. O'Brien CA, Jia D, Plotkin LI, et al. Glucocorticoids act directly on osteoblasts and osteocytes to induce their apoptosis and reduce bone formation and strength. *Endocrinology* 2004;145:1835–1841.

26. Plotkin LI, Weinstein RS, Parfitt AM, et al. Prevention of osteocyte and osteoblast apoptosis by bisphosphonates and calcitonin. *J Clin Invest* 1999;104:1363–1374.

27. Jilka RL, Weinstein RS, Bellido T, et al. Increased bone formation by prevention of osteoblast apoptosis with parathyroid hormone. *J Clin Invest* 1999;104:439–446.

28. Borah B, Dufresne TE, Chmielewski PA, et al. Risedronate preserves bone architecture in postmenopausal women with osteoporosis as measured by three-dimensional microcomputed tomography. *Bone* 2004;34:736–746.

29. Parfitt AM. Use of bisphosphonates in the prevention of bone loss and fractures. *Am J Med* 1991;91(5B):42S–46S.

30. Roschger P, Rinnerthaler S, Yates J, et al. Alendronate increases degree and uniformity of mineralization in cancellous bone and decreases the porosity in cortical bone of osteoporotic women. *Bone* 2001;29:185–191.

31. Boivin G, Meunier PJ. Changes in bone remodeling rate influence the degree of mineralization of bone. *Connect Tissue Res* 2002;43:535–537.

32. Delmas PD, Seeman E. Changes in bone mineral density explain little of the reduction in vertebral or nonvertebral fracture risk with anti-resorptive therapy. *Bone* 2004;34:599–604.

33. Cummings SR, Karpf DB, Harris F, et al. Improvement in spine bone density and reduction in risk of vertebral fractures during treatment with antiresorptive drugs. *Am J Med* 2002;112:281–289.

34. Heaney RP. Is the paradigm shifting? *Bone* 2003;33:457–465.

## 2

# Pathophysiology of Systemic Bone Loss in Rheumatologic Disorders: The Role of Inflammatory Cytokines

*Steven R. Goldring and Tania N. Crotti*

## INTRODUCTION

### Inflammatory Disease Associated with Bone Loss

Inflammation of articular and periarticular tissues is the hallmark of rheumatic diseases such as rheumatoid arthritis (RA), systemic lupus erythematosus (SLE), and the seronegative spondyloarthropathies (SpA). In these disorders, not only may skeletal tissues be involved at juxtaarticular and subchondral sites, but also there is evidence that many of these conditions may produce effects on bone remodeling that affect the entire skeleton. This review covers the inflammatory rheumatologic disorders that target the articular and periarticular tissues with particular focus on the adverse effects of these conditions on systemic skeletal remodeling and the pathogenic mechanisms leading to increased risk of osteoporosis.

### Physiologic Bone Remodeling

Physiologic bone remodeling enables the skeleton to adapt to changing local biomechanical forces, repairs damage to the bone microarchitecture, and, in certain instances, provides a system for regulation of mineral ion homeostasis by releasing calcium and phosphate ions during the phase of bone resorption. The remodeling of human skeletal tissues is mediated by the reciprocal activities of osteoclasts and osteoblasts. Under physiologic conditions skeletal remodeling is a tightly coupled process in which an exquisite balance is maintained between bone resorption and formation. In pathological states associated with several of the inflammatory rheumatologic diseases, there is a shift in the equilibrium state such that net bone resorption exceeds bone formation. This disequilibrium leads to a progressive loss of bone mass and deterioration of skeletal architecture and strength, resulting in increased risk of fracture.

Multiple mechanisms contribute to the bone loss associated with inflammatory joint disease. Not only are these conditions associated with increased systemic bone resorption but under certain conditions there may also be suppression of coupled bone formation. In many patients, this suppression of bone formation is related to concomitant use of glucocorticosteroids, but additional factors such as poor nutrition, inactivity, and the systemic effects of inflammatory cytokines may also suppress osteoblast activity or survival.

## ROLE OF CYTOKINES IN BONE REMODELING

Multiple hormones and cytokines are involved in the regulation of bone remodeling. The factors controlling bone resorption act via regulation of osteoclast differentiation, activation, survival, and function. These factors include parathyroid hormone (PTH), vitamin D, parathyroid-related protein (PTHrP), prostaglandin $E_2$ ($PGE_2$), interleukin (IL)-1$\alpha$ and 1$\beta$, IL-6, IL-7, IL-11, IL-15, IL-17, tumor necrosis factor-$\alpha$ (TNF-$\alpha$,) oncostatin-M, macrophage-colony stimulating factor (M-CSF), and receptor activator nuclear factor $\kappa$B ligand (RANKL) (Table 2.1) (1–8). These factors either act directly on osteoclasts or osteoclast precursors, or produce their effects indirectly by acting on bone-lining cells, marrow stromal cells, or other cell types that in turn release the primary osteoclast-inducing factors. Only a restricted number of these factors participate in physiologic bone remodeling. Many of these factors, however, are abundantly produced in the RA synovium and act locally to produce increased bone resorption. It is possible that, under certain circumstances, they are released from the inflamed synovium and then enter the circulation where they act in an endocrine fashion to enhance systemic bone resorption.

Cytokines have also been shown to act as inhibitors of osteoclastic bone resorption. These include, for example, IL-4, IL-12, IL-18, granulocyte monocyte-colony stimulating factor (GM-CSF) and interferon-$\gamma$ (IFN-$\gamma$) (9–14). If these inhibitory cytokines act systemically to modulate bone remodeling in inflammatory arthritis is not known. However, exploiting the activities of these cytokines or their signal pathways does represent a rational therapeutic approach for inhibiting both articular and systemic bone loss in inflammatory arthritides.

## PRIMARY MEDIATORS OF OSTEOCLAST DIFFERENTIATION AND ACTIVATION: THEIR ROLE IN SYSTEMIC AND LOCAL BONE RESORPTION

Recent studies have demonstrated the role of RANKL in regulating osteoclast-mediated bone resorption. RANKL is essential for osteoclast differentiation and activation as well as dendritic cell survival, lymphocyte development, and lymph node organogenesis (15). RANKL interacts with its receptor, receptor activator of nuclear factor $\kappa$B (RANK), which is present on preosteoclasts, osteoclasts, B cells, and T cells. The interaction between RANKL and RANK can be inhibited by the soluble decoy receptor osteoprotegerin (OPG). OPG can also interact with TNF-related apoptosis-inducing ligand (TRAIL) to inhibit its apoptosis-inducing capability (16). Changes in the regulation of the OPG to RANKL ratio are likely to play a major role in controlling both localized articular and systemic bone resorption and may act in physiologic and pathologic conditions.

A recent review extensively covers the primary mediators of bone resorption in physiological and pathological conditions and discusses recent treatments that target these molecules (17). Of particular significance are clinical studies in postmenopausal women that have demonstrated the profound effect OPG has on inhibiting bone resorption by osteoclasts (18). OPG or related therapeutic strategies that interfere with RANKL activity may offer a novel therapeutic approach for the treatment of osteoporosis and other diseases associated with increased bone resorption such as RA.

## RHEUMATOID ARTHRITIS

Among the rheumatic disorders, RA represents an excellent model for gaining insights into the effects of local as well as systemic consequences of inflammatory processes on skeletal tissue remodeling. Three principal forms of bone disease have been described in RA: marginal joint erosions, juxtarticular osteoporosis, and generalized axial and appendicular osteoporosis distant from the joints. This review focuses on the systemic pattern of bone loss in RA.

### Generalized Axial and Appendicular Osteoporosis Distant from the Joints

The presence of generalized axial and appendicular osteoporosis at sites that are distant from inflamed joints has been well established using different techniques (19–23). There is compelling evidence that this reduction is associated with an increased risk of hip and vertebral fracture (24–27). The conflicting data concerning the effects of RA

### TABLE 2.1
### FACTORS REGULATING LOCAL BONE RESORPTION

| Stimulatory | Inhibitory |
|---|---|
| RANKL | OPG |
| M-CSF | IL-4 |
| Oncostatin-M | IL-12 |
| $PGE_2$ | IL-18 |
| TNF-$\alpha$ | GM-CSF |
| IL-1-$\alpha$ and $\beta$ | IFN-$\gamma$ |
| IL-6 | |
| IL-7 | |
| IL-15 | |
| IL-17 | |
| PTH | |
| PTHrP | |
| Vitamin D | |

RANKL, receptor activator nuclear factor-$\kappa$B ligand; M-CSF, macrophage-colony stimulating factor; oncostatin-M; $PGE_2$, prostaglandin $E_2$; TNF-$\alpha$, tumor necrosis factor-$\alpha$; IL, interleukin; PTH, parathyroid hormone; PTHrP, PTH-related protein; OPG, osteoprotegerin; GM-CSF, granulocyte monocyte-colony stimulating factor; IFN-$\gamma$ interferon-$\gamma$.

on skeletal mass are in part related to the fact that most observations have been based on cross-sectional studies and have focused on patients late in the evolution of their disease when factors such as disability and glucocorticoid and other treatments may confound the analyses.

## Systemic Bone Remodeling in RA

Although earlier studies using histomorphometric analysis of bone biopsies from patients with RA indicate that, in the absence of glucocorticoid use, the cellular basis of the generalized reduction in bone mass is related to a decrease in bone formation rather than an increase in bone resorption (28–30), more recent studies support the contention that the generalized bone loss in RA is principally caused by increased osteoclast activity. Biochemical markers of bone turnover have been used to study patients with RA and the results of these studies indicate that there is increased bone resorbing activity. Higher rates of bone resorption were associated with more severe disease activity, especially in patients receiving chronic corticosteroids (31–35). Further evidence indicating an association between RA disease activity and systemic bone remodeling is provided in studies by D'Elia et al. (36). In these studies, the Larsen score in hands, wrists, and forefeet was determined in RA patients not on bisphosphonate treatment or hormone replacement therapy (HRT). The cartilage remodeling marker, serum levels of cartilage oligomeric matrix protein (COMP) and bone anabolic factor, insulin-like growth factor (IGF)-1 were determined by radioimmunoassay. Serum bone remodeling markers of bone resorption, carboxyterminal crosslinked telopeptide of Type I collagen (CTx), and of bone formation, carboxyterminal propeptide of Type I procollagen (PICP) were also measured. High IGF-1 levels negatively correlated with erosion score (Larsen), suggesting that women with lower erosion scores (and presumably less active RA) had higher bone formation rates. Reduced COMP and increased CTx correlated with erosion, suggesting that more active disease was associated with increased systemic resorption. Consistent with the results of this study, the Larsen score was shown to be the strongest disease-related determinant of bone mass in the forearm, total hip, and femoral neck.

## Determinants of Systemic Bone Mass in RA

Several factors have emerged as important determinants of bone mass in patients with RA: increased age, low body mass index (BMI) and menopausal status, reduced mobility, disease activity, the influence of antirheumatic therapy (especially glucocorticosteroids), and disease duration (36–43). Assessment of postmenopausal women, not on bisphosphonate or hormone therapy, has shown higher levels of osteoporosis in RA patients relative to healthy age-matched postmenopausal women (36). Recently the Oslo-

Truro-Amsterdam study confirmed an association between high disease activity (measured by the Larsen score) and low bone mineral density (BMD). The disease activity was found to be an independent determinant of vertebral deformity after correction for center, age, BMI, and BMD (43). These findings supported a large longitudinal prospective study by Gough and coworkers (39), which concluded that significant amounts of generalized skeletal bone was lost early in RA and that this loss was associated with disease activity. Similar findings have been reported by Als et al (44) who noted a significant decrease in bone mass during the early phases of RA. Caution must be taken when interpreting these studies because the selection of patients, the site at which BMD was assessed and the diverse equipment used for assessment of bone measurements, may yield different conclusions. For instance, the BMD of the lumbar spine may be less influenced by RA than the BMD of the forearm, total hip, and femoral neck (36,45,46).

## Glucocorticoids and RA

The use of glucocorticoid treatments and their influence on the progression of bone loss in RA is still controversial. In part, this is related to the tendency to use these medications in patients with more severe disease. Some authors suggest that if steroids satisfactorily suppress inflammation and maintain mobility, the deleterious effects of glucocorticosteroids may be outweighed (39,40). Results from the recent Combinatietherapie Bij Reumatoide Artritis (COBRA) trial in which high-dose prednisolone was used as a component of an induction therapy using disease modifying agents indicate that glucocorticosteroids may reduce development of focal bone erosions (34). Interestingly, patients enrolled in this protocol developed transient bone loss in the lumbar spine that may have been related to the effects of glucocorticosteroids on reducing bone formation. Presently, however, it is premature to generally advocate the use of glucocorticosteroids in patients with RA because there is considerable evidence that their chronic use is associated with many potentially serious extraskeletal complications (47). This cautionary note is supported by the findings of Saag and coworkers who found that low-dose, long-term prednisone use, equal to or greater than 5 mg/day, was correlated in a dose-dependent fashion with the development of several adverse reactions, including fracture (25). In a recent study, van Everdingen et al. (48) examined the relationship between low-dose glucocorticosteroids use and fracture risk. Subjects were given prednisone 10 mg/day or placebo. These results indicated an increased risk of fracture that in part could be attributed not only to the effects of RA on bone mass but also to the adverse effects of glucocorticosteroids on bone quality and strength. Additional cross-sectional studies agree that the cumulative dose of prednisolone is an important determinant of osteopenia in RA (38,41,49).

## Systemic Levels of Cytokines in RA

As discussed previously, considerable evidence indicates that cytokines produced locally in the inflamed synovium enter the general circulation where they can act via an endocrine mechanism to modulate systemic bone remodeling. For example, in a recent cross-sectional study, D'Elia et al. detected high levels of IL-6 and soluble IL6 receptor in the peripheral blood of post-menopausal RA women (36). They also found an association of elevated cytokine levels with joint destruction (measured by the Larsen score). This is in accord with earlier studies that showed levels of IL-6 and IL-6 receptor in patients with RA correlated with disease activity (50) and radiologic joint damage.

## RANKL and OPG in RA

While many of the inflammatory mediators present in the RA joint are involved in stimulating osteoclast-mediated bone resorption, their major effects may be mediated indirectly through stimulation of RANKL production (2,5,51,52). Since its detection in RA synovium by Kong et al. (53), particular attention has focused on RANKL because of its potent osteoclastogenic activity. Further evidence implicating RANKL as an essential regulatory mediator of articular bone loss is derived from several different animal models of inflammatory arthritis, in which treatment with the inhibitor OPG results in marked suppression of bone erosions (53–55). There is also evidence that blocking RANKL activity with OPG decreases systemic bone loss in TNF-$\alpha$ transgenic mice (56).

RANKL, its receptor RANK, and OPG mRNA are expressed in cells isolated from human RA joints, and there is a significant correlation between the number of resorption pits formed by cells extracted from these tissues and the ratio of RANKL mRNA to OPG mRNA (52). Semiquantitative and quantitative analysis of OPG protein in the synovial tissue, detected by immunostaining, reveal that OPG expression was markedly decreased in RA patients with active synovitis compared with inactive RA patients, osteoarthritis (OA), and normal controls (57). This was in accordance with the decreased OPG levels detected in RA synovial fluid compared with OA using an enzyme-linked immunoassay (ELISA) (58). In contrast, higher levels of RANKL protein have been detected in synovial tissue in RA patients with active synovitis and in some patients with SpA compared with OA and normal controls, suggesting that an increase in RANKL in the inflamed joints of RA patients is likely to be an important cause of joint erosions in RA (59).

## Local and Systemic RANKL and OPG Levels in RA

The local concentrations of soluble RANKL and OPG detected in joint synovial fluid are higher in the joint than in peripheral circulation (58,60). Although the levels are lower in serum compared to synovial fluids, higher levels (but similar ratio) of serum OPG and soluble RANKL are present in RA patients when compared with controls (60). Despite these observations, the level of serum OPG may not be a useful biochemical marker for disease activity assessment and drug monitoring in patients with RA. In a recent study evaluating the effects of the bisphosphonate etidronate in RA patients, investigators found that serum OPG levels were not related to biochemical markers of bone formation or resorption (61). At baseline and at study termination, serum OPG levels correlated significantly with age. At baseline, the mean serum OPG level was higher in patients receiving 5–10 mg/day prednisone compared with those receiving less than 5 mg/day or with those receiving no prednisone. Based on their data, the authors postulated that serum OPG measurements, perhaps because of the multiplicity of factors regulating its production, would be difficult to use in the evaluation of antiresorptive therapy. They also concluded that low-dose, corticosteroid-associated osteoporosis is probably not mediated by inhibition of OPG.

## BONE LOSS AND SPONDYLOARTHROPATHY

The spondyloarthropathies (SPAs) are a heterogeneous group of disorders including ankylosing spondylitis (AS), psoriatic arthritis, inflammatory bowel disease–related arthritis, reactive arthritis, and undifferentiated spondyloarthropathy/spondyloarthritis (62). Several studies have documented an increased incidence of spinal compression fractures in patients with AS (63–66). This increase in fracture incidence has been attributed to decreased axial bone mass. The chronic back pain experienced by many patients with AS and the high incidence of paraspinal calcifications and syndesmophytes, which artificially elevates BMD, has led to an underestimation of the fracture incidence in these patients. The decrease in axial bone density has also been attributed to the effects of immobilization of the spine associated with the progressive ankylosis, although systemic inflammation, as in RA, may also be a contributing factor (67,68).

In addition to increased bone resorption, there is also evidence of decreased bone formation. For example, women with AS have been found to have significantly lower bone formation rates based on serum osteocalcin (OC) and bone-specific alkaline phosphatase (BALP) levels, compared with age- and sex-matched controls (69). Osteopenia and osteoporosis in the hip is significantly more frequent in patients with advanced AS compared to individuals with more mild forms of the disease, whereas the frequency of osteopenia and osteoporosis of the spine as assessed by anteroposterior lumbar Dual Energy X-ray Absorptiometry (DEXA) is similar in both groups. This suggests a hip DEXA may be a more reliable indicator of actual vertebral and total body BMD and, therefore, may be the preferred measurement for identifying patients with decreased BMD who are at risk of fracture (70). Alternatively, quantitative ultrasound (QUS) of the calcaneus is a potential method of prescreening for vertebral and nonvertebral fractures and in discriminating osteoporotic from normal bone density in patients with AS (66). The presence of syndesmophytes and calcified ligaments in the later stages may explain why studies have not found significant correlations of BMD with disease duration or disease activity nor correlations between QUS and BMD (69).

## Bone Turnover in Spondyloarthropathy

Psoriatic arthritis (PsA) is an inflammatory joint disease that is associated with aggressive bone resorption. In contrast to RA, there is also evidence of increased new bone formation (often in the same joint) suggesting that the effects of joint inflammation in RA and PsA results in differential effects on bone formation. Interestingly, the increase in local articular osteoclast-mediated bone resorption is accompanied by detection of higher numbers of tartrate-resistant acid phosphatase (TRAP)–positive preosteoclasts in unstimulated peripheral blood mononuclear cells from PsA patients with erosive disease compared with normal controls (71).

## The Production of Cytokines in Spondyloarthropathy

The increased production of cytokines in the chronic inflammatory axial or peripheral joint lesions of patients with AS (72,73) is likely responsible for the adverse effects of SpA on systemic bone remodeling. IL-6 and TNF-α serum levels, but not IL-1β and IFN-γ serum levels, have been found to be significantly higher in patients with AS than in patients with noninflammatory back pain. Patients with RA have higher serum levels of IL-6, TNF-α and IFN-γ than both AS and noninflammatory back pain patients. Gratacos et al. found that IL-6 levels closely correlated with the activity of the disease (72). More recent studies have shown peripheral blood cells from patients with psoriatic arthritis secrete higher basal levels of TNF-α and IFN-γ than cells from healthy controls (71). A recent study investigating cytokine gene polymorphisms found a significant association between IFN-γ and -β gene polymorphisms and the age of psoriasis onset and the presence and progression of joint erosions in early PsA. The results of this study support the use of anti-TNF treatment in severe progressive PsA (74).

## RANKL and OPG Levels Associated with Spondyloarthropathy

Recent studies have shown increased RANKL protein in synovial tissue of PsA patients (71). Results obtained using immunohistochemical analyses were confirmed using replacement therapy Polymerase Chain Reaction (PCR), which demonstrated RANKL mRNA in tissue retrieved from patients with erosive PsA. RANKL protein and mRNA were absent in the sample from a nonerosive patient. In this study, OPG expression was restricted to the endothelium (71).

## ANGIOGENIC FACTORS IN RHEUMATOID ARTHRITIS AND SPONDYLOARTHROPATHY

Angiogenesis facilitates the development and persistence of chronic inflammatory joint diseases such as RA and SpAs. Vascular endothelial growth factor (VEGF) has been detected in RA synovial fluids, and serum levels have been found to correlate with disease activity (75).

The enthesitis and synovitis that are hallmarks of RA and SpA are associated with intense neovascularization (76). Evidence suggests that proangiogenic factors, such as the angiopoietins (Ang) and VEGF, could potentially be used as markers of disease activity in SpA. Ang2 and Ang1 mRNA and protein can be detected early in the course of PsA, with significantly greater levels of Ang2 detected in the PsA synovial membrane infiltrate compared with RA. Levels of VEGF in both the synovial membrane infiltrate and synovial fluid are significantly greater in the PsA than the RA (77). In addition to these findings, serum VEGF levels have been found to be significantly higher in patients with SpA and RA than in control patients and correlate with disease activity parameters (76). The higher levels of VEGF in SpA compared with RA may be associated with its role in stimulating osteoblast activity (78).

## BONE LOSS ASSOCIATED WITH SYSTEMIC LUPUS ERYTHEMATOSUS

Although not associated with focal bone erosions, generalized bone loss is also a significant clinical problem in patients with systemic lupus erythematosus (SLE). A particularly high prevalence of osteoporosis and reduced BMD has been reported in prednisolone-treated patients with SLE (79), and reductions in both cortical as well as trabecular bone mass have been found, even in the absence of glucocorticoid treatment (79–82). As in patients with RA, the effects of systemic inflammation, decreased physical activity, nutritional factors, glucocorticoid use, and drug treatments all likely contribute to the adverse effects on generalized bone mass. Similar factors contribute to the reduced bone mass, delayed skeletal linear growth, and increased incidence of fractures in patients with a history of juvenile chronic (rheumatoid) arthritis (JRA) (83–85). Patients with JRA, for example, have a significantly lower BMD than healthy controls, which appears to be related to glucocorticoid use rather than disease activity (86).

## CONCLUSION

Systemic bone loss and increased risk of fracture complicate many of the inflammatory rheumatic disorders. Although the mechanisms of bone loss are multifactorial, systemic effects of proinflammatory cytokines produced at sites of joint inflammation likely play an important pathological role. Recent insights into the role of RANKL in regulating osteoclast-mediated bone resorption have helped to identify this molecule as a potential target for preventing systemic as well as articular bone loss in RA and other inflammatory disorders.

## REFERENCES

1. Ogata Y, Kukita A, Kukita T, et al. A novel role of IL-15 in the development of osteoclasts: inability to replace its activity with IL-2. *J Immunol* 1999;162(5):2754–2760.
2. Kotake S, Udagawa N, Takahashi N, et al. IL-17 in synovial fluids from patients with rheumatoid arthritis is a potent stimulator of osteoclastogenesis. *J Clin Invest* 1999;103(9):1345–1352.
3. Manolagas SC, Jilka RL. Bone marrow, cytokines, and bone remodeling. Emerging insights into the pathophysiology of osteoporosis. *N Engl J Med* 1995;332(5):305–311.
4. Suda T, Takahashi N, Udagawa N, et al. Modulation of osteoclast differentiation and function by the new members of the tumor necrosis factor receptor and ligand families. *Endocr Rev* 1999;20(3):345–357.
5. Weitzmann MN, Cenci S, Rifas L, et al. Interleukin-7 stimulates osteoclast formation by up-regulating the T- cell production of soluble osteoclastogenic cytokines. *Blood* 2000;96(5):1873–1878.
6. Goldring SR, Gravallese EM. Pathogenesis of bone erosions in rheumatoid arthritis. *Curr Opin Rheumatol* 2000;12(3):195–199.
7. Duong LT, Rodan GA. Regulation of osteoclast formation and function. *Rev Endocr Metab Disord* 2001;2(1):95–104.
8. Kudo O, Sabokbar A, Pocock A, et al. Interleukin-6 and interleukin-11 support human osteoclast formation by a RANKL-independent mechanism. *Bone* 2003;32(1):1–7.
9. Horwood NJ, Udagawa N, Elliott J, et al. Interleukin 18 inhibits osteoclast formation via T cell production of granulocyte macrophage colony-stimulating factor. *J Clin Invest* 1998;101:595–603.
10. Horwood NJ, Elliott J, Martin TJ, Gillespie MT. IL-12 alone and in synergy with IL-18 inhibits osteoclast formation in vitro. *J Immunol* 2001;166:4915–4921.
11. Takayanagi H, Ogasawara K, Hida S, et al. T-cell-mediated regulation of osteoclastogenesis by signalling cross-talk between RANKL and IFN-gamma. *Nature* 2000;408:600–605.
12. Udagawa N, Horwood NJ, Elliott J, et al. Interleukin-18 (interferon-gamma-inducing factor) is produced by osteoblasts and acts via granulocyte/macrophage colony-stimulating factor and not via interferon-gamma to inhibit osteoclast formation. *J Exp Med* 1997;185(6):1005–1012.
13. Makiishi-Shimobayashi C, Tsujimura T, Iwasaki T, et al. Interleukin-18 up-regulates osteoprotegerin expression in stromal/osteoblastic cells. *Biochem Biophys Res Commun* 2001;281:361–366.
14. Wei S, Wang M-H, Teitelbaum S, Ross F. Interleukin-4 reversibly inhibits osteoclastogenesis via inhibition of NF-kb and mitogen-activated protein kinase signaling. *J Biol Chem* 2002;277:6622–6630.
15. Kong YY, Yoshida H, Sarosi I, et al. OPGL is a key regulator of osteoclastogenesis, lymphocyte development and lymph-node organogenesis. *Nature* 1999;397(6717):315–323.
16. Emery JG, McDonnell P, Burke MB, et al. Osteoprotegerin is a receptor for the cytotoxic ligand TRAIL. *J Biol Chem* 1998;273(23):14363–14367.
17. Bolon B, Shalhoub V, Kostenuik PJ, et al. Osteoprotegerin, an endogenous antiosteoclast factor for protecting bone in rheumatoid arthritis. *Arthritis Rheum* 2002;46(12):3121–3135.
18. Becker PJ, Holloway D, Nakanishi A, et al. The effect of a single dose of osteoprotegerin in postmenopausal women. *J Bone Miner Res* 2001;16(2):348–360.
19. Joffe I, Epstein S. Osteoporosis associated with rheumatoid arthritis: pathogenesis and management. *Semin Arthritis Rheum* 1991;20:256–272.
20. Peel NF, Eastell R, Russell RGG. Osteoporosis in rheumatoid arthritis—the laboratory perspective. *Br J Rheum* 1991;30:84–85.
21. Woolf AD. Osteoporosis in rheumatoid arthritis—the clinical viewpoint. *Br J Rheum* 1991;30:82–84.
22. Neva MH, Isomaki P, Hannonen P, et al. Early and extensive erosiveness in peripheral joints predicts atlantoaxial subluxations in patients with rheumatoid arthritis. *Arthritis Rheum* 2003;48(7):1808–1813.
23. Neva MH, Kotaniemi A, Kaarela K, et al. Atlantoaxial disorders in rheumatoid arthritis associate with the destruction of peripheral and shoulder joints, and decreased bone mineral density. *Clin Exp Rheumatol* 2003;21(2):179–184.
24. Beat AM, Bloch DA, Fries JF. Predictors of fractures in early rheumatoid arthritis. *J Rheumatol* 1991;18:804–808.
25. Saag K, Rochelle K, Caldwell J, et al. Low dose longterm corticosteroid therapy in rheumatoid arthritis; an analysis of serious adverse events. *Am J Med* 1994;96:115–123.
26. Spector TD, Hall GM, McCloskey EV, Kanis JA. Risk of vertebral fracture in women with rheumatoid arthritis. *Br Med J* 1993;306:558.
27. Verstraeten A, Dequeker J. Vertebral and peripheral bone density content and fracture incidence in postmenopausal patients with rheumatoid arthritis; effects of low-dose corticosteroids. *Ann Rheum Dis* 1986;45:852–857.
28. Mellish RWE, O'Sullivan MM, Garrahan NJ, Compston JE. Iliac crest trabecular bone mass and structure in patients with non-steroid treated rheumatoid arthritis. *Ann Rheum Dis* 1987;46:830–836.
29. Compston JE, Vedi S, Croucher PI, et al. Bone turnover in non-steroid treated rheumatoid arthritis. *Ann Rheum Dis* 1994;53:163–166.
30. Kroger H, Arnala I, Alhava EM. Bone remodeling in osteoporosis associated with rheumatoid arthritis. *Calcif Tiss Int* 1991;49:S90.
31. Gough AK, Peel NF, Eastell R, et al. Excretion of pyridinium crosslinks correlates with disease activity and appendicular bone loss in early rheumatoid arthritis. *Ann Rheum Dis* 1994;53:14–17.
32. Hall GM, Spector TD, Delmas PD. Markers of bone metabolism in postmenopausal women with rheumatoid arthritis. Effects of corticosteroids and hormone replacement therapy. *Arthritis Rheum* 1995;38:902–906.
33. Gough A, Sambrook P, Devlin J, et al. Osteoclastic activation is the principal mechanism leading to secondary osteoporosis in rheumatoid arthritis. *J Rheumatol* 1998;7:1282–1289.
34. Garnero P, Landewe R, Boers M, et al. Association of baseline levels of markers of bone and cartilage degradation with long-term progression of joint damage in patients with early rheumatoid arthritis: the COBRA study. *Arthritis Rheum* 2002;46(11):2847–2856.
35. Iwamoto J, Takeda T, Ichimura S. Urinary cross-linked N-telopeptides of type I collagen levels in patients with rheumatoid arthritis. *Calcif Tissue Int* 2003;72(4):491–497.
36. D'Elia HF, Larsen A, Waltbrand E, et al. Radiographic joint destruction in postmenopausal rheumatoid arthritis is strongly associated with generalised osteoporosis. *Ann Rheum Dis* 2003;62(7):617–623.
37. Sambrook P, Cohen M, Eisman J, et al. Effects of low-dose corticosteroid on bone mass in rheumatoid arthritis: a longitudinal study. *Ann Rheum Dis* 1989;48:535.
38. Laan R, van Riel P, van Erning L, et al. Vertebral osteoporosis in rheumatoid arthritis patients; effects of low-dose prednisone therapy. *Br J Rheumatol* 1992;31:91–96.
39. Gough AK, Lilley J, Eyre S, et al. Generalized bone loss in patients with rheumatoid arthritis. *Lancet* 1994;344:23–27.
40. Kirwan JR. The effects of glucocorticoids on joint destruction in rheumatoid arthritis. *N Engl J Med* 1995;333:142–146.
41. Kroger H, Honkanen R, Saarikoski S, Alhava E. Decreased axial bone mineral density in perimenopausal women with rheumatoid arthritis. *Ann Rheum Dis* 1994;53:18–23.
42. Sambrook P, Birmingham J, Champion D, et al. Postmenopausal bone loss in rheumatoid arthritis: effects of estrogens and androgens. *J Rheumatol* 1992;19:357–361.

43. Lodder MC, Haugeberg G, Lems WF, et al. Radiographic damage associated with low bone mineral density and vertebral deformities in rheumatoid arthritis: the Oslo-Truro-Amsterdam (OSTRA) collaborative study. *Arthritis Rheum* 2003;49(2):209–215.

44. Als OS, Gotfredsen A, Riis BJ, Christisnsen C. Are disease duration and degree of functional impairment determinants of bone loss in rheumatoid arthritis? *Ann Rhem Dis* 1985;44:406–411.

45. Orstavik RE, Haugeberg G, Uhlig T, et al. Vertebral deformities in 229 female patients with rheumatoid arthritis: associations with clinical variables and bone mineral density. *Arthritis Rheum* 2003;49(3):355–360.

46. Haugeberg G, RE OR, Uhlig T, et al. Comparison of ultrasound and X-ray absorptiometry bone measurements in a case control study of female rheumatoid arthritis patients and randomly selected subjects in the population. *Osteoporos Int* 2003;14(4):312–319.

47. Fries JF, Williams CA, Ramsey DR, Bloch DA. The relative toxicity of disease-modifying antirheumatic drugs. *Arthritis Rheum* 1993;44:406–411.

48. van Everdingen AA, Siewertsz van Reesema DR, Jacobs JW, Bijlsma JW. Low-dose glucocorticoids in early rheumatoid arthritis: discordant effects on bone mineral density and fractures? *Clin Exp Rheumatol* 2003;21(2):155–160.

49. Sinigaglia L, Nervetti A, Mela Q, et al. A multicenter cross sectional study on bone mineral density in rheumatoid arthritis. Italian Study Group on Bone Mass in Rheumatoid Arthritis. *J Rheumatol* 2000;27(11):2582–2589.

50. Dasgupta B, Corkill M, Kirkham B, et al. Serial estimation of interleukin 6 as a measure of systemic disease in rheumatoid arthritis. *J Rheumatol* 1992;19(1):22–25.

51. Nakashima T, Kobayashi Y, Yamasaki S, et al. Protein expression and functional difference of membrane-bound and soluble receptor activator of NF-kappaB ligand: modulation of the expression by osteotropic factors and cytokines. *Biochem Biophys Res Commun* 2000;275(3):768–775.

52. Haynes DR, Crotti TN, Loric M, et al. Osteoprotegerin and receptor activator of nuclear factor kappaB ligand (RANKL) regulate osteoclast formation by cells in the human rheumatoid arthritic joint. *Rheumatology (Oxf)* 2001;40(6):623–630.

53. Kong YY, Feige U, Sarosi I, et al. Activated T cells regulate bone loss and joint destruction in adjuvant arthritis through osteoprotegerin ligand. *Nature* 1999;402(6759):304–309.

54. Romas E, Sims N, Hards D, et al. Osteoprotegerin reduces osteoclast numbers and prevents bone erosion in collagen-induced arthritis. *Am J Pathol* 2002;161:1419–1427.

55. Redlich K, Hayer S, Maier A, et al. Tumor necrosis factor-a-mediated joint destruction is inhibited by targeting osteoclasts with osteoprotegerin. *Arthritis Rheum* 2002;46:785–792.

56. Schett G, Redlich K, Hayer S, et al. Osteoprotegerin protects against generalized bone loss in tumor necrosis factor-transgenic mice. *Arthritis Rheum* 2003;48(7):2042–2051.

57. Haynes DR, Barg E, Crotti TN, et al. Osteoprotegerin expression in synovial tissue from patients with rheumatoid arthritis, spondyloarthropathies and osteoarthritis and normal controls. *Rheumatology (Oxf)* 2003;42(1):123–134.

58. Kotake S, Udagawa N, Hakoda M, et al. Activated human T cells directly induce osteoclastogenesis from human monocytes: possible role of T cells in bone destruction in rheumatoid arthritis patients. *Arthritis Rheum* 2001;44(5):1003–1012.

59. Crotti TN, Smith MD, Weedon H, et al. Receptor activator NF-kappaB ligand (RANKL) expression in synovial tissue from patients with rheumatoid arthritis, spondyloarthropathy, osteoarthritis, and from normal patients: semiquantitative and quantitative analysis. *Ann Rheum Dis* 2002;61(12):1047–1054.

60. Ziolkowska M, Kurowska M, Radzikowska A, et al. High levels of osteoprotegerin and soluble receptor activator of nuclear factor kappa B ligand in serum of rheumatoid arthritis patients and their normalization after anti-tumor necrosis factor alpha treatment. *Arthritis Rheum* 2002;46(7):1744–1753.

61. Valleala H, Mandelin J, Laasonen L, et al. Effect of cyclical intermittent etidronate therapy on circulating osteoprotegerin levels in patients with rheumatoid arthritis. *Eur J Endocrinol* 2003;148(5):527–530.

62. Braun J, Sieper J. Building consensus on nomenclature and disease classification for ankylosing spondylitis: results and discussion of a questionnaire prepared for the International Workshop on New Treatment Strategies in Ankylosing Spondylitis, Berlin, Germany, 18–19 January 2002. *Ann Rheum Dis* 2002;61(Suppl 3):61–67.

63. Will R, Bhalla A, Palmer R, et al. Osteoporosis in early ankylosing spondylitis; a primary pathological event? *Lancet* 1989;23:1483–1485.

64. Ralston SH, Urquhart GD, Brzeski M, Sturrock RD. Prevalence of vertebral compression fractures due to osteoporosis in ankylosing spondylitis. *BMJ* 1990;300:563–565.

65. Hitchons PW, From AM, Brenton MD, et al. Fractures of the thoracolumbar spine complicating ankylosing spondylitis. *J Neurosurg* 2002;97:218–222.

66. Jansen TL, Aarts MH, Zanen S, Bruyn GA. Risk assessment for osteoporosis by quantitative ultrasound of the heel in ankylosing spondylitis. *Clin Exp Rheumatol* 2003;21(5):599–604.

67. Dos Santos FP, Constantin A, Laroche M, et al. Whole body and regional bone mineral density in ankylosing spondylitis. *J Rheumatol* 2001;28:547–549.

68. Maillefert JF, Aho LS, Maghraoui A, et al. Changes in bone density in patients with ankylosing spondylitis: a two year follow-up study. *Osteoporos Int* 2001;12:605–609.

69. Speden DJ, Calin AI, Ring FJ, Bhalla AK. Bone mineral density, calcaneal ultrasound, and bone turnover markers in women with ankylosing spondylitis. *J Rheumatol* 2002;29(3):516–521.

70. Capaci K, Hepguler S, Argin M, Tas I. Bone mineral density in mild and advanced ankylosing spondylitis. *Yonsei Med J* 2003;44(3):379–384.

71. Ritchlin CT, Haas-Smith SA, Li P, et al. Mechanisms of TNF-alpha- and RANKL-mediated osteoclastogenesis and bone resorption in psoriatic arthritis. *J Clin Invest* 2003;111(6):821–831.

72. Gratacos J, Collado A, Filella X, et al. Serum cytokines (IL-6, TNF-alpha, IL-1 beta and IFN-gamma) in ankylosing spondylitis: a close correlation between serum IL-6 and disease activity and severity. *Br J Rheumatol* 1994;33(10):927–931.

73. Allali F, Breban M, Porcher R, et al. Increase in bone mineral density of patients with spondyloarthropathy treated with anti-tumour necrosis factor alpha. *Ann Rheum Dis* 2003;62(4):347–349.

74. Balding J, Kane D, Livingstone W, et al. Cytokine gene polymorphisms: association with psoriatic arthritis susceptibility and severity. *Arthritis Rheum* 2003;48(5):1408–1413.

75. Lee SS, Joo YS, Kim WU, et al. Vascular endothelial growth factor levels in the serum and synovial fluid of patients with rheumatoid arthritis. *Clin Exp Rheumatol* 2001;19(3):321–4.

76. Drouart M, Saas P, Billot M, et al. High serum vascular endothelial growth factor correlates with disease activity of spondylarthropathies. *Clin Exp Immunol* 2003;132(1):158–162.

77. Fearon U, Griosios K, Fraser A, et al. Angiopoietins, growth factors, and vascular morphology in early arthritis. *J Rheumatol* 2003;30(2):260–268.

78. Deckers MM, Karperien M, van der Bent C, et al. Expression of vascular endothelial growth factors and their receptors during osteoblast differentiation. *Endocrinology* 2000;141(5):1667–1674.

79. Boyanov M, Robeva R, Popivanov P. Bone mineral density changes in women with systemic lupus erythematosus. *Clin Rheumatol* 2003;22(4–5):318–323.

80. Dhillon VB, Davies MC, Hall ML, et al. Assessment of the effect of oral corticosteroids on bone mineral density in systemic lupus erythematosus; a preliminary study with dual energy xray absorptiometry. *Ann Rheum Dis* 1990;49:624–626.

81. Kalla AA, Fataar AB, Jessop SJ, Bewerunge L. Loss of trabecular bone mineral density in systemic lupus erythematosus. *Arthritis Rheum* 1993;36:1726–1734.

82. Becker A, Fischer R, Scherbaum WA, Schneider M. Osteoporosis in systemic lupus erythematosus: impact of disease duration and organ damage. *Lupus* 2001;10:809–814.

83. Varonos S, Ansell BM, Reeve J. Vertebral collapse in juvenile chronic arthritis; its relationship with glucocorticoid therapy. *Calcif Tiss Int* 1987;41:75–78.

84. Loftus J, Allen R, Hesp R, et al. Randomized, double-blind trial of deflazacort versus prednisone in juvenile chronic (or rheumatoid) arthritis: a relatively bone-sparing effect of deflazacort. *Pediatrics* 1991;88:428–436.

85. French AR, Mason T, Nelson AM, et al. Osteopenia in adults with a history of juvenile rheumatoid arthritis. A population based study. *J Rheumatol* 2002;29:1065–1070.

86. Celiker R, Bal S, Bakkaloglu A, et al. Factors playing a role in the development of decreased bone mineral density in juvenile chronic arthritis. *Rheumatol Int* 2003;23(3):127–129.

# Pathogenesis of Focal Bone Loss in Inflammatory Arthritis

## 3

*Allison R. Pettit    Ellen M. Gravallese*

Bone is a target organ in many diseases including arthritis, malignancy, and periodontal disease. Technological developments in molecular and cellular biology in the last decade have lead to important advances in our understanding of the mechanisms involved in bone remodeling in disease states. Rheumatoid arthritis (RA) is the prototype of a chronic inflammatory arthritis that can lead to disabling bone loss in diarthrodial joints. Recent evidence has established an important role of the osteoclasts (OC), the cell responsible for resorption in physiologic bone remodeling in RA-associated bone erosion. Additionally, elucidation of the principal role of the receptor activator of NF-κB (RANK)/RANK ligand (RANKL)/osteoprotegerin (OPG) system in regulating both physiologic bone remodeling and certain immune responses has stimulated research into the potential role of this system, as well as other immune modulators, in pathologic bone loss. Clear delineation of the pathways involved in RA-associated pathologic bone loss may well provide new avenues for the design of directed therapies for the prevention of bone loss in inflammatory arthritis.

## RHEUMATOID ARTHRITIS

Patients with RA develop a chronic inflammatory process in synovial tissues (synovitis) that is mediated by both the innate and adaptive immune responses and is accompanied by destruction of joint cartilage and bone. Protection from bone destruction is an important therapeutic goal in RA, as continued radiographic deterioration is associated with poor prognosis (1). The pathologic changes seen in rheumatoid synovitis include angiogenesis, cellular infiltration into both the synovial tissue and fluid, and subsequent marked synovial hyperplasia. The cellular infiltrate in RA synovial tissues is heterogeneous and includes monocytes and macrophages, T and B cells, plasma cells, dendritic cells, and mast cells (2–4).

The cytokines expressed in synovial tissues in RA are predominantly of macrophage-fibroblast origin, including tumor necrosis factor (TNF)-α and interleukin (IL)-1 (5–7). A T helper 1 (Th1) phenotype has also been described (5,6). The local production of proinflammatory cytokines induces the expression of matrix degrading enzymes, including matrix metalloproteinases (MMPs), which are involved in cartilage degradation (8). Mounting evidence supports the hypothesis that the proinflammatory environment in RA also favors the generation and activation of OCs and that these cells are primarily responsible for removal of the mineralized bone matrix (bone erosion) in RA. This chapter discusses the evidence supporting the role of OCs in RA-associated focal bone erosion and reviews the factors in this inflammatory environment that may regulate OC differentiation and activation.

## OSTEOCLASTOGENESIS

OCs are derived from hematopoietic precursor cells of the monocyte-macrophage lineage and are differentiated multinucleated cells that have acquired unique characteristics enabling them to resorb bone. Precursor cells can branch from the monocyte-macrophage lineage to the OC differentiation pathway at various points along this lineage and include early CD34+ bone marrow or peripheral blood (PB) precursor cells and CD14+ PB monocytes (9–12). It has also been demonstrated that tissue macrophages can be induced to differentiate into OCs (13). The most common PB OC precursors are CD11b$^{high}$c-fms+ and require exposure to macrophage-colony stimulating factor (M-CSF) for survival, expansion, and expression of RANK, a receptor essential for the further differentiation of these cells to OCs (9,14–16).

RANKL, the ligand for RANK, has been demonstrated to be a required factor for osteoclastogenesis in the presence of M-CSF (17,18). Exposure of RANK+ OC precursors to RANKL diverts these cells along the OC pathway. RANKL also efficiently stimulates migration, cell fusion, OC activation, function, and survival and, therefore, induces the formation of mature OCs with bone resorption capabilities (17,19–22). OPG was originally described as a novel soluble factor that regulated bone mass (23) and has subsequently been identified as a soluble decoy receptor for RANKL. Thus, OPG blocks all of the proosteoclastogenic actions of RANKL (23–26). The current paradigm is that the RANKL to OPG expression ratio is the critical determinant of the degree of OC differentiation and function in bone remodeling (27,28). The essential role of the RANKL/RANK/OPG system in the differentiation of OCs and, subsequently, in OC-mediated bone resorption has been clearly illustrated by the phenotype of mice in which these genes have been genetically altered (18,23,29–34). In physiologic bone remodeling, the cellular source of RANKL and OPG is bone lining (osteoblast-lineage) cells and expression of these factors by bone lining cells accounts for much of the coupling between bone resorption and bone formation (35).

The RANKL/RANK/OPG system also plays a role in regulating immune responses. RANKL has been demonstrated to increase the survival and stimulatory capacity of dendritic cells (DC) and, thus, enhances and prolongs T cell responses (36,37). Activated T cells and activated B cells can express RANKL and have the capacity to stimulate osteoclastogenesis in vitro (36,38–41) and in vivo (27,42). Interestingly, reintroduction of RANKL expression only in T and B lymphocytes partially rescues the osteopetrotic phenotype in RANKL–/– mice (33). In addition, the osteoporotic phenotype in CTLA-4–/– mice is dependent on RANKL expression by activated T cells (27). These observations provide evidence that the immune system can directly influence bone homeostasis in vivo and suggest that lymphocytes in particular could potentially stimulate pathologic osteolysis.

## CONTRIBUTION OF OSTEOCLASTS TO FOCAL BONE EROSION IN RA

Marginal and subchondral focal bone erosions are common features of RA and contribute, at least in part, to the significant functional morbidity that is associated with this

disease over time (1). Recent research has demonstrated that OCs are likely to be the critical cell responsible for focal bone erosion in RA, including studies examining the role of RANKL or the requirement of OC precursors in this process. Cells with the phenotypic features of OCs have been demonstrated at sites of bone erosion in RA joint tissues (43,44) and in animal models of arthritis (27,45–47). RANKL mRNA and protein expression has been demonstrated in synovial fibroblasts and activated CD4+ T cells in RA tissue sections and in cells cultured from RA tissues (27,40,41,48–51). Additionally, it has been demonstrated that these cells can stimulate osteoclastogenesis in vitro (40,41,49,52). Furthermore, synovial tissue–derived macrophages can be differentiated into OCs in vitro in the presence of RANKL and M-CSF (41,53), and fully mature OCs can spontaneously generate in cultures of digested RA synovial tissue (51,54). This OC formation is inhibited by OPG, and the ratio of RANKL to OPG mRNA levels in digested RA tissue cultures correlates with the number of resorption pits formed (51). These observations demonstrate that the RA synovial environment contains all the necessary components required for, and likely favors, OC differentiation and activation, and that synovial expression of RANKL is likely to be an integral step in this process.

Seminal studies by Kong et al. using the rat adjuvant–induced arthritis model (AIA) provided definitive evidence for the central role of RANKL-directed osteoclastogenesis in the pathogenesis of bone resorption associated with inflammatory arthritis (27). In this model, expression of RANKL was demonstrated in the inflammatory infiltrate, particularly in activated T cells. RANKL blockade, using OPG treatment from disease onset, substantially protected animals from cortical and trabecular bone loss and was accompanied by a dramatic reduction in OC numbers in affected joints. Gross inflammation appeared to be unaffected by OPG treatment (27). In kinetic studies examining various OPG doses and treatment schedules, OPG decreased the number of OCs and inhibited bone destruction in a dose-dependent manner (55).

RA is a heterogeneous disease and the pathogenic mechanism(s) involved in disease initiation and perpetuation are not yet fully delineated. Therefore, confirmation of the observations of Kong et al. in animal models of inflammatory arthritis with different pathogenic mechanisms would strengthen the hypothesis that RANKL-stimulated osteoclastogenesis plays a central role in bone erosion in RA (27). The AIA model used by Kong et al. is predominantly a T cell-driven experimental arthritis; therefore, there is the potential for RANKL blockade in AIA to result in subtle modulation of the immune response that may result in a secondary protective effect on bone. This motivated our research group to examine a model of arthritis with a different disease mechanism, one in which the osteoclastogenic effects of RANKL could be isolated from its effects on immune responses. The K/BxN (KRN/B6 X

NOD) spontaneous arthritis model elegantly demonstrates the ability of a systemic autoimmune antibody response to provoke inflammatory arthritis (56). Transfer of serum containing pathogenic antibodies from K/BxN arthritic mice results in the development of an arthritis in recipient mice (serum transfer arthritis, STA) that represents the tissue destructive "effector" phase of the parent spontaneous arthritis. Importantly, STA does not require T cells or B cells, as their primary role in the spontaneous arthritis is in the production of pathogenic antibody (56). This model, therefore, provided an opportunity to determine the role of RANKL in osteoclastogenesis and bone erosion in the setting of inflammatory arthritis, independent of the role of RANKL in T and B cell mediated immune responses. We used the STA model to further examine and validate the role of RANKL-driven osteoclastogenesis in arthritic focal bone erosion, by transferring this arthritis to RANKL-/- OC-deficient mice (57). RANKL-/- mice with STA were dramatically protected from bone erosion despite ongoing inflammation, and TRAP+ multinucleated OC-like cells were completely absent in the arthritic RANKL-/- mice. This study provided further support for the hypothesis that RANKL is required for osteoclastogenesis and subsequently for bone erosion in inflammatory arthritis.

In collagen-induced arthritis (CIA), an arthritis model that involves both innate and adaptive immune responses, treatment of arthritic mice with OPG resulted in a greater than 75% reduction in OC numbers in juxtaarticular bone, an absence of OCs in pannus tissue, and protection from bone erosion. OPG therapy did not result in a change in paw swelling in treated compared to untreated arthritic mice (58). The human TNF transgenic (hTNFtg) mouse is yet another model of inflammatory arthritis. This mouse develops spontaneous arthritis that is driven by the systemic overexpression of the proinflammatory cytokine TNF-α. Treatment with OPG in this animal model yielded similar results, as inflammation was unaffected while the area of bone erosion was reduced by 56% if OPG was used alone and by 81% when OPG was used in combination with a bisphosphonate (pamidronate) with corresponding reductions in OC number (59). Finally, when the hTNFtg mouse was crossed with the c-fos deficient mouse, the latter of which completely lacks functional OCs because of the requirement of c-fos in OC differentiation, the resulting hTNFtg/c-fos-/- mice developed inflammation that was equivalent to the arthritic hTNFtg mice in severity, cellular distribution, and MMP expression. However, arthritic hTNFtg/c-fos-/- mice were fully protected from bone erosion with continued absence of OCs in this inflammatory environment (60). These studies provide considerable evidence that OCs are the primary cells mediating bone erosion in inflammatory arthritis and that RANKL is a critical signal driving the formation and activation of OCs in inflamed joints.

The use of bisphosphonates is an established therapeutic method to regulate OC-mediated bone resorption. High-dose bisphosphonate treatment decreased bone loss in animal models of arthritis (59,61,62). In RA, however, bisphosphonates have been shown to inhibit generalized bone loss but not focal bone erosion (63). This observation could be the result of insufficient drug dosage or insufficient drug delivery to sites of focal bone erosion or alternatively may reflect differences between the mechanisms of bone erosion in RA versus in animal models of arthritis. Therefore, further trials with new generation, more potent bisphosphonates including close assessment of drug availability and efficacy in both the generalized skeleton and affected joints is required before the full benefit of this therapeutic approach can be determined.

There is still the possibility that other cell types, including activated macrophages and synovial fibroblasts, may be directly contributing to bone erosion in inflammatory arthritis, independent of OCs. However, the ability of activated fibroblasts and macrophages to directly resorb bone in both in vitro and in vivo models is limited compared to the resorptive capabilities of OCs in the same assay systems (64,65). It is likely, however, that activated macrophages and synovial fibroblasts do contribute indirectly to focal bone resorption in inflammatory arthritis by expression of factors such as cathepsin K and MMPs that can enhance bone resorption (66,67). Although the contribution of cells other than OCs to focal bone erosion is worthy of further investigation, the data in animal models suggests that the independent contribution of these cells is limited. The accumulating evidence thus supports the hypothesis that OCs are key mediators of bone loss in inflammatory arthritis, independent of the underlying pathogenic mechanism driving the disease.

## FACTORS EXPRESSED IN RA SYNOVIAL TISSUES THAT MAY REGULATE OSTEOCLASTOGENESIS

The above discussion focuses on the role of the RANK/RANKL/OPG system in regulating osteoclastogenesis in inflammatory arthritis. However, cells within the RA synovium also produce many other cytokines and factors that have the potential to influence bone resorption via direct and indirect effects on OC differentiation and function. The net outcome of the RA inflammatory environment on bone is an increase in resorption over formation. However, review of the components of the inflammatory response reveals a complex hierarchy of signals that could provide both stimulatory and inhibitory input for bone resorption. Clearly defining the order and hierarchy of these regulatory factors, and the key cellular sources of these factors, will be critical to our further understanding of the pathways regulating OCs in RA.

The proinflammatory cytokines TNF-α and IL-1 have been identified as critical regulators of the inflammatory cascade in RA (5) and are likely to play a prominent role in regulating OC formation and activation and subsequent

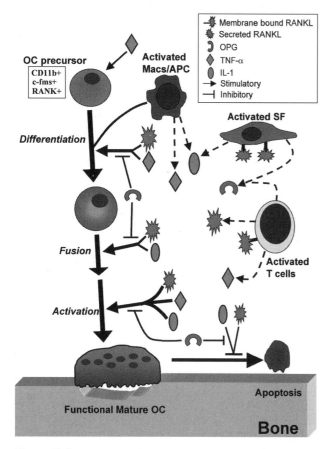

**Figure 3.1** Potential pathways involving the RANK/RANKL/OPG system, IL-1 and TNF-α in osteoclastogenesis in RA. The mechanisms leading to osteoclastogenesis in RA have not been definitively characterized. However, from both in vitro and in vivo observations the following paradigm outlining potential key components can be formulated: Several possible OC precursor populations have been identified including CD11b$^{high}$ c-fms$^+$ RANK$^+$ cells (16) and synovial tissue macrophages (Macs/APC [41,53]). Cytokines that are likely to have the most dominant effect on osteoclastogenesis in RA are RANKL, TNF-α, and IL-1. Cellular sources of RANKL in RA include synovial fibroblasts and activated CD4$^+$ T cells (27,40,41,48–51). In addition, T cells can express both membrane-bound and soluble forms of RANKL and could, therefore, stimulate synovial OC differentiation by both contact-dependent and -independent mechanisms (89). RANKL directly stimulates OC differentiation, activation, fusion, and survival (17,19–21,27). Both synovial fibroblasts and T cells are also potential sources of OPG, that could counteract the actions of RANKL (40). Activated tissue macrophages are the major source of TNF-α and IL-1 in RA, activated T cells can also produce TNF-α (6,100,113) and synovial fibroblasts can produce IL-1 (7). TNF-α directly stimulates OC differentiation and activation in synergy with RANKL and may also increase the available pool of CD11b$^{high}$ OC precursor cells (16). IL-1 directly stimulates OC fusion, activation, and survival. Studies in-vitro and in animal models suggest that TNF-α and IL-1 are able to modulate the degree of OC differentiation and/or function and may act in this manner in RA. This modulation may occur both directly, as illustrated in the current figure or indirectly through regulation of the expression ratio of RANKL/OPG in other cell types (Table 3.1 and references 59,81,114).

bone erosion. Figure 3.1 illustrates the pathways leading to OC differentiation and activation and the potential cellular sources and postulated actions of RANKL, TNF-α, and IL-1

on OC differentiation and activation in RA. TNF-α is known to directly stimulate OC differentiation and activation in synergy with RANKL, and IL-1 directly enhances OC activity and survival (68–72). Recent data suggest that an additional effect of TNF-α in promoting osteoclastogenesis in inflammatory arthritis may be its ability to mobilize a CD11b$^{high}$ population of immediate OC precursor cells, thus, increasing the number of OC precursor cells available in the periphery (blood and spleen) (16). In the arthritic hTNFtg mouse, an increase in CD11b$^{high}$ cells in the periphery correlated with the appearance of systemic TNF-α expression and with the onset of inflammatory arthritis. Blockade of the biological effects of TNF-α was able to reverse this increase in peripheral OC precursor cell number (16).

Blockade of TNF-α or IL-1 in animal models of arthritis has generally been shown to result in a significant reduction in measures of disease activity and/or joint destruction (73–76). The availability and success of therapies targeting TNF-α and IL-1 in RA have further established the central role of these cytokines in human disease (77–80). However, despite the success of these biological-response modifying drugs, a portion of patients do not respond adequately to these therapies, few patients achieve complete remission, and relapse is almost universal when therapy is ceased. It is, therefore, important to consider alternative new therapeutic strategies, including combination therapy, for maximizing clinical benefit, particularly protection from joint destruction. Supporting the usefulness of combination strategies, Redlich et al. compared the OC-targeted therapies OPG and bisphosphonates (pamidronate), or a combination of both, in the hTNFtg arthritis model (59). These therapies did not result in improvement in parameters of inflammation but did significantly decreases OC number and the size of bone erosions, with the combined therapy being the most effective (59). The same group recently demonstrated that in arthritic hTNFtg mice, anti-TNF plus OPG therapy was more effective at blocking both inflammation and joint destruction than either agent as a single therapy and showed similar efficacy to the combination of TNF plus IL-1 blockade or triple therapy with all of these agents (81). Combination therapy, therefore, is one potential strategy that may provide better therapeutic efficacy and prevention from joint destruction in RA

In addition to TNF-α, IL-1, and the RANK/RANKL/OPG system, many other cytokines and factors that are components of the inflammatory cascade in RA have been demonstrated to have effects (both direct and indirect) on osteoclastogenesis and/or OC function and therefore have the potential to modulate OC generation and activation in RA (Table 3.1). Because of the complex cytokine milieu that exists in RA, numerous pathways are likely to influence OC number and function. Therapeutic approaches designed to target multiple pathways and potentially also stimulate repair of damaged joints are currently being tested in animal models of arthritis (82).

**TABLE 3.1**

**FACTORS PRODUCED IN THE RA SYNOVIUM THAT COULD POTENTIALLY REGULATE OSTEOCLASTOGENESIS**

| Cytokine | Cellular Source | Cellular Target | RANKL/ OPG Ratio | Effects on Osteoclastogenesis and Function |
|---|---|---|---|---|
| M-CSF | OB, Mac, SF, T cells (88, 89) | Pre-OC | NA | Differentiation, proliferation, activation, and survival (15) |
| VEGF | Macs, SF (88, 90) | Pre-OC | NA | Differentiation, migration, resorption, and survival (22,91) |
| FGF-2 | OB, MC, Syn, Pannus (92, 93) | OB | $\uparrow$/– (93) | All RANKL effects |
| | | Pre-OC | NA | Inhibitory—counteracts M-CSF signaling (93) |
| TGF-$\beta$ | SF, Mac, bone matrix (94, 95) | Pre- and Imm-OC | NA | Differentiation, activation, and survival (95–97) |
| | | T cells | $\uparrow$/– (98) | All RANKL effects |
| | | OB | $\downarrow$/$\uparrow$ (35, 99) | OPG effects |
| TNF-$\alpha$ | Mac, T cells | Pre- and Imm-OC | NA | Differentiation and activation (68) |
| | | OB | $\uparrow\uparrow$/$\uparrow$ (35) | All RANKL effects |
| IL-1 | Mac, SF (7) | Imm-OC and OC | NA | Activation and survival (70) |
| | | OB | $\uparrow\uparrow$/$\uparrow$ (35) | All RANKL effects |
| IFN-$\gamma$ | T cells (100) | Pre-OC | NA | Inhibits differentiation in RANKL-naïve Pre-OC (101, 102) |
| | | Mac | NA | Increase TNF-$\alpha$ and IL-1 production (8) |
| PTHrP | SF (103) | OB | $\uparrow$/– (35, 104) | All RANKL effects |
| PGE$_2$ | OB, SF (105,106) | OB | $\uparrow$/$\downarrow$ (35) | All RANKL effects |
| IL-6 | OB, SF (88,107) | OB | $\uparrow$/– (108) | All RANKL effects |
| IL-17 | T cells (109) | OB, T cells, SF | $\uparrow$/– (110) | All RANKL effects |
| IL-7 | SF (111) | T cells | $\uparrow$/– (112) | All RANKL effects, TNF-$\alpha$ expression |

Imm-OC, immature osteoclast; T cells, CD4+ T cells; OB, bone-lining cells; Mac, macrophages; SF, synovial fibroblasts; VEGF, vascular endothelial growth factor; FGF-2, fibroblast growth factor-2; TGF-$\beta$, transforming growth factor-$\beta$; PTHrP, parathyroid hormone-related peptide; PGE$_2$, prostaglandin E$_2$; Syn, macrophage-like and/or fibroblast like-synoviocytes; MC, mast cells; $\uparrow$, increased expression; $\downarrow$, decreased expression; –, undetermined or no change in expression.

## BONE EROSION IN OTHER INFLAMMATORY ARTHRITIDIES

Psoriatic arthritis (PsA) is a polyarticular inflammatory arthritis that is associated with a predominance of Th1 cytokine production (83) and extensive bone destruction. Similar to its contribution in RA, TNF-$\alpha$ has also been suggested to play a critical role in PsA, and TNF-$\alpha$ blockade is currently in therapeutic use for the treatment of PsA (83–85). The pattern of bone destruction in RA and PsA differs, however, suggesting that both overlapping and distinct pathologic mechanisms may be at work in these diseases. Recently OC-like cells were demonstrated at the bone-pannus junction and at sites of subchondral bone erosion in PsA. Additionally, the number of OC precursor cells (CD11b$^{high}$) was increased in the blood of PsA patients, especially those with evident bone erosions, and treatment with a TNF-$\alpha$ blocking agent (infliximab) markedly diminished the number of OC precursor cells in vivo. The RANKL to OPG expression ratio was found to be upregulated in PsA synovial tissues, and synovial fibroblasts were identified as a major source of RANKL expression. The data suggest that in PsA there is an increase in potential OC precursor cell numbers and that the synovial microenvironment is biased in favor of OC differentiation and activation through expression of RANKL and TNF-$\alpha$ (84). Therefore, therapies targeting TNF-$\alpha$ and/or OC activity may protect against bone destruction in PsA.

Bone destruction is also associated with juvenile idiopathic arthritis (JIA) (86). As in RA, bone destruction is often an early feature of JIA, occurs in several forms (focal, juxtaarticular osteopenia, and generalized osteoporosis), and is associated with more severe polyarticular disease (86). Recently, large numbers of CD11b$^+$RANK$^+$ cells were demonstrated in JIA synovial fluid, indicating that potential OC-precursor cells are present within the JIA synovium. T cells isolated from JIA synovial fluid were also shown to express RANKL (87) and, therefore, may potentially play a role in the generation of functional OCs and subsequent joint destruction in JIA. More detailed investigation into the role of OCs in JIA-associated joint destruction is warranted. An important implication of the aforementioned observations is that in several forms of inflammatory arthritis with varying pathogenic mechanisms, the disease processes appear to converge on common downstream pathways resulting in increased OC activity and subsequent pathologic bone erosion.

## CONCLUSIONS

The new biologic armamentarium now available to the rheumatologist is testimony to the success of the dissection of the cellular and molecular mechanisms of inflammatory arthritis and subsequent design and application of targeted therapies. Recent studies have provided considerable evidence that OCs are important mediators of focal bone erosion in inflammatory arthritis and have provided insight into the pathways leading to OC generation and activation in inflamed joints. These observations support the hypothesis that therapies targeting OC differentiation and activity may be useful in protecting against joint destruction in RA. Protection from joint destruction is a key goal of RA therapy, a goal that is often not fully achieved by current therapeutic regimens, which primarily target inflammation. The combination of OC-targeted therapies with therapies that target the inflammatory cascade may enhance current therapeutic strategies by achieving optimal blockade of both inflammation and joint destruction.

## REFERENCES

1. Scott DL. Prognostic factors in early rheumatoid arthritis. *Rheumatology (Oxf)* 2000;39(Suppl 1):24–9.
2. Pettit AR, MacDonald KP, O'Sullivan B, Thomas R. Differentiated dendritic cells expressing nuclear RelB are predominantly located in rheumatoid synovial tissue perivascular mononuclear cell aggregates. *Arthritis Rheum* 2000;43(4):791–800.
3. Storgard CM, Stupack DG, Jonczyk A, et al. Decreased angiogenesis and arthritic disease in rabbits treated with an alphaVpbeta3 antagonist. *J Clin Invest* 1999;103(1):47–54.
4. Kraan MC, Haringman JJ, Post WJ, et al. Immunohistological analysis of synovial tissue for differential diagnosis in early arthritis. *Rheumatology (Oxf)* 1999;38(11):1074–1080.
5. Arend WP, Dayer J-M. Inhibition of the production and effects of interleukin-1 and tumor necrosis factor a in rheumatoid arthritis. *Arthritis Rheum* 1995;38:151–160.
6. Dolhain RJ, van der Heiden AN, ter Haar NT, et al. Shift toward T lymphocytes with a T helper 1 cytokine-secretion profile in the joints of patients with rheumatoid arthritis. *Arthritis Rheum* 1996;39(12):1961–1969.
7. Ritchlin C. Fibroblast biology. Effector signals released by the synovial fibroblast in arthritis. *Arthritis Res* 2000;2(5):356–360.
8. Klimiuk PA, Yang H, Goronzy JJ, Weyand CM. Production of cytokines and metalloproteinases in rheumatoid synovitis is T cell dependent. *Clin Immunol* 1999;90(1):65–78.
9. Arai F, Miyamoto T, Ohneda O, et al. Commitment and differentiation of osteoclast precursor cells by the sequential expression of c-Fms and receptor activator of nuclear factor kappa B (RANK) receptors. *J Exp Med* 1999;190:1741–1754.
10. Lean JM, Matsuo K, Fox SW, et al. Osteoclast lineage commitment of bone marrow precursors through expression of membrane-bound TRANCE. *Bone* 2000;27(1):29–40.
11. Shalhoub V, Elliott G, Chiu L, et al. Characterization of osteoclast precursors in human blood. *Br J Haematol* 2000;111(2):501–512.
12. Quinn JM, Whitty GA, Byrne RJ, et al. The generation of highly enriched osteoclast-lineage cell populations. *Bone* 2002;30(1):164–170.
13. Danks L, Sabokbar A, Gundle R, Athanasou NA. Synovial macrophage-osteoclast differentiation in inflammatory arthritis. *Ann Rheum Dis* 2002;61(10):916–921.
14. Quinn JM, Elliott J, Gillespie MT, Martin TJ. A combination of osteoclast differentiation factor and macrophage-colony stimulating factor is sufficient for both human and mouse osteoclast formation in vitro. *Endocrinology* 1998;139(10):4424–4427.
15. Tanaka S, Takahashi N, Udagawa N, et al. Macrophage colony-stimulating factor is indispensable for both proliferation and differentiation of osteoclast progenitors. *J Clin Invest* 1993;91(1):257–263.
16. Li P, Schwarz EM, O'Keefe RJ, et al. Systemic tumor necrosis factor alpha mediates an increase in peripheral CD11bhigh osteoclast precursors in tumor necrosis factor alpha-transgenic mice. *Arthritis Rheum* 2004;50(1):265–276.
17. Lacey DL, Timms E, Tan HL, et al. Osteoprotegerin ligand is a cytokine that regulates osteoclast differentiation and activation. *Cell* 1998;93(2):165–176.
18. Kong YY, Yoshida H, Sarosi I, et al. OPGL is a key regulator of osteoclastogenesis, lymphocyte development and lymph-node organogenesis. *Nature* 1999;397(6717):315–323.
19. Jimi E, Akiyama S, Tsurukai T, et al. Osteoclast differentiation factor acts as a multifunctional regulator in murine osteoclast differentiation and function. *J Immunol* 1999;163(1):434–442.
20. Burgess TL, Qian Y, Kaufman S, et al. The ligand for osteoprotegerin (OPGL) directly activates mature osteoclasts. *J Cell Biol* 1999;145(3):527–538.
21. Lacey DL, Tan HL, Lu J, et al. Osteoprotegerin ligand modulates murine osteoclast survival in vitro and in vivo. *Am J Pathol* 2000;157(2):435–448.
22. Henriksen K, Karsdal M, Delaisse JM, Engsig MT. RANKL and vascular endothelial growth factor (VEGF) induce osteoclast chemotaxis through an ERK1/2-dependent mechanism. *J Biol Chem* 2003;278(49):48745–48753.
23. Simonet WS, Lacey DL, Dunstan CR, et al. Osteoprotegerin: a novel secreted protein involved in the regulation of bone density. *Cell* 1997;89(2):309–319.
24. Yasuda H, Shima N, Nakagawa N, et al. Identity of osteoclastogenesis inhibitory factor (OCIF) and osteoprotegerin (OPG): a mechanism by which OPG/OCIF inhibits osteoclastogenesis in vitro. *Endocrinology* 1998;139(3):1329–1337.
25. Shalhoub V, Faust J, Boyle WJ, et al. Osteoprotegerin and osteoprotegerin ligand effects on osteoclast formation from human peripheral blood mononuclear cell precursors. *J Cell Biochem* 1999;72(2):251–261.
26. Hakeda Y, Kobayashi Y, Yamaguchi K, et al. Osteoclastogenesis inhibitory factor (OCIF) directly inhibits bone-resorbing activity of isolated mature osteoclasts. *Biochem Biophys Res Commun* 1998;251(3):796–801.
27. Kong YY, Feige U, Sarosi I, et al. Activated T cells regulate bone loss and joint destruction in adjuvant arthritis through osteoprotegerin ligand. *Nature* 1999;402(6759):304–309.
28. Fazzalari NL, Kuliwaba JS, Atkins GJ, et al. The ratio of messenger RNA levels of receptor activator of nuclear factor kappaB ligand to osteoprotegerin correlates with bone remodeling indices in normal human cancellous bone but not in osteoarthritis. *J Bone Miner Res* 2001;16(6):1015–1027.
29. Mizuno A, Amizuka N, Irie K, et al. Severe osteoporosis in mice lacking osteoclastogenesis inhibitory factor/osteoprotegerin. *Biochem Biophys Res Commun* 1998;247(3):610–615.
30. Bucay N, Sarosi I, Dunstan CR, et al. Osteoprotegerin-deficient mice develop early onset osteoporosis and arterial calcification. *Genes Dev* 1998;12(9):1260–1268.
31. Dougall WC, Glaccum M, Charrier K, et al. RANK is essential for osteoclast and lymph node development. *Genes Dev* 1999;13: 2412–2424.
32. Li J, Sarosi I, Yan XQ, Morony S, et al. RANK is the intrinsic hematopoietic cell surface receptor that controls osteoclastogenesis and regulation of bone mass and calcium metabolism. *Proc Natl Acad Sci U S A* 2000;97(4):1566–1571.
33. Kim N, Odgren PR, Kim DK, et al. Diverse roles of the tumor necrosis factor family member TRANCE in skeletal physiology revealed by TRANCE deficiency and partial rescue by a lymphocyte-expressed TRANCE transgene. *Proc Natl Acad Sci U S A* 2000;97(20):10905–10910.
34. Min H, Morony S, Sarosi I, et al. Osteoprotegerin reverses osteoporosis by inhibiting endosteal osteoclasts and prevents vascular calcification by blocking a process resembling osteoclastogenesis. *J Exp Med* 2000;192(4):463–474.
35. Hofbauer LC, Khosla S, Dunstan CR, et al. The roles of osteoprotegerin and osteoprotegerin ligand in the paracrine regulation of bone resorption. *J Bone Miner Res* 2000;15(1):2–12.

36. Wong BR, Josien R, Lee SY, et al. TRANCE (tumor necrosis factor [TNF]-related activation-induced cytokine), a new TNF family member predominantly expressed in T cells, is a dendritic cell-specific survival factor. *J Exp Med* 1997;186(12):2075–2080.

37. Josien R, Li HL, Ingulli E, et al. TRANCE, a tumor necrosis factor family member, enhances the longevity and adjuvant properties of dendritic cells in vivo. *J Exp Med* 2000;191(3):495–502.

38. Choi Y, Woo KM, Ko SH, et al. Osteoclastogenesis is enhanced by activated B cells but suppressed by activated CD8(+) T cells. *Eur J Immunol* 2001;31(7):2179–2188.

39. Yun TJ, Chaudhary PM, Shu GL, et al. OPG/FDCR-1, a TNF receptor family member, is expressed in lymphoid cells and is up-regulated by ligating CD40. *J Immunol* 1998;161(11):6113–6121.

40. Horwood NJ, Kartsogiannis V, Quinn JMW, et al. Activated T lymphocytes support osteoclast formation in vitro. *Biochem Biophys Res Commun* 1999;265(1):144–150.

41. Kotake S, Udagawa N, Hakoda M, et al. Activated human T cells directly induce osteoclastogenesis from human monocytes: possible role of T cells in bone destruction in rheumatoid arthritis patients. *Arthritis Rheum* 2001;44(5):1003–1012.

42. Ukai T, Hara Y, Kato I. Effects of T cell adoptive transfer into nude mice on alveolar bone resorption induced by endotoxin. *J Periodontal Res* 1996;31(6):414–422.

43. Bromley M, Woolley DE. Chondroclasts and osteoclasts at subchondral sites of erosion in the rheumatoid joint. *Arthritis Rheum* 1984;27(9):968–975.

44. Gravallese EM, Harada Y, Wang JT, et al. Identification of cell types responsible for bone resorption in rheumatoid arthritis and juvenile rheumatoid arthritis. *Am J Pathol* 1998;152(4):943–951.

45. Kuratani T, Nagata K, Kukita T, et al. Induction of abundant osteoclast-like multinucleated giant cells in adjuvant arthritic rats with accompanying disordered high bone turnover. *Histol Histopathol* 1998;13(3):751–759.

46. Suzuki Y, Nishikaku F, Nakatuka M, Koga Y. Osteoclast-like cells in murine collagen induced arthritis. *J Rheumatol* 1998;25(6):1154–1160.

47. Lubberts E, Oppers-Walgreen B, Pettit AR, et al. Increase in expression of receptor activator of nuclear factor kappaB at sites of bone erosion correlates with progression of inflammation in evolving collagen-induced arthritis. *Arthritis Rheum* 2002;46(11):3055–3064.

48. Gravallese EM, Manning C, Tsay A, et al. Synovial tissue in rheumatoid arthritis is a source of osteoclast differentiation factor. *Arthritis Rheum* 2000;43:250–258.

49. Takayanagi H, Iizuka H, Juji T, et al. Involvement of receptor activator of nuclear factor kappa-B ligand/osteoclast differentiation factor in osteoclastogenesis from synoviocytes in rheumatoid arthritis. *Arthritis Rheum* 2000;43:259–269.

50. Crotti TN, Smith MD, Weedon H, et al. Receptor activator NF-kappaB ligand (RANKL) expression in synovial tissue from patients with rheumatoid arthritis, spondyloarthropathy, osteoarthritis, and from normal patients: semiquantitative and quantitative analysis. *Ann Rheum Dis* 2002;61(12):1047–1054.

51. Haynes DR, Crotti TN, Loric M, et al. Osteoprotegerin and receptor activator of nuclear factor kappaB ligand (RANKL) regulate osteoclast formation by cells in the human rheumatoid arthritic joint. *Rheumatology (Oxf)* 2001;40(6):623–630.

52. Shigeyama Y, Pap T, Kunzler P, et al. Expression of osteoclast differentiation factor in rheumatoid arthritis. *Arthritis Rheum* 2000;43(11):2523–2530.

53. Itonaga I, Fujikawa Y, Sabokbar A, et al. Rheumatoid arthritis synovial macrophage-osteoclast differentiation is osteoprotegerin ligand–dependent. *J Pathol* 2000;192(1):97–104.

54. Suzuki Y, Tsutsumi Y, Nakagawa M, et al. Osteoclast-like cells in an in vitro model of bone destruction by rheumatoid synovium. *Rheumatology (Oxf)* 2001;40(6):673–682.

55. Campagnuolo G, Bolon B, Feige U. Kinetics of bone protection by recombinant osteoprotegerin therapy in Lewis rats with adjuvant arthritis. *Arthritis Rheum* 2002;46(7):1926–1936.

56. Korganow AS, Ji H, Mangialaio S, et al. From systemic T cell self-reactivity to organ-specific autoimmune disease via immunoglobulins. *Immunity* 1999;10(4):451–461.

57. Pettit AR, Ji H, von Stechow D, et al. TRANCE/RANKL knockout mice are protected from bone erosion in a serum transfer model of arthritis. *Am J Pathol* 2001;159(5):1689–1699.

58. Romas E, Gillespie MT, Martin TJ. Involvement of receptor activator of NFkappaB ligand and tumor necrosis factor-alpha in bone destruction in rheumatoid arthritis. *Bone* 2002;30(2):340–346.

59. Redlich K, Hayer S, Maier A, et al. Tumor necrosis factor alpha-mediated joint destruction is inhibited by targeting osteoclasts with osteoprotegerin. *Arthritis Rheum* 2002;46(3):785–792.

60. Redlich K, Hayer S, Ricci R, et al. Osteoclasts are essential for TNF-alpha-mediated joint destruction. *J Clin Invest* 2002;110(10):1419–1427.

61. Pysklywec MW, Moran EL, Bogoch ER. Zoledronate (CGP 42'446). a bisphosphonate, protects against metaphyseal intracortical defects in experimental inflammatory arthritis. *J Orthop Res* 1997;15:858–861.

62. Francis MD, Hovancik K, Boyce RW. NE-58095: a diphosphonate which prevents bone erosion and preserves joint architecture in experimental arthritis. *Int J Tiss Reac* 1989;11:239–252.

63. Eggelmeijer F, Papapoulos SE, van Paassen HC, et al. Increased bone mass with pamidronate treatment in rheumatoid arthritis; results of a three-year randomized double-blind trial. *Arthritis Rheum* 1996;39:396–402.

64. Pap T, Claus A, Ohtsu S, et al. Osteoclast-independent bone resorption by fibroblast-like cells. *Arthritis Res Ther* 2003;5(3):R163–R173.

65. Chambers TJ, Horton MA. Failure of cells of the mononuclear phagocyte series to resorb bone. *Calcif Tissue Int* 1984;36(5):556–558.

66. Hummel KM, Petrow PK, Franz JK, et al. Cysteine proteinase cathepsin K mRNA is expressed in synovium of patients with rheumatoid arthritis and is detected at sites of synovial bone destruction. *J Rheumatol* 1998;25(10):1887–1894.

67. Hou WS, Li W, Keyszer G, et al. Comparison of cathepsins K and S expression within the rheumatoid and osteoarthritic synovium. *Arthritis Rheum* 2002;46(3):663–674.

68. Fuller K, Murphy C, Kirstein B, et al. TNF-alpha potently activates osteoclasts, through a direct action independent of and strongly synergistic with RANKL. *Endocrinology* 2002;143(3):1108–1118.

69. Lam J, Takeshita S, Barker JE, et al. TNF-alpha induces osteoclastogenesis by direct stimulation of macrophages exposed to permissive levels of RANK ligand. *J Clin Invest* 2000;106(12):1481–1488.

70. Jimi E, Nakamura I, Duong LT, et al. Interleukin 1 induces multinucleation and bone-resorbing activity of osteoclasts in the absence of osteoblasts/stromal cells. *Exp Cell Res* 1999;247(1):84–93.

71. Jimi E, Nakamura I, Ikebe T, et al. Activation of NF-kappaB is involved in the survival of osteoclasts promoted by interleukin-1. *J Biol Chem* 1998;273(15):8799–8805.

72. Azuma Y, Kaji K, Katogi R, et al. Tumor necrosis factor-alpha induces differentiation of and bone resorption by osteoclasts. *J Biol Chem* 2000;275(7):4858–4864.

73. Wooley PH, Dutcher J, Widmer MB, Gillis S. Influence of a recombinant human soluble tumor necrosis factor receptor FC fusion protein on type II collagen-induced arthritis in mice. *J Immunol* 1993;151(11):6602–6607.

74. Lewthwaite J, Blake S, Hardingham T, et al. Role of TNF alpha in the induction of antigen induced arthritis in the rabbit and the anti-arthritic effect of species specific TNF alpha neutralising monoclonal antibodies. *Ann Rheum Dis* 1995;54(5):366–374.

75. Joosten LAB, Helsen MMA, Saxne T, et al. IL-1 alpha beta blockade prevents cartilage and bone destruction in murine type II collagen–induced arthritis, whereas TNF-alpha blockade only ameliorates joint inflammation. *J Immunol* 1999;163(9):5049–5055.

76. Bendele A, McAbee T, Sennello G, et al. Efficacy of sustained blood levels of interleukin-1 receptor antagonist in animal models of arthritis: comparison of efficacy in animal models with human clinical data. *Arthritis Rheum* 1999;42(3):498–506.

77. Moreland LW, Schiff MH, Baumgartner SW, et al. Etanercept therapy in rheumatoid arthritis; a randomized, controlled trial. *Ann Intern Med* 1999;130(6):478–486.

78. Maini R, St Clair EW, Breedveld FC, et al. Infliximab (chimeric anti-tumour necrosis factor alpha monoclonal antibody) versus placebo in rheumatoid arthritis patients receiving concomitant methotrexate: a randomised phase III trial. ATTRACT Study Group. *Lancet* 1999;354:1932–1939.

79. Bresnihan B, Cobby M. Clinical and radiological effects of anakinra in patients with rheumatoid arthritis. *Rheumatology (Oxf)* 2003;42(Suppl 2):ii22–ii28.

80. Cohen SB, Woolley JM, Chan W. Interleukin 1 receptor antagonist anakinra improves functional status in patients with rheumatoid arthritis. *J Rheumatol* 2003;30(2):225–231.

81. Zwerina J, Hayer S, Tohidast-Akrad M, et al. Single and combined inhibition of tumor necrosis factor, interleukin-1, and RANKL pathways in tumor necrosis factor-induced arthritis: Effects on synovial inflammation, bone erosion, and cartilage destruction. *Arthritis Rheum* 2004;50(1):277–290.

82. Redlich K, Gortz B, Hayer S, et al. Repair of local bone erosions and reversal of systemic bone loss upon therapy with anti-tumor necrosis factor in combination with osteoprotegerin or parathyroid hormone in tumor necrosis factor-mediated arthritis. *Am J Pathol* 2004;164(2):543–555.

83. Danning CL, Illei GG, Hitchon C, et al. Macrophage-derived cytokine and nuclear factor kappaB p65 expression in synovial membrane and skin of patients with psoriatic arthritis. *Arthritis Rheum* 2000;43(6):1244–1256.

84. Ritchlin CT, Haas-Smith SA, Li P, et al. Mechanisms of TNF-alpha- and RANKL-mediated osteoclastogenesis and bone resorption in psoriatic arthritis. *J Clin Invest* 2003;111(6):821–831.

85. Victor FC, Gottlieb AB, Menter A. Changing paradigms in dermatology: tumor necrosis factor alpha (TNF-alpha) blockade in psoriasis and psoriatic arthritis. *Clin Dermatol* 2003;21(5):392–397.

86. Mason T, Reed AM, Nelson AM, et al. Frequency of abnormal hand and wrist radiographs at time of diagnosis of polyarticular juvenile rheumatoid arthritis. *J Rheumatol* 2002;29(10):2214–2218.

87. Varsani H, Patel A, van Kooyk Y, et al. Synovial dendritic cells in juvenile idiopathic arthritis (JIA) express receptor activator of NF-kappaB (RANK). *Rheumatology (Oxf)* 2003;42(4):583–590.

88. Inoue H, Takamori M, Shimoyama Y, et al. Regulation by PGE2 of the production of interleukin-6, macrophage colony stimulating factor, and vascular endothelial growth factor in human synovial fibroblasts. *Br J Pharmacol* 2002;136(2):287–295.

89. Weitzmann MN, Cenci S, Rifas L, et al. T cell activation induces human osteoclast formation via receptor activator of nuclear factor kappaB ligand-dependent and -independent mechanisms. *J Bone Miner Res* 2001;16(2):328–337.

90. Kasama T, Shiozawa F, Kobayashi K, et al. Vascular endothelial growth factor expression by activated synovial leukocytes in rheumatoid arthritis: critical involvement of the interaction with synovial fibroblasts. *Arthritis Rheum* 2001;44(11):2512–2524.

91. Niida S, Kaku M, Amano H, et al. Vascular endothelial growth factor can substitute for macrophage colony- stimulating factor in the support of osteoclastic bone resorption. *J Exp Med* 1999;190(2):293–298.

92. Qu Z, Huang XN, Ahmadi P, et al. Expression of basic fibroblast growth factor in synovial tissue from patients with rheumatoid arthritis and degenerative joint disease. *Lab Invest* 1995;73(3):339–346.

93. Chikazu D, Katagiri M, Ogasawara T, et al. Regulation of osteoclast differentiation by fibroblast growth factor 2: stimulation of receptor activator of nuclear factor kappaB ligand/osteoclast differentiation factor expression in osteoblasts and inhibition of macrophage colony-stimulating factor function in osteoclast precursors. *J Bone Miner Res* 2001;16(11):2074–2081.

94. Chu CQ, Allard S, Abney E, et al. Detection of cytokines at the cartilage/pannus junction in patients with rheumatoid arthritis; implications for the role of cytokines in cartilage destruction and repair. *Br J Rheumatol* 1992;32:653–661.

95. Fuller K, Lean JM, Bayley KE, et al. A role for TGFbeta(1) in osteoclast differentiation and survival. *J Cell Sci* 2000;113 (Pt 13):2445–2453.

96. Kaneda T, Nojima T, Nakagawa M, et al. Endogenous production of TGF-beta is essential for osteoclastogenesis induced by a combination of receptor activator of NF-kappa B ligand and macrophage-colony-stimulating factor. *J Immunol* 2000;165(8):4254–4263.

97. Quinn JM, Itoh K, Udagawa N, et al. Transforming growth factor beta affects osteoclast differentiation via direct and indirect actions. *J Bone Miner Res* 2001;16(10):1787–1794.

98. Wang R, Zhang L, Zhang X, et al. Regulation of activation-induced receptor activator of NF-kappaB ligand (RANKL) expression in T cells. *Eur J Immunol* 2002;32(4):1090–1098.

99. Takai H, Kanematsu M, Yano K, et al. Transforming growth factor-beta stimulates the production of osteoprotegerin/osteoclastogenesis inhibitory factor by bone marrow stromal cells. *J Biol Chem* 1998;273(42):27091–27096.

100. Canete JD, Martinez SE, Farres J, et al. Differential Th1/Th2 cytokine patterns in chronic arthritis: interferon gamma is highly expressed in synovium of rheumatoid arthritis compared with seronegative spondyloarthropathies. *Ann Rheum Dis* 2000;59(4):263–268.

101. Takayanagi H, Ogasawara K, Hida S, et al. T-cell-mediated regulation of osteoclastogenesis by signalling cross-talk between RANKL and IFN-gamma. *Nature* 2000;408(6812):600–605.

102. Huang W, O'Keefe RJ, Schwarz EM. Exposure to receptor-activator of NFkappaB ligand renders pre-osteoclasts resistant to IFN-gamma by inducing terminal differentiation. *Arthritis Res Ther* 2003;5(1):R49–R59.

103. Yoshida T, Sakamoto H, Horiuchi T, et al. Involvement of prostaglandin E(2) in interleukin-1alpha-induced parathyroid hormone-related peptide production in synovial fibroblasts of patients with rheumatoid arthritis. *J Clin Endocrinol Metab* 2001;86(7):3272–3278.

104. Funk JL, Chen J, Downey KJ, et al. Blockade of parathyroid hormone-related protein prevents joint destruction and granuloma formation in streptococcal cell wall-induced arthritis. *Arthritis Rheum* 2003;48(6):1721–1731.

105. Sugiyama T. Involvement of interleukin-6 and prostaglandin E2 in periarticular osteoporosis of postmenopausal women with rheumatoid arthritis. *J Bone Miner Metab* 2001;19(2):89–96.

106. Yano K, Nakagawa N, Yasuda H, et al. Synovial cells from a patient with rheumatoid arthritis produce osteoclastogenesis inhibitory factor/osteoprotegerin: reciprocal regulation of the production by inflammatory cytokines and basic fibroblast growth factor. *J Bone Miner Metab* 2001;19(6):365–372.

107 Chenoufi HL, Diamant M, Rieneck K, et al. Increased mRNA expression and protein secretion of interleukin-6 in primary human osteoblasts differentiated in vitro from rheumatoid and osteoarthritic bone. *J Cell Biochem* 2001;81(4):666–678.

108. Horowitz MC, Xi Y, Wilson K, Kacena MA. Control of osteoclastogenesis and bone resorption by members of the TNF family of receptors and ligands. *Cytokine Growth Factor Rev* 2001;12(1):9–18.

109. Lubberts E, van den Bersselaar L, Oppers-Walgreen B, et al. IL-17 promotes bone erosion in murine collagen-induced arthritis through loss of the receptor activator of NF-kappa B ligand/osteoprotegerin balance. *J Immunol* 2003;170(5):2655–2662.

110. Miossec P. Interleukin-17 in rheumatoid arthritis: if T cells were to contribute to inflammation and destruction through synergy. *Arthritis Rheum* 2003;48(3):594–601.

111. Harada S, Yamamura M, Okamoto H, et al. Production of interleukin-7 and interleukin-15 by fibroblast-like synoviocytes from patients with rheumatoid arthritis. *Arthritis Rheum* 1999;42(7):1508–1516.

112. Toraldo G, Roggia C, Qian WP, et al. IL-7 induces bone loss in vivo by induction of receptor activator of nuclear factor kappa B ligand and tumor necrosis factor alpha from T cells. *Proc Natl Acad Sci U S A* 2003;100(1):125–130.

113. Chu CQ, Field M, Feldmann M, Maini RN. Localization of tumor necrosis factor alpha in synovial tissues and at the cartilage-pannus junction in patients with rheumatoid arthritis. *Arthritis Rheum* 1991;34(9):1125–1132.

114. Ji H, Pettit A, Ohmura K, et al. Critical roles for interleukin 1 and tumor necrosis factor alpha in antibody-induced arthritis. *J Exp Med* 2002;196(1):77–85.

# Measurement Tools in Osteoporosis and Arthritis

# Biochemical Markers of Bone and Cartilage Turnover

*Apurva K. Srivastava*    *David J. Baylink*

Biochemical markers are useful in clinical practice because (i) they can indicate disease status prior to overt damage, (ii) they can identify those at higher risk for disease progression, and (iii) they can assess the efficacy of intervention therapy in a timely manner. The concept of using biochemical markers to assess both bone and cartilage turnover is an old one. Assays such as serum alkaline phosphatase (1) and urinary hydroxyproline (2) have been used to assess bone and arthritis diseases for many decades; however, those tests were not sufficiently specific and precise enough to assess osteoporosis or arthritis. Over the last two decades, new sensitive marker assays have been developed that are more specific for bone and cartilage matrix. In addition, because these new assay technologies are more reliable, rapid, and cost effective, they have already had an impact on the clinical management of bone diseases. As a result of the progress made in the development of bone markers with improved sensitivity and specificity, clinicians are now beginning to use markers in clinical practice for the management of osteoporosis (3).

For a marker analysis to be reliable, it is necessary that its concentration is a specific indicator of metabolic status of the bone or joint tissues and not other tissues. In addition, marker levels should be independent of variation in the biological fluid in which it is measured and rate of clearance by liver, kidneys, or synovial fluids, etc. An understanding of the nature and origin of the markers, their processing, and whether their presence is indicative of synthesis or degradation is key to insure their careful application in the clinical management of bone and cartilage diseases. In this article, we briefly overview markers of bone and cartilage turnover and discuss their clinical utility in the management of osteoporosis and joint diseases.

## MARKERS OF BONE TURNOVER

Although bone markers have been in research for long time, recent studies indicate that markers can now play a very important role in the management of osteoporosis. The diagnosis of osteoporosis is made by determining that the patient has low bone mineral density (BMD), usually by a dual energy x-ray absorptiometry (DXA) measurement. Low bone density places the patient at increased risk for fracture, which is the ultimate adverse effect and main source of morbidity and mortality from disease osteoporosis. Thus, BMD is accepted as surrogate for fracture risk (4). Recent studies emphasize, however, that the risk for fracture is determined by bone quality (5), as well as the amount of bone, that is, the bone density. In this regard, it is of particular interest that one can get some indirect assessment of bone quality by measurement of biochemical markers (Table 4.1). The reason for this is that the biochemical markers measure bone turnover or remodeling, and, in general, the higher the bone turnover, the worse the bone quality (Fig. 4.1). Therefore, best assessment of fracture risk can be made by bone density measurement along with the measurement of a bone marker.

In the management of osteoporosis, bone density generally provides assessments about every 2 years, whereas biochemical markers can provide dynamic information on the effectiveness of therapeutic agents within 3–6 months.

| **TABLE 4.1** MARKERS OF BONE TURNOVER | |
|---|---|
| **Resorption Markers** | **Formation Markers** |
| Free and total deoxypyridinoline (DPD) | Serum osteocalcin (sOC) |
| Free and total deoxypyridinoline (PYD) | Urine osteocalcin (uOC) |
| Serum and urine collagen type I cross-linked N-telopeptide (sNTx & uNTx) | Serum bone specific alkaline phosphatase (bone ALP) |
| Serum and urine collagen type I cross-linked C-telopeptide (sCTx & uCTx) | Serum procollagen I carboxyterminal propeptide (PICP) |
| Serum carboxyterminal telopeptide of type I collagen (ICTP) | Serum procollagen type I N-terminal propeptide (PINP) |
| Tartrate resistant acid-phosphatase (TRAP) | Bone sialoprotein (BSP) |
| Galactosyl hydroxylysine (Gal-Hyl) | |
| Glucosylgalactosyl hydroxylysine (Glc-Gal-Hyl) | |

Importantly, currently available osteoporosis therapies such as bisphosphonates, estrogens, selective estrogen receptor modulators (SERMS), and calcitonins act by reducing the bone marker levels; hence, markers are useful in monitoring therapy. The BMD is an excellent index of fracture risk; however, changes in BMD during therapy poorly reflect percent reduction in fracture risk. The reduction in fracture risk explained by the observed changes in BMD by alendronate (6), raloxifene (7), and risedronate (8) therapy is approximately 16%, 4%, and 28%, respec-

tively; indicating that other factors contribute to bone strength and change with treatment. Recently, it has been shown that decrease in bone turnover markers can account for a major fraction (40%–50%) of the observed antifracture efficacy of these drugs (9). Finally, there is evidence that long-term compliance of patients to continue osteoporosis treatment benefits from physician reinforcement using bone turnover markers. In a recent study (10), the effect of physician reinforcement was assessed using bone turnover markers on persistence with risedronate treatment. Patients with a good marker response had improved compliance; thus, the authors concluded that monitoring osteoporosis treatment using marker data should be encouraged. The foregoing suggests that biochemical markers have an important role in the clinical management of osteoporosis.

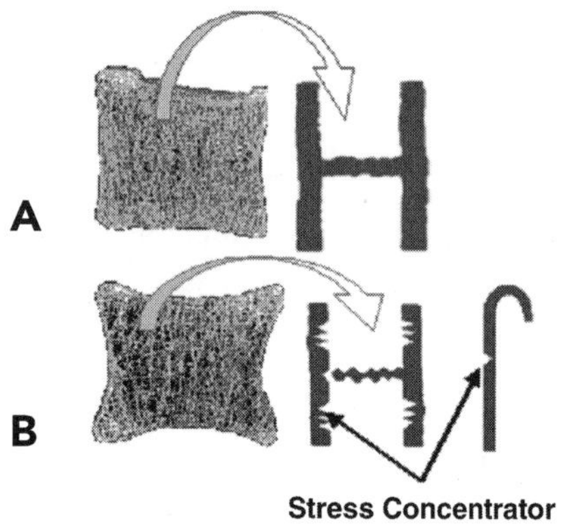

**Figure 4.1**   Small changes in bone turnover make large changes in bone strength. (A) Cross section of a vertebral body from a normal person showing the pattern of spinal trabecular bone, and (B) that of a patient with osteoporosis showing the "thinning" and loss of spinal trabecular bone, which compromises the overall mechanical strength of the bone. On the right hand panels, the illustrations show how high bone turnover affects trabecular bone microarchitecture and causes fractures. Normal bone turnover process creates resorption cavities, which are smoothed off by osteoblasts (A). In osteoporosis patients, the osteoclasts create more and excessively deep cavities (B) causing loss of trabecular connectivity. Small areas of clustered deep cavities on thin, unsupported vertical trabeculae act as stress concentrators (Einhorn TA. Bone strength: the bottom line. *Calcif Tissue Int*. 1992;51[5]: 333–339). The stress concentrators represent a focal weakness, which significantly decreases the stress required for fracture (as shown in the example of walking stick). This concept also illustrates that small local losses of bone don't decrease as much of bone density but markedly decreases the bone strength.

## BONE MARKERS

Adult bone is remodeled throughout life. This remodeling or bone turnover occurs via a coupled process of bone resorption, initiated by osteoclasts, followed by bone formation, by osteoblasts. Approximately 20% of bone tissue is replaced annually by this remodeling process, which occurs over approximately 4 to 8 months, with a range of 3 months to 2 years. Osteoporosis occurs when resorption is more active than formation, resulting in a net bone loss. The utility of biochemical markers is based on the fact that the rate of bone turnover can be assessed by measurement of a variety of proteins and peptides that are generated during the remodeling process and are released into serum and urine (Table 4.1). These markers include osteocalcin, skeletal alkaline phosphatase, and procollagen peptides that are secreted by osteoblasts and represent bone formation markers. On the other hand, degradation products of type-I collagen peptides (90% of organic osteoid matrix is type-I collagen) such as pyridinoline crosslinks, N-telopeptides (NTx), and C-telopeptide (CTx) are mainly generated during osteoclastic bone resorption and referred as bone resorption markers. Because bone resorption and formation are coupled, an increase in either process increases marker levels. In chronic steady state conditions, most markers reflect both formation and resorption because only a small imbalance exists. In addition, biochemical markers are not disease specific but reflect alterations in skeletal metabolism regardless of the underlying cause.

## CLINICAL UTILITY OF BONE MARKERS

### Bone Markers Assess Risk of Rapid Bone Loss

Bone mineral density in osteoporotic patients is a result of both peak bone density and subsequent postmenopausal, or age-related, bone loss. Longitudinal studies of postmenopausal women have demonstrated two characteristic groups, those losing a significant amount of bone mineral density (the high bone turnover group) and those losing a minor amount of bone mineral density (the normal or low bone turnover group). Biochemical assays are useful to identify those subjects who are losing bone most rapidly. This is particularly important, because patients with rapid bone loss show the greater stabilization and increase in bone density in response to antiresorptive medications. Longitudinal studies of cohorts (11) who have not undergone treatment for postmenopausal osteoporosis suggest that baseline bone marker levels are associated with those who lose bone most rapidly. Figure 4.2 shows how baseline levels of a urinary resorption marker, NTx, are associated with subsequent rapid bone loss measured after 1 year. A high baseline NTx, above 67 units, indicated a 17.3 times higher risk of BMD loss if not treated.

In summary, the fast bone losers appear to have elevated concentrations of biochemical markers compared to slow bone losers; consequently, measurement of biochemical markers can be used to identify fast bone losers. Elevated markers, however, do not always indicate bone loss. Important exceptions include the growth period during early life or during treatment with parathyroid hormone (PTH) when accelerated formation exceeds resorption, and, thus, increased bone marker value indicates bone gain.

### High Rate of Bone Turnover Is Associated with Increased Risk of Fracture

There is evidence that high bone turnover, as measured by bone markers, is associated with increased fracture risk. The relationship between biochemical markers and fracture risk has been investigated in retrospective studies comparing markers in patients with osteoporotic fractures and in controls and, more recently, in prospective studies in which markers were measured before the occurrence of fractures. In a prospective study (12) with 7,598 healthy women of more than 75 years of age, the authors demonstrated that increased rates of bone turnover might identi-

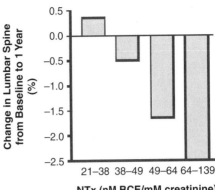

**Figure 4.2  Bone markers predict rapid bone loss.** Baseline data on N-terminal telopeptides of Type-I collagen (NTx, expressed as ratio of creatinine), in a randomized placebo-controlled trial in younger postmenopausal women predicts loss in lumbar spine BMD (L1–L4) after 1 year. The authors averaged four NTx values at baseline and, during the course of study, found that subjects with highest NTx values experienced the greatest spinal BMD loss (adapted from Chesnut CH 3rd, Bell NH, Clark GS, et al. Hormone replacement therapy in postmenopausal women: urinary N-telopeptide of type I collagen monitors therapeutic effects and predicts response of bone mineral density. *Am J Med* 1997;102(1):29–32.

fy those patients at highest risk for hip fracture as indicated by increased excretion of urinary resorption marker (CTx) with an odds ratio of 2.2 per standard deviation (SD) increase in CTx level. Women with both a low femoral neck bone mineral density and increased urinary CTx levels were at greater risk of hip fracture with an odds ratio of 4.8 per SD. In another example of how bone markers are associated with increased fracture risk, a meta-analysis by Hochberg and coworkers (13) of 18 clinical trials of antiresorptive therapy indicated that a 70% reduction in resorption markers would be associated with a 40% reduction in nonvertebral fractures, and a 50% reduction in formation markers would be associated with 44% reduction in fracture risk. Despite this promising evidence, the ability of markers to predict fractures has not been fully established; thus, bone markers are neither substitutes nor surrogates for BMD measurements in predicting bone fractures. Additional studies involving markers as the primary outcome variable are required to confirm some of these findings.

### Bone Markers Predict Response to Therapy Before Evidence of BMD Changes

Bone density is comparatively less effective in terms of measuring acute changes because bone density measures net balance between bone resorption and bone formation, which is typically less than 2% per year or a maximum of less than 1% for 3–6 months, in response to therapy (Table 4.2). However, less than 1% changes are difficult to measure because of precision limitations of BMD technologies. In contrast, osteoporosis therapies such as hormone replacement, SERMs (7), bisphosphonates (6,8),

### TABLE 4.2

#### DECREASE IN COLLAGEN CROSSLINK MARKERS IN RESPONSE TO ANTIRESORPTIVE THERAPY

| Treatment | Decrease in NTx, CTx, and Total DPD (%) | Time When Maximum Changes Observed (months) |
|---|---|---|
| Bisphosphonates | 50–70 | 3 |
| HRT | 40–60 | 6–12 |
| SERMs | 30–40 | 6–12 |
| Nasal Calcitonin | 20–40 | 6–12 |

and calcitonin (14) act by reducing the bone markers levels by 40%–70% within 3–6 months. Even though bone density is much more precise than bone biochemical assays, it is still easier to detect a 50% change with a biochemical assay than a 1% change with a bone densitometry after 3–6 months of therapy (Fig. 4.3). The rapid changes in bone markers allow making important therapeutic decisions for optimal management of osteoporosis patients, particularly if osteoporosis is severe (Fig. 4.4).

### Variability of Bone Markers

In the past, practical utilization of markers was limited by diurnal and longitudinal variation in bone markers, which was considered too great for diagnostic use in individual patients. New assays are better and improved understanding of biological variation has led to more intelligent application of markers in clinical trials (15,16). For monitoring response to treatment in individual patients, use of least significant change (LSC) defines a true biological

change in a marker. For example, to monitor therapy, a posttreatment value in bone marker is compared with baseline values determined before initiating therapy. If percent change in posttreatment value is greater than LSC (Fig. 4.3), then it is considered a true biological change as a result of therapy and not because of long-term variation (LSC) in an individual. Changes in marker levels are generally greater than LSC for most of the drugs currently used for the treatment of osteoporosis.

### Conclusion

The aim of bone marker analysis is to individualize treatment, and the consensus of experts in this area is that measurement of bone turnover markers provides potentially useful information to supplement BMD measurement. As described in a clinical algorithm (Fig. 4.4), which is used by the authors in clinical practice, there are two main areas where bone markers are particularly useful.

1. In classifying patients with low or intermediate bone density into low- and high-remodeling groups to individualize therapy and reduce fracture risk. This is particularly important because patients with rapid bone loss show greater stabilization and increase in bone density in response to antiresorptive medications.
2. In predicting response to therapy before evidence of BMD changes can be seen, which is comparatively less effective in terms of measuring acute changes because changes are small and difficult to measure because of precision limitations of BMD technologies. The rapid changes in bone markers allow making important therapeutic decisions for optimal management of osteoporosis patients, particularly if osteoporosis is severe. The best management of patients with osteoporosis who have a low bone turnover is not clear at this time. Biochemical marker data suggest that these patients would be the least likely to respond favorably to antiresorptive therapy. However, this issue needs to be investigated further. Such patients could be eligible for PTH 1-34 treatment (an anabolic agent), which is now commercially available.

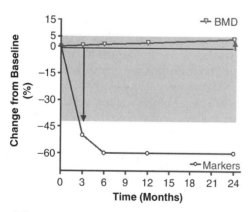

**Figure 4.3** Changes in BMD and bone markers in response to bisphosphonate therapy of osteoporosis patients. A precision error of 1%–1.5% in BMD measurements means that 2 years of treatment may be needed between testing to observe a significant change in BMD. However, a 50% change in marker means a significant change in response to treatment can be seen after only 3 months. The shaded area shows minimum change required in decrease in some urinary resorption markers and increase in BMD to be considered a true biologic change.

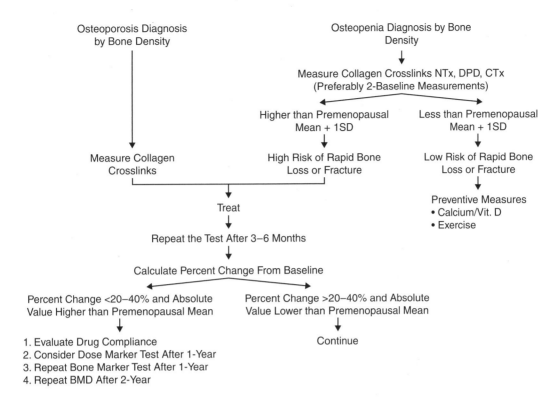

**Figure 4.4**    A clinical algorithm for using bone markers in treatment and management of osteoporosis.

## MARKERS OF ARTHRITIS

Studies of cartilage turnover markers in joint disease are following a pattern seen in the development and application of bone markers, albeit with several years delay. The major clinical manifestation of rheumatoid arthritis (RA) or osteoarthritis (OA) is cartilage tissue destruction resulting in joint damage, pain, and immobility. The gold standard in noninvasive assessment of functional and structural damage of joint disease is joint space width (JSW) measurement by radiography (17,18), which represents the best surrogate for cartilage deterioration in OA or RA of the hip and/or knee. However, the slow progressive destruction of joints makes radiographic assessment difficult within 1–2 years of progression or reduction by treatment. The possibility that markers can be utilized to improve early diagnoses of joint diseases or to predict disease progression is based on the knowledge (i) that metabolic changes in cartilage tissue occur significantly earlier than detection of loss of tissue by radiography, and (ii) that measurement of various biomolecules generated from the cartilage metabolism (degradation or synthesis of matrix components) is now possible in blood and urine. The goal of cartilage markers is to detect destruction of articular cartilage and eventually to detect an imbalance between degradation and repair. Early detection of cartilage destruction is particularly important because arthritis patients may have a window of opportunity to benefit from aggressive treatment at early

stages. Because markers can provide information on molecular events occurring over a short time, they are also ideal tools for monitoring drug therapy in a longitudinal manner. Recent progress made in our understanding of cartilage matrix proteins has led to the development of several new markers of OA and RA. To introduce cartilage turnover markers, we first review how these markers are biologically generated in cartilage and synovium tissues and released into circulation, and we then discuss evidence on how their measurements may be useful in the clinical investigations and eventually clinical management of the joint diseases.

### Markers of Cartilage Matrix Synthesis and Breakdown

Articular cartilage is a highly organized avascular tissue composed of chondrocytes embedded within an extracellular matrix of collagens, proteoglycans, and noncollagenous proteins. The two major structural proteins generated by chondrocytes are type-II collagen and aggrecans (a large proteoglycan). The aggrecans are held in the tissue within a fibrous network of triple-helical, type-II collagen fibrils, which are crosslinked and provide cartilage with its tensile strength. Together, these two macromolecules make up approximately 25% of the wet weight of cartilage, with water accounting for most of the remainder. The aggrecan component is continuously remodeled while type-II collagen

## TABLE 4.3

### SELECTED MARKERS OF OSTEOARTHRITIS (OA) AND RHEUMATOID ARTHRITIS (RA)

| Aggrecan-Based Markers | Type-II Collagen Based Markers | Minor Component of Cartilage Matrix | Inflammation Markers |
|---|---|---|---|
| Cartilage proteoglycan aggrecan core protein | C-telopeptide (CTx-II) | Cartilage oligomeric protein (COMP) | C-reactive protein (CRP) |
| Keratan sulfate (KS) epitopes | C-Terminal propeptide | GP-39/YKL-40 | Cytokines (IL-6, IL-1) |
| Chondroitin sulfate (CS) epitopes | | Type III collagen (N- and C-terminal propeptides) | TNF-alpha receptors |
| Aggrecan core protein cleavage neoepitopes | | | |
| Hyaluronic acid (HA) | | | |

is essentially maintained throughout life. In our discussion, we divide markers of cartilage destruction into three categories: (i) aggrecan, (ii) type-II collagen markers, and (iii) minor constituents of cartilage (Table 4.3). Aggrecan and type-II collagen are the two major structural molecules involved in cartilage turnover, whereas our third group of markers are minor constituents of cartilage including cartilage oligomeric protein (COMP) biglycan; collagen types VI, IX, and XI; and a range of cartilage-specific matrix glycoproteins.

## Aggrecan Based Markers

Aggrecan (Fig. 4.5) is found in huge multimolecular aggregates, comprising up to 100 monomers bound to hyaluronan (HA). Aggrecan monomer is a multidomain proteoglycan with a core protein of about 220 kD. The aggrecan structure is made of three domains, the N-terminal G1 domain, which consists of three subdomains, the interglobular G2 domain (IGD), the glycosaminoglycan-bearing domains, which includes glycosaminoglycan (GAG) chains keratan sulfate region and chondroitin sulfate region, and the C-terminal G3 domain. The chondroitin sulphate GAG is made up of 40–50 repeating disaccharide units of glucuronate and N-acetylglucosamine in the basic structure carrying a sulphate at carbon 6 or 4. In most tissues, each chain contains variable stretches of one or the other sulphate variant.

## Markers of Aggrecan Core Protein Degradation

A prominent feature of joint disease is a loss of aggrecan, which is degraded by enzymes metalloproteinases and aggrecanase at two major cleavage sites that are present in the IGD-domain that separates the G1 and G2 domains. By far the major portion of aggrecan released appears to be cleaved by aggrecanase (which also acts during normal turnover). The serum levels of aggrecan fragments

(frequently called epitopes in the literature because these fragments are detected by various antibodies used in the assays) are 30%–40% elevated in OA/RA compared to controls. These assays include keratan sulfate (19) and chondroitin sulfate (20,21). Keratan sulfate is indicative of

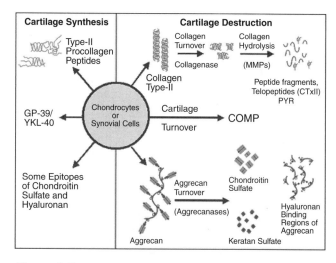

**Figure 4.5** Molecular markers generated by turnover of key cartilage matrix proteins. Chondrocytes maintain articular cartilage by replacing degraded matrix component via local matrix synthesis. In arthritic disease this equilibrium is shifted towards degradation. Chondrocytes and synovial cells upon activation secrete matrix components such as aggrecan, type-II collagen, and GP-39 as well as enzymes that degrade matrix components such as aggrecanase, matrix metalloproteinase (MMPs), collagenases, etc. These enzymes promote rapid degradation of aggrecan and type-II collagen, releasing products such as keratan and chondroitin sulfate, hyaluronan, and fragments of type-II collagen including C-telopeptide. All these markers can be measured in blood where their levels correlate with cartilage destruction. Elevated level of another matrix component, cartilage oligomeric matrix protein (COMP), is also a specific indicator of cartilage destruction. Type-II collagen is synthesized as a procollagen peptide and assays specific for propeptide such as C-terminal propeptide measure cartilage matrix synthesis. Some epitopes of chondroitin sulfate and hyaluronan also indicate new synthesis of aggrecan. These matrix synthesis assays can be used to measure the balance between cartilage destruction and synthesis.

cartilage degradation, but common chondroitin sulfate assays are taken as indicative of newly synthesized aggrecan. In addition, several new assays against recently generated fragments, called neopeptides (22), have been developed that show increased concentration of these peptides in RA.

## Hyaluronan

Hyaluronan (HA) is a constituent of extracellular matrix and is present in abundance in synovium and cartilage. Aggrecan molecules are bound to hyaluronan by G1 domain and a link protein to form large aggregates. HA can be detected by various assays (23) specific for HA and by those specific for the G1 domain or link protein of aggrecan molecule. Serum HA shows significant correlations with joint counts, joint inflammation, and disease progression in RA and is persistently elevated in OA patients who have rapid disease progression. The major clinical drawbacks of the HA assay for joint disease is that serum HA has a large diurnal variation and that its concentration can be affected by physical activity.

## Type-II Collagen Turnover Markers

Type-II collagen constitutes the largest component of the organic matrix in the articular cartilage matrix. Measurements of type-II collagen offer clear opportunities to detect an imbalance in cartilage degradation and synthesis because assays are available that can clearly distinguish between these two processes (Fig. 4.5). Assays for degradation products such as C-telopeptide (24) of type-II collagen (CTx-II), which is generated by collagenase, represent a highly specific index of cartilage degradation, as CTxII levels are significantly upregulated in OA.

The type-II collagen is synthesized as a procollagen that contains amino and carboxyl propeptides. These are removed extracellularly by single cleavages of amino (N-terminal) and carboxyl (C-terminal) proteinases as collagen is incorporated into the fibril. Thus, procollagen peptide-based markers are specific indicators of cartilage matrix synthesis. An assay for C-terminal procollagen peptide has been developed (25), and its content and release from the cartilage is directly correlated with collagen synthesis in both OA and RA. This could eventually become an important clinical research assay because it may reflect the repair process in arthritic joints.

## Additional Markers of Cartilage Matrix Degradation

### Cartilage Oligomeric Protein

Apart from aggrecan and type-II collagen, the two major components of cartilage matrix, several other cartilage matrix proteins have received attention as biomarkers because of their proposed specificity. Cartilage oligomeric protein (COMP) is the most effective of these markers. COMP is an abundant cartilage macromolecule and a member of the thrombospondin family. Although its exact function is not clear, COMP can bind to cells, collagen, and other matrix components, and its release indicates lack of retention by degenerative matrix (26). COMP levels are increased in blood in OA. In studies of OA patients, an increase in serum COMP was associated with rapid disease progression. Serum COMP levels show strong correlation with joint space width at baseline and with yearly mean joint space narrowing.

### GP-39/YKL-40

GP-39/YKL-40 is a glycoprotein that is a member of the chitinase family, and its serum and synovial fluid (SF) level is a marker (27) of active RA. This protein is not made by normal chondrocytes but is produced by chondrocytes and synovial cells in arthritic joints undergoing degradation, reflecting new synthesis. The elevated levels of YKL-40 correlate with inflammatory markers in RA suggesting it mainly reflects inflammation. More studies are needed to establish clinical usefulness of this test.

### Type-III Collagen Amino (N) Propeptides

Although the type-III collagen propeptides are minor components of cartilage matrix, their blood levels are directly correlated with matrix synthesis. Increases in C-terminal procollagen peptide content are observed in SF following knee injury and RA, and a decrease in propeptide levels is observed in OA. Therefore, the N-terminal, type-III collagen propeptide is a marker (28) of matrix synthesis. This marker, however, is also elevated in inflamed synovium; therefore, the increase seen in OA may also reflect synovitis.

In summary, a number of biochemical markers have been developed and investigated. Because of their abundance and specificity, aggrecan, type-II collagen, and COMP are most relevant in terms of clinical utility; hence, more published data is available about the clinical efficacy of these particular markers than others.

## Clinical Utility of Cartilage Markers

### Are Markers of Cartilage Destruction Associated with Disease Severity or Progression?

In studying arthritis disease activity, markers often have sufficient power to differentiate groups of patients with arthritis from normal individuals. In addition, there are indications that markers can distinguish patients when grouped according to disease severity. Clark et al. (29) in radiographic examination of knee or hip OA demonstrated that COMP levels correlated with severity of OA in The

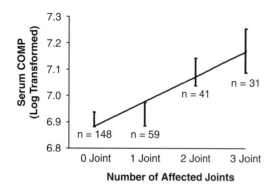

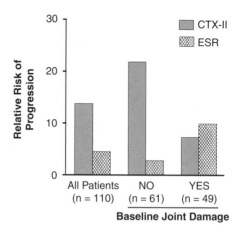

**Figure 4.6** Levels of cartilage turnover marker correlate with disease severity. In a fairly large trial, the Johnston County Osteoarthritis Study, involving 291 participants with 143 affected with radiographic knee or hip osteoarthritis (OA) (29), demonstrated that cartilage oligomeric protein (COMP) levels increased steadily with the number of OA joint involvement. The mean COMP levels showed a significant correlation with the number of affected joints with an r-value of 0.96 (p<0.05). The bars indicate mean±SD.

**Figure 4.7** Cartilage turnover markers can predict disease progression. Garnero and coworkers (24) investigated the relationship between baseline levels of cartilage turnover marker, type-II collagen degradation product (CTX-II), in 110 patients with early RA participating in the COBRA trial, over a 4-year follow-up period. The predictive value of radiological progression of CTX-II was significantly greater than erythrocyte sedimentation rate (ESR) when patients were grouped according to the presence (n = 49) or absence (n = 61) of joint damage at baseline. CTX-II levels were predictive in those patients that did not show baseline joint damage. The authors suggest that an increase in bone and cartilage metabolism occurs very early in the disease process in some, but not all, RA patients, and the marker could be useful in identifying these patients.

Johnston County Osteoarthritis Study involving 291 participants with 143 affected. Not only can serum levels of COMP distinguish an OA-affected subgroup from the unaffected group, but also COMP levels increased steadily with each additional joint affected (Fig. 4.6). If only one joint were affected, however, distinction with the unaffected group was difficult because of poor sensitivity. This study indicates that serum concentrations of cartilage macromolecules have the potential for segregating patients according to disease severity in clinical research studies.

One of the biggest challenges to the rheumatologist is to predict early cartilage destruction because RA can cause destruction of the joints if not treated early and aggressively. Garnero et al (24) investigated the relationship between baseline levels of telopeptide of type-I and type-II (CTX-II) collagen and disease progression in 110 patients with early RA participating in the Combinatietherapie Bij Reumatoide Artritis (COBRA) trial over 4 years. Interestingly, the serum CTX-II levels were predictive of disease progression in those patients that showed no joint damage at baseline (Fig. 4.7). CTX-II levels in the highest tertile were the strongest predictors of radiological progression, independent of erythrocyte sedimentation rate (ESR) and baseline joint damage (Sharp score). The authors conclude that an increase in bone and cartilage metabolism occurs very early in the disease process in some, but not all, RA patients; therefore, markers may be useful in differentiating these patients.

Another approach to explore the utility of markers is to look for cartilage degradation and its relationship to biosynthesis. This approach may offer more valuable indications than measurement of either process alone because OA is characterized by the degeneration of articular cartilage, accompanied by a response of the tissue to repair this damage, which involves enhanced matrix synthesis and turnover. This approach has been used by Garnero et al. (25) in patients with OA. In this study, the authors observed that increased degradation of cartilage matrix (determined by CTx-II) was accompanied by decreased synthesis of propeptide (type-II collagen) in patients with rapid progression, suggesting that it is the imbalance between matrix synthesis and degradation that more clearly reflects rapid progression of joint degeneration than cartilage matrix degradation alone.

In summary, data from several clinical trials indicate that a strong potential exists for biomarkers in predicting disease progression or identifying severity of disease. However, at present, the large variation and overlap between control and disease groups observed in these studies indicate that these assays cannot yet be applied in individual patients in clinical management.

## Can Markers of Cartilage Turnover Be Used to Monitor Treatment?

Markers are highly desirable for monitoring drug therapy in joint diseases because (1) radiographic assessment is largely ineffective at early stages of treatment, (2) there is large variability in patients' response to a given dose of a drug, and (3) there may be a window of opportunity for effective treatment of RA during the early stages of the disease, which needs to be identified. Thus, molecular markers offer the potential for eventually improving clinical assessment. So far, markers of arthritis have made only a modest contribution (30,31) in the evaluation of therapy in clinical trials. Markers such as COMP (32) show small but rapid reduction within 3–6 months after initiation of treatment. Studies employing matrix metalloproteinase inhibitors that inhibit cartilage metabolism have also demonstrated significant reduction in aggrecan or type-II collagen turnover markers. In general, markers show significant suppression within 3–12 months after initiation of treatment. However, there are two main limitations in the published studies:

1. There is a large variation in a single individual from day to day and from week to week in bone markers. It seems likely that the cartilage metabolism markers may show similar large intrapatient variation such that without defining this variation, estimating whether or not a given suppression in a marker by a therapeutic agent is a true biological change is difficult.
2. Little is known about how these markers correlate with long-term changes in joint disease as assessed by radiography.

Hopefully, large prospective clinical trials with markers and precise radiographic assessment as end points using therapeutic agents that can reduce disease activity in arthritis will further indicate the utility of marker for monitoring treatment.

## CONCLUSION

Theoretically, it should be feasible to identify analytes and measure them with the precision required to assist in the diagnosis and the management of joint disease. In sharp contrast to metabolic bone diseases, however, joint diseases are often local as opposed to generalized skeletal diseases and as a result, more sensitive assays are required. The sensitivity of current assays is insufficient to apply to individual patients. Two types of assays that have shown promise with respect to monitoring joint destruction are the COMP assays and the collagen type-II assays. These assays, and perhaps one or two of the other assays mentioned earlier, are useful in studying groups of patients for clinical research studies.

In The Johnston County Osteoarthritis Study, the COMP assay changes in a linear fashion in response to total amount of total joint destruction. There is a large individual variation in this response, however, which needs to be explored in detail before we can ever hope to apply this otherwise promising assay to individual patients.

## REFERENCES

1. Shifrin LZ. Correlation of serum alkaline phosphatase with bone formation rates. *Clin Orthop* 1970;70:212–215.
2. Wize J, Sopata I, Gietka J, et al. Hydroxyproline levels and collagenolytic activity in synovial fluids of patients with rheumatic diseases. *Scand J Rheumatol* 1975;4:65–72.
3. Miller PD, Baran DT, Bilezekian J, et al. Practical clinical applications of biochemical markers of bone turnover. *J Clin Densitom* 1999;2(3):323–342.
4. WHO Study Group. Assessment of fracture risk and its application to screening for postmenopausal osteoporosis: Report of a WHO Study Group. *WHO Technical Report Series* 843, Geneva, Switzerland: World Health Organization, 1994:1–129.
5. Genant HK, Cooper C, Poor G, et al. Interim report and recommendations of the World Health Organization Task-Force for Osteoporosis. *Osteoporos Int* 1999;10:259–264.
6. Black DM, Thompson DE, Bauer DC, et al. Fracture risk reduction with alendronate in women with osteoporosis: the Fracture Intervention Trial. FIT Research Group. *J Clin Endocrinol Metab* 2000;85(11):4118–4124.
7. Ettinger B, Black DM, Miltak BH, et al. Reduction of vertebral fracture risk in postmenopausal women with osteoporosis treated with raloxifene: results from a 3-year randomized clinical trial. Multiple Outcomes of Raloxifene Evaluation (MORE) Investigators. *JAMA* 1999;282(7):637–645.
8. Reginster JY, Minne HW, Sorenson OH, et al. Randomized trial of the effects of risedronate on vertebral and non-vertebral fractures in women with postmenopausal osteoporosis: a randomized controlled trial. Vertebral Efficacy with Risedronate Therapy (VERT) Study Group. *JAMA* 1999;282(14):1344–1352.
9. Eastell R, Barton I, Hannon RA, et al. Relationship of early changes in bone resorption to the reduction in fracture risk with risedronate. *J Bone Miner Res* 2003;18(6):1051–1056.
10. Delmas PD, Vrijens B, Roux C, et al. A reinforcement message based on bone turnover marker response influences long-term persistence with risedronate in osteoporosis: The IMPACT Study. *J Bone Miner Res* 2003;18(Supp-1):M330.
11. Ross PD, Knowlton W. Rapid bone loss is associated with increased levels of biochemical markers. *J Bone Miner Res* 1998;13(2):297–302.
12. Garnero P, Hausherr E, Chapuy MC, et al. Markers of bone resorption predict hip fracture in elderly women: the EPIDOS Prospective Study. *J Bone Miner Res* 1996;11(10):1531–1538.
13. Hochberg MC, Greenspan S, Wasnich RD, et al. Changes in bone density and turnover explain the reductions in incidence of non-vertebral fractures that occur during treatment with antiresorptive agents. *J Clin Endocrinol Metab* 2002;87(4):1586–1592.
14. Chesnut CH, Silverman S, Andriano K, et al. A randomized trial of nasal spray salmon calcitonin in postmenopausal women with established osteoporosis: the prevent recurrence of osteoporotic fractures study. PROOF Study Group. *Am J Med* 2000; 109: 267–276.
15. Hannon R, Blumsohn A, Naylor K, et al. Response of biochemical markers of bone turnover to hormone replacement therapy: impact of biological variability. *J Bone Miner Res* 1998;13(7): 1124–1133.
16. Vesper HW, Deners LM, Eastell R, et al. Assessment and recommendations on factors contributing to preanalytical variability of urinary pyridinoline and deoxypyridinoline. *Clin Chem* 2002;48(2):220–235.
17. Buckland-Wright JC. Radiographic assessment of osteoarthritis: comparison between existing methodologies. *Osteoarthritis Cartilage* 1999;7:430–433.
18. Buckland-Wright JC, Macfarlane DG, Lynch JA, et al. Joint space width measures cartilage thickness in osteoarthritis of the knee: high resolution plain film and double contrast macroradiographic investigation. *Ann Rheum Dis* 1995;54:263–268.
19. Caterson B, Christner JE, Baker JR. Identification of a monoclonal antibody that specifically recognizes corneal and skeletal keratan sulfate. Monoclonal antibodies to cartilage proteoglycan. *J Biol Chem* 1983;258:8848–8854.
20. Glant TT, Mikecz K, Roughley PJ, et al. Age-related changes in protein-related epitopes of human articular-cartilage proteoglycans. *Biochem J* 1986; 236:71–75.
21. Lohmander LS, Ionescu M, Jugessur H, et al. Changes in joint cartilage aggrecan after knee injury and in osteoarthritis. *Arthritis Rheum* 1999; 42:534–544.
22. Hughes CE, Caterson B, Fosang AJ, et al. Monoclonal antibodies that specifically recognize neoepitope sequences generated by

"aggrecanase" and matrix metalloproteinase cleavage of aggrecan: Application to catabolism in situ and in vitro. *Biochem J* 1995;305:799–804.

23. Laurent TC, Laurent UB, Fraser JR. Serum hyaluronan as a disease marker. *Ann Med* 1996;28:241–253.
24. Garnero P, Landewe R, Boers M, et al. Association of baseline levels of markers of bone and cartilage degradation with long-term progression of joint damage in patients with early rheumatoid arthritis: the COBRA study. *Arthritis Rheum* 2002;46:2847–2856.
25. Garnero P, Ayral X, Rousseau JC, et al. Uncoupling of type-II collagen synthesis and degradation predicts progression of joint damage in patients with knee osteoarthritis. *Arthritis Rheum* 2002;46:2613–2624.
26. Saxne T, Heinegård D. Cartilage oligomeric matrix protein: a novel marker of cartilage turnover detectable in synovial fluid and blood. *Br J Rheumatol* 1992;31:583–591.
27. Johansen JS, Stoltenberg M, Hansen M, et al. Serum YKL-40 concentrations in patients with rheumatoid arthritis: relation to disease activity. *Rheumatology* 1999;38:618–626.
28. Sharif M, George E, Dieppe PA. Synovial fluid and serum concentrations of aminoterminal propeptide of type-III procollagen in healthy volunteers and patients with joint disease. *Ann Rheum Dis* 1996;55:47–51.
29. Clark AG, Jordan JM, Vilim V, et al. Serum cartilage oligomeric matrix protein reflects osteoarthritis presence and severity. *Arthritis Rheum* 1999;42:2356–2364.
30. Den Broeder AA, Joosten LA, Saxne T, et al. Long term antitumour necrosis factor alpha monotherapy in rheumatoid arthritis: effect on radiological course and prognostic value of markers of cartilage turnover and endothelial activation. *Ann Rheum Dis* 2002; 61:311–318.
31. Sharif M, Salisbury C, Taylor DJ, et al. Changes in biochemical markers of joint tissue metabolism in a randomized controlled trial of glucocorticoid in early rheumatoid arthritis. *Arthritis Rheum* 1998;41:1203–1209.
32. Crnkic M, Månsson B, Larsson L, et al. Serum cartilage oligomeric matrix protein (COMP) decreases in rheumatoid patients treated with infliximab or etanercept. *Arthritis Res Ther* 2003; 5: R181–R185.

# Measurement of Bone Mineral Density: DXA and QCT

*Dorothy A. Nelson*     *Jean M. Weigert*     *Angelia D. Mosley-Williams*

Low bone mass is a key characteristic used by the World Health Organization (WHO) in the consensus definition of osteoporosis (1). Although the definition also incorporates architectural deterioration, the WHO's diagnostic categories for osteoporosis are based on bone mass measurements (1). Furthermore, the indications for drugs approved for osteoporosis prevention and treatment include a low bone mass measurement, obtained through any of a variety of techniques. Bone densitometry, therefore, has come to play a major role in both the diagnosis and follow-up of patients with osteoporosis. In this chapter, we discuss the principles of operation and appropriate clinical applications of dual-energy, x-ray absorptiometry (DXA) and quantitative computed tomography (QCT).

## HISTORICAL CONTEXT FOR DXA AND QCT

In the early 1960s, the forerunner of DXA, a technique based on single-energy photon absorptiometry (SPA), was introduced (2). The underlying principle of this method is the absorption by bone of the energy emitted by a decaying radioactive isotope. This method is useful in appendicular skeletal sites (such as the forearm and calcaneus), because the thickness of bone and soft tissue must be relatively uniform. Over the next several decades, data amassed with SPA instruments helped to describe patterns of the gain and loss of bone mineral over a lifetime and the effects of menopause and some diseases on bone loss. Studies also showed differences between men and women and between African-Americans and whites (3). Results were reported as mass per area, which was loosely referred to as "bone mineral density" (BMD). Most providers of this test expressed results in standard deviation units, which would later become the conventional method endorsed by the WHO task force.

An extension of this technology, based on dual-energy photon absorptiometry (DPA), was soon developed to allow the measurement of bone density in the spine and hip, where osteoporotic fractures often occur. This method utilized a radioactive isotope that emits photon energy at two different photoelectric peaks. The attenuation of the photon beam by soft tissue and bone affect the two peaks differently, so that the soft tissue contribution can be mathematically subtracted (4). This technological advancement allowed the systematic study of bone density in the central skeleton, as well as in the entire skeleton, but this advantage was offset by the fluctuations in accuracy and precision caused by the decay of the isotope over time. The same disadvantage was encountered with SPA, and both methods were essentially replaced with x-ray–based instruments, single energy, x-ray absorptiometry (SXA) and dual-energy, x-ray absorptiometry (DXA). The underlying principles are the same, but there is no confounding effect of the decaying isotope as seen in SPA and DPA; therefore, x-ray–based absorptiometric methods, especially DXA, have become the gold standard in bone densitometry. We must reiterate that DXA provides an estimate of bone density that is expressed as mass per area ($g/cm^2$).

Quantitative computed tomography (QCT) was developed in the late 1970s by comparing bone to a series of liquid standards in a phantom for which bone density equivalence had been established. Most systems today utilize solid phantoms, although there is a phantom-less system using muscle and fat in the patient as a comparative standard. In comparison to DXA, QCT provides a true volumetric measurement of bone and is measured in milligrams per centimeter cubed ($mg/cm^3$). Also in contrast to DXA, QCT can measure trabecular bone density separately from cortical bone (5).

In a two-dimensional QCT scan, the calibration phantom is placed under the patient's back while the body is scanned. A computed radiographic localizer view is obtained to determine the levels of L1 to L3 and each vertebral body is imaged with a 1.0-cm section thickness. BMD is then calculated by comparing the spine scan results to the calibrated standards. While accurate, the reproducibility (precision) can be diminished by variability in sampling through the center of the vertebral body (6,7). With the advent of spiral CT scanners and three-dimensional (3-D) software that acquires true volumetric imaging, reproducibility has been significantly improved. Patient positioning errors, artifacts from bowel gas, or increased image noise from gantry angulation are eliminated. Precision has been measured at a coefficient of variation (CV) of 0.9% on average in normal and osteoporotic bone (range 0.7%–1.1%) (8). There is now software for measuring the proximal femur, which provides DXA-equivalent clinical data for the hip. Most, if not all, DXA instruments use a reference database for the proximal femur that is based on, or consistent with, the hip BMD data provided by the National Health and Nutrition Examination Survey III (NHANES III) (9). These advancements in bone densitometry of the hip allow relatively standardized results regardless of the method or manufacturer. Measuring the hip by QCT can also separate the cortical and trabecular bone envelopes in addition to calculating total bone density in a region of interest (10,11).

## DUAL-ENERGY X-RAY ABSORPTIOMETRY

BMD as measured by DXA is not a true density measurement, because it does not provide an estimate of bone volume. (Some manufacturers provide a surrogate for this in the spine by combining anterior-posterior and lateral data

to estimate volume.) The use of only two dimensions for a given skeletal site does not control entirely for variation in bone size among individuals. The practical implication of this limitation is that men have higher BMD on average than women, based on a larger bone size. There are also ramifications for pediatric bone densitometry using DXA, because bones grow and change in size and shape and at different rates. As discussed below, QCT provides a volumetric measure of BMD that ameliorates the problems of differences in bone size.

The practitioner must recognize that results from DXA instruments vary among manufacturers because of differences in software and hardware. They use different approaches to producing two distinct photoelectric peaks from a wide range of energies, different edge-detection algorithms and regions of interest definitions, different modes of data acquisition (pencil versus fan beam), and a variety of other software features that affect the calculation of bone mineral content (BMC) and area. Thus, different manufacturers' instruments produce different results and are not interchangeable. Furthermore, each manufacturer provides reference data specific to their instruments. The populations from which the reference data are obtained, the sample sizes, and the methods used to identify normal subjects can be very different. The exception to this generalization is the relative uniformity of hip bone density reference data made possible by the results of NHANES III (9) (Fig. 5A.1). The NHANES III data provide reference data for a wide age range in men and women and in white, African-American, and Mexican-American groups. As discussed below, the availability of reference data is critical for generating standardized scores for use in the diagnosis of osteoporosis.

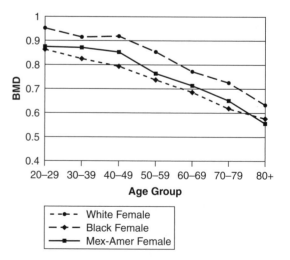

**Figure 5A.1** Illustrative data from NHANES III; Femoral neck BMD for females, by ethnic group and age group (9).

## Diagnostic Categories Based on WHO Definition

The WHO developed diagnostic categories for osteoporosis and low bone mass (osteopenia) based on bone density measurements that could be used for epidemiologic research (1). They were developed for white women only and were defined by the number of standard deviation (SD) units below peak bone mass for this group. These categories were quickly put to use in the clinical setting and sometimes extended to men and nonwhite ethnic groups. The categories are as follows:

- *Normal:* A value for BMD that is within 1 SD of the young adult reference mean.
- *Low bone mass (osteopenia):* A value for BMD that is more than 1 SD below the young adult mean but less than 2.5 SD below this value.
- *Osteoporosis:* A value for BMD that is 2.5 SD or more below the young adult mean.
- *Severe osteoporosis (established osteoporosis):* A value for BMD more than 2.5 SD below the young adult mean in the presence of one or more fragility fractures.

The standardized score that expresses the number of SD above or below the young adult mean has come to be called the "T score." It is calculated using the following formula:

$$\text{T score} = \frac{(\text{patient's BMD} - \text{reference BMD})}{\text{reference SD}}$$

## T Scores and Z Scores

The T score is used for the diagnostic categories described above and refers only to BMD measurements in patients who are past the age of peak bone mass. However, standardized scores that are based on age-matched reference data, called "Z scores," are also useful. These describe a patient's BMD result in relation to the normal range for normal subjects of the same age.

As previously mentioned, the WHO categories were designed for epidemiologic studies, not for individual patient care. However, the WHO criteria have become the standard for use in clinical practice. Thus, the output from most commercially available bone densitometers provides not only bone density measurements but also T scores and Z scores. The use of these categories for groups other than white women or for methods of bone mass measurement that were not included in the WHO report is not clear. The reference data used to calculate standardized scores has been assumed to be specific to sex and ethnic group, but there is ongoing discussion on this topic (12). Unfortunately, the availability of reference databases for nonwhite populations is somewhat limited and variable among manufacturers. We advise determining whether appropriate reference data are available for any given patient before proceeding with the bone density test.

T scores have a strong relationship to increasing fracture risk. A number of large studies have demonstrated that for each −1 SD, the risk of fracture increases by approximately 1.5–2.7 fold (13). This relationship is not linear but exponential ($T^{-n}$). For example, if the patient's T score in the spine is −3, her risk of spine fracture is approximately 8 times that of an aged-matched woman with a T score of 0.

Using the WHO criteria for QCT measurements is problematic. Because the WHO guidelines are based on absorptiometric measurements, they cannot technically be applied to QCT bone density values. Just as with DXA, data obtained by QCT are compared with a reference database. However, if the WHO criteria for T scores are used for QCT results to diagnose osteoporosis, a substantially higher number of individuals will be diagnosed as osteoporotic because BMD measured with QCT shows a faster rate of loss with age than DXA. For example, 50% of patients over the age of 60 will have a QCT-derived T score of −2.5 (14). Some research would suggest using different cutoff points for QCT, but more research is needed to settle these issues (14).

## Monitoring BMD

Serial measurements of BMD are performed to monitor the natural history of bone loss or to assess effects of therapy. To ascertain that a change in bone mineral density is a true biological change and not simply a statistical variation of the measurement, knowledge of the precision error is essential. To determine the average precision error, each center must perform a precision analysis by measuring 15 patients 3 times or 30 patients 2 times and repositioning each patient after each scan. The least significant change (LSC) at 95% confidence interval is calculated by multiplying 2.77 times the precision error (15). For example, if the precision error at the lumbar spine is 1%, the LSC is then 2.77%. A difference less than this would not be significant and would not indicate a need to alter treatment.

## QUANTITATIVE COMPUTED TOMOGRAPHY

QCT may be used as the primary modality for assessing bone density in several situations. In particular, it may be useful in obese patients; in patients with severe degenerative change, compression fractures, or scoliosis; and for following patients on therapy (11,16). The problem of areal measurement of BMD versus true volumetric measurement may affect the accuracy of DXA imaging because of its dependence on the size of the bone being measured (17). This discrepancy in the calculation of BMD may be a significant factor in evaluating children as well as people of different statures (18).

In the obese patient, DXA measurements of areal bone density ($g/cm^2$) are reported to be higher in the spine and the proximal femur compared to age-matched controls (19). This observation has been attributed to the increased mechanical forces placed on the weight-bearing skeleton in obese patients or to the possibility of increased circulating estrogen in body fat (20, 21). Variability in overlying tissue composition is known to affect the results of DXA studies but is not included in most reports (22, 23).

Although the possible inaccuracies in DXA measurements caused by soft tissue variations have been determined in studies in vitro or in phantoms, little in-vivo data exist that compare bone density measured by DXA with bone density measured using techniques that are not affected by the composition of overlying tissue such as QCT. In one study, BMD was measured in the spine and proximal femur of 6 obese women and 18 age-matched control patients using DXA and 3-D QCT (16). Results of this study suggest that DXA of both the spine and hip overestimate BMD in obese women and that such results should be interpreted with caution. In addition, because DXA assumes that soft tissue lying in the path of the beam is of constant composition, variation in the fat to lean ratio may cause inaccuracies in BMD values. Large patients can also cause an increase in beam hardening and scatter (24,25). For these reasons, 3-D QCT, which is not affected to a significant degree by overlying soft tissue, should be the preferred method to measure BMD for accurate diagnostic measurements in the obese patient.

Peripheral quantitative computed tomography (pQCT) is a bone densitometry technique that provides volumetric BMD values of the cortical and trabecular envelopes separately, or in total, in regions of the appendicular skeleton. The advantages include low radiation (1 μSv) and high sensitivity and reproducibility (26). Normal reference curves have been established in postmenopausal women measured at 4% of the ulnar length proximal to the wrist ("ultradistal" region) for total, trabecular, and cortical bone density. There is a continuously significant ($p < 0.0001$), age-dependent decline in bone density in both trabecular and cortical envelopes (27,28). This technology has been used particularly in the pediatric population assessing various metabolic disease processes and other drug exposures or conditions that affect bone growth (29,30).

## RADIATION DOSE

A comparison of radiation doses delivered by DXA and QCT of various skeletal regions, along with other common sources of radiation, is provided in Table 5A.1. The radiation dose from QCT, although higher than pencil beam DXA, is still quite modest when performed correctly. For example, it is no greater than the exposure from dental x-rays and much less than a mammogram. Because the image quality is not important in QCT bone densitometry, the radiation dose can be maintained at a low level, approximately 60 μSv with 120 milliamperes per second (MAS) (Table 5A.1) (31–35). The newer fan beam DXA systems deliver a higher radiation dose to some areas of the

## TABLE 5A.1

**TYPICAL EFFECTIVE X-RAY DOSAGES (ICRP 60) FROM COMMONLY USED PROCEDURES AND NATURAL SOURCES[4]**

| Source | Dose in μSv |
| --- | --- |
| Annual natural background exposure | 2,400 |
| Round trip transcontinental flight | 60 |
| Lateral lumbar spine x-ray | 700 |
| Mammogram | 450 |
| Dental x-ray | 100 |
| Chest x-ray | 50 |
| QCT with localizer | 30–100 |
| DXA PA-spine (fan beam) | 30–50 |
| DXA hip (premenopausal) | 6 |
| DXA PA-spine (pencil beam) | 3 |
| DXA lateral spine | 2.5 |
| DXA wrist or heel | <1 |

(Reproduced with permission from Mindways Software, Inc.)

body than the pencil bean instruments. For example, a fan beam DXA scan of the spine is roughly equivalent to QCT of the spine, and both are at least 10 times higher than a pencil beam measurement of the spine (Table 5A.1).

## EFFECTS ON BMD OF DEGENERATIVE DISEASE AND SCOLIOSIS

Severe degenerative changes of the lumbar spine and the presence of compression fractures are also shown to result in false elevation of DXA BMD measurements. Studies have shown that with increasing osteophytosis of the spine, the DXA measurement increases while QCT measurements of the same spine stay constant (36–38). In patients with even minimal degenerative changes, particularly in their facet joints (those with facet arthropathy or spondylolisthesis), DXA may measure a higher BMD (Fig. 5A.2A and Table 5A.2), even though the trabecular bone could be far less. With severe degenerative changes even the hip may not be accurate. Scoliosis has been shown to be an independent risk factor for osteoporosis. However, there is significant difficulty in measuring bone density in a scoliotic spine DXA (Fig. 5A.2B and Table 5A.2). Utilizing QCT and in particular 3-D QCT technology (Fig. 5A.3) we can untorque the spine and measure an area of unaffected bone density in its true volumetric measurement.

## RELATIONSHIP OF BMD TO FRACTURE RISK

QCT measurements of vertebral BMD have been shown to have the strongest ability to discriminate between healthy postmenopausal women and those with vertebral fractures (36,39–42). This is due, in part, to the fact that trabecular bone is metabolically more active than cortical bone and

## TABLE 5A.2
### BMD AND T SCORES FOR VERTEBRAE IN FIGURES 5A.2A AND B.*

| Vertebra(e) | Figure 5A.2A (Focal Areas of High BMD) | | Figure 5A.2B (Vertebral body compression and Scoliosis) | |
|---|---|---|---|---|
| | BMD | T score | BMD | T score |
| L1 | 0.981 | −1.2 | 1.022 | −0.9 |
| L2 | 1.037 | −1.4 | 1.016 | −1.5 |
| L3 | 1.434 | 2.0 | 1.325 | 1.0 |
| L4 | 1.540 | 2.8 | 1.426 | 1.9 |
| L1–L4 | 1.266 | 0.7 | 1.222 | 0.4 |
| L1–L2 | 1.010 | −1.2 | 1.005 | −1.1 |

*(65)
(Redrawn with permission from The Humana Press, Inc.)

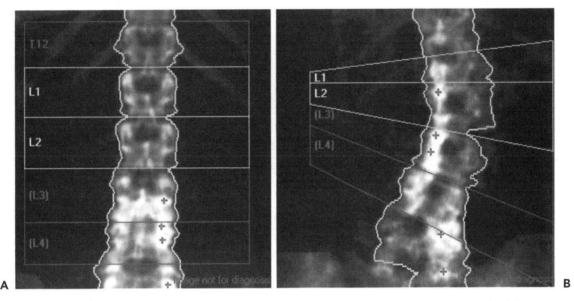

A        B

**Figure 5A.2** DXA images of lumbar spine showing (A) focal areas of high BMD, probably the result of degenerative changes and (B) vertebral body compression and scoliosis, which elevate BMD (Table 5A.2) (65). (Reproduced with permission from The Humana Press, Inc.)

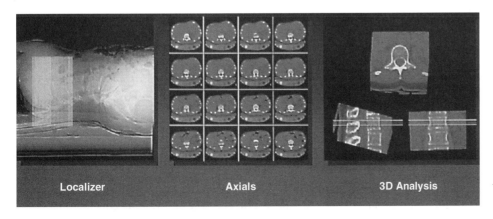

Localizer      Axials      3D Analysis

**Figure 5A.3** 3-D QCT-BMD analysis from reconstructed images in the axial, coronal, and sagittal planes. (Reproduced with permission from Mindways Software Inc.)

has more surface area, so it is a sensitive indicator of early bone loss in vertebral fracture risk. Spinal trabecular BMD also correlates with trochanteric fracture risk (43).

## WHO SHOULD HAVE A BONE DENSITY TEST?

The simplest way to determine who should have a bone density test is to decide in each case whether the results will influence a clinical decision. There are some categories of patients who do *not* need a bone density test, for example, healthy premenopausal women, healthy young men, and very elderly or frail patients (44). Anyone who has a disease or condition or who is taking certain drugs that potentially induce bone loss is a candidate for a bone density measurement. Prolonged corticosteroid use is a risk factor in any age, sex, or ethnic group and is a major consideration in the population of patients seen by the rheumatologist. For postmenopausal women, other considerations include indecision about or refusal to take therapy or an incidental finding of a vertebral deformity on a radiograph (45).

### Guidelines from the International Society for Clinical Densitometry

The International Society for Clinical Densitometry's (ISCD) recent position statement (12) recommends bone density testing for the following groups:

- Women aged 65 and older
- Postmenopausal women under age 65 with risk factors
- Men aged 70 and older
- Adults with a fragility fracture
- Adults with a disease or condition associated with low bone mass or bone loss
- Adults taking medications associated with low bone mass or bone loss
- Anyone being considered for pharmacologic therapy
- Anyone being treated to monitor treatment effect
- Anyone not receiving therapy in whom evidence of bone loss would lead to treatment

### Guidelines from the American College of Rheumatology

The American College of Rheumatology (ACR) issued a position statement in 1997 that is currently available on its website (46). The ACR endorsed the use of bone densitometry for the diagnosis of low bone mass, as an assessment of future fracture risk for therapeutic management and decision making, and for monitoring bone mass when assessing treatment efficacy. These guidelines are consistent with the ISCD's recommendations, but they provide further detail regarding patients in whom bone density measurement for diagnosis and follow-up is appropriate.

- Women at or after menopause, if the result of the study influences the decision for estrogen replacement therapy or other potential interventional therapy.
- Women who have a family history of osteoporosis, who have early onset of menopause, who have had surgical menopause, or who have low body weight.
- Women with aberrations of the menstrual cycle, including female athletes who have ceased to have menstrual periods or have irregular menstrual periods, or women with luteal phase deficiencies.
- Individuals with vertebral abnormalities or x-ray evidence of osteopenia.
- Individuals receiving long-term drug therapy known to predispose to osteoporosis including glucocorticoid therapy, phenytoin therapy, or heparin therapy.
- Individuals who have been on excessive doses of thyroid replacement.
- Men with hypogonadism.
- Individuals suspected of being estrogen malabsorbers or nonresponders.
- Individuals with chronic malabsorption or documented calcium malabsorption.
- Individuals with asymptomatic primary hyperparathyroidism.
- Individuals with a recent fracture of the spine, long bone, hip, or pelvis and the fracture is suspected to be associated with osteoporosis.

## PEDIATRIC BONE DENSITOMETRY

Measurements in children are problematic for a number of reasons. First, there are inadequate reference data for children. Second, there is tremendous variability in developmental age at any given chronological age, so age-specific reference data may not be appropriate for assessing children's bone mineral status. Third, DXA has inherent limitations for pediatric use because of its inability to measure the bone size in three dimensions. It is important to appreciate that bones with the same volumetric measurement of BMD (mg/cc) but with different areas have significantly different areal BMD measurements (g/cm$^2$) based on DXA. Larger bones have a greater calculated (areal) BMD than smaller bones (47,48). This causes problems with pediatric measurements in children of different sizes and in whom bone size is expected to change during growth. Recent research has also shown this to be a factor in terms of sex, ethnicity, and fracture risk (49–51). Caution must be used, therefore, in interpreting BMD in children based on nonvolumetric measurements (18,52–54).

To ameliorate this problem, whole-body bone mineral content is sometimes recommended for pediatric measurements (55). One must verify before ordering a test for a child that there are appropriate reference data available for pediatric patients. Also, the Z score, rather than the T score, is the appropriate measure for assessing bone mineral status.

The T score implies a loss of bone mass after peak bone mass has been achieved. There are no data legitimizing the use of T scores in children who have not yet achieved their peak level.

One appropriate use of DXA in pediatric populations, whether or not reference data are available, is to use serial measurement for detection of change in bone mineral status. Bone mineral content would be preferable to BMD because of the problems with changing bone size and shape during growth.

QCT can assess both the volume and the true density of bone in axial and appendicular skeletons without influence from body or skeletal size, making it a useful tool in pediatric bone densitometry (18,56,57). This technology has been used in preterm infants, as well as in adolescents in whom increases in DXA areal spine BMD are more likely to reflect vertebral size than actual changes in density. QCT may, therefore, be a better method for measuring changes in bone density as a result of various pathologic processes that may affect the children and their growing skeletons. This includes patients with osteogenesis imperfecta or long-term corticosteroid use or those who have undergone radiation and/or chemotherapy for malignancies, and other bone disorders (58,59).

## WHICH SKELETAL SITES SHOULD BE MEASURED?

There has been much debate over the past decade on the relative utility of measuring the peripheral or the central skeleton. During the first two decades that photon absorptiometry was available, most bone mass data were collected from forearm measurements. Methods for measuring the forearm are still available, but measurements of the hip and spine are preferred by most clinicians and/or researchers for assessing the adverse effects of various diseases and drug exposures as well as for determining the efficacy of osteoporosis drugs. There are several reasons for this preference. The most serious osteoporotic fractures occur in the spine and hip, and both sites appear to be sensitive to bone resorption and, therefore, to antiresorptive therapies (60). The forearm, mainly cortical bone in the shaft, is considered to be less responsive to changes in bone and mineral metabolism than the more highly trabecular sites, such as vertebral bodies. However, results from a study of 179,471 women participating in the National Osteoporosis Risk Assessment (NORA) project indicate that peripheral BMD measured by DXA and/or quantitative ultrasound (QUS) successfully identified women with an increased risk of osteoporotic fracture (61). In this study, self-reported fracture data reported after 12 months indicated a four-fold higher fracture rate among women whose T scores were less than or equal to −2.5 SD. For diagnostic purposes, the ISCD recommends measurement of both the posterior-anterior (PA) spine and the

hip in all patients selected for testing (12). The forearm should be measured when the spine and/or hip cannot be measured or interpreted, when hyperparathyroidism is suspected, or in very obese patients. In the spine, all evaluable vertebrae (at least 2) from L1 through L4 should be used. In the hip, the femoral neck, total proximal femur, or trochanteric regions should be used. When the forearm is measured, the 33% site (radial shaft) is recommended.

## BONE MASS MEASUREMENT ACT AND REIMBURSEMENT ISSUES

Most FDA-approved bone densitometers are sufficiently reliable to be used for a single time-point assessment of an individual's global fracture risk. That is, a bone density result from almost any skeletal site can be used in conjunction with relevant clinical data to detect low bone mass with an increased fracture risk. The Bone Mass Measurement Act provides Medicare coverage for a baseline test by any FDA-approved modality (with the exception of DPA) as well as a follow-up baseline test using a second method that is to be used for following the patient (62). So, for example, a physician may have a peripheral instrument that measures the forearm or heel for the initial assessment of the patient, but he or she can also refer the patient for a spine and hip DXA. Both measurements would be covered, and the patient can be followed with serial spine and hip measurements. The Bone Mass Measurement Act allows follow-up measurements every 2 years but will reimburse for shorter intervals in some circumstances such as high-dose corticosteroid use.

The following indications for bone mass measurements are provided under the Bone Mass Measurement Act (62).

1. An estrogen-deficient woman who, based on a clinical evaluation of medical history or other findings, is at risk for osteoporosis.
2. An individual who has radiographic evidence of osteoporosis, low bone mass, or vertebral abnormalities (i.e., fractures).
3. An individual receiving or expecting to receive long-term glucocorticoid therapy of at least 7.5 mg of prednisone/day for more than 3 months.
4. An individual with hyperparathyroidism.
5. An individual receiving an FDA-approved osteoporosis drug who is being monitored to assess response to therapy.

Private insurers such as Blue Cross and Blue Shield plans, commercial insurers, and various managed care plans, provide health insurance coverage with benefits that vary tremendously from company to company and from contract to contract. Medicaid is a joint federal-state program designed to provide health insurance to low-income individuals. Because eligibility requirements are set by each state, Medicaid benefits vary tremendously. It is best to check the individual insurance policy for coverage and copayment status.

## CONSIDERATIONS IN REPORTING BONE DENSITY RESULTS

Most instruments provide output that includes graphic as well as quantitative data, including T scores, for the selected skeletal sites and a variety of regions of interest. These results must be reviewed and interpreted by a properly trained professional to ensure the following:

- Technical quality of the measurements
- Proper identification of skeletal regions of interests
- Identification of anatomic variations (some pathological)
- May require clinical follow-up (e.g., x-rays or biochemical tests)
- May invalidate the BMD results for that region
- Appropriate use of guidelines for diagnosis and intervention

Given the importance of expert review of the output, a report should accompany the results from a bone density test. This report should at least minimally comment on the technical quality of the scans, anomalies noted in the images, and the significance of the results for clinical care (e.g., whether or not indicative of diagnosis of low bone mass or osteoporosis and whether or not intervention should be considered). If the output is not appended to the report, then the BMC, area, BMD, and standardized scores must be provided. In addition to these basic components, reports can be as comprehensive as one desires. Bone density providers either devise their own reporting method or use sample report forms that can be obtained from the manufacturer in some cases or from various websites. The take-home message is that referring physicians should expect an interpretive report of the bone density results to be provided by an expert bone density provider.

## IMPROVING THE PRACTICE OF BONE DENSITOMETRY

It should be clear from the discussion in this chapter that there are many issues to consider when ordering, interpreting, or reporting bone density tests. Appropriate training and education of bone densitometry providers, as well as referring physicians, plays a key role in quality assurance in this field. Lenchik (63) has recommended five objectives for improving the practice of bone densitometry;

1. A provider should know the strengths and limitations of the equipment,
2. Technologists should be properly trained to use the equipment.
3. Physicians or other clinical caregivers should learn how to use the output data to diagnose osteoporosis, estimate fracture risk, and monitor response to therapy.
4. Providers should recognize common pitfalls in bone density interpretation.

5. Information given in interpretive reports should be clinically relevant to the referring physicians.

In addition, one must know which method should be used to give valid information regarding the specific patient. As with any clinical test, bone densitometry should be performed only when it has an impact on good patient care.

## SUMMARY

DXA is often considered the state-of-the-art method for measuring bone density. It has become increasingly available in most communities and is suitable for use in the diagnosis and follow-up of patients with low bone mass or osteoporosis. DXA has also been widely used in clinical trials and epidemiologic studies, providing tremendous insight into skeletal health and disease in a variety of populations worldwide. There are some limitations, however, of this method, discussed throughout the chapter, including the inability to measure mass per volume (true bone *density*), the inclusion of both trabecular and cortical bone in the measurements, and the varying effects of bone size, artifacts, anatomic variations, and positioning on BMD results. QCT can overcome many of these problems but is less widely available than DXA. Nonetheless, bone density data acquired with QCT have added substantially to the osteoporosis literature and provide valuable insights into trabecular bone density across populations and diseases.

Many professional organizations, including the ISCD and the ACR, have provided clinical guidelines for the appropriate use of bone densitometry. The Bone Mass Measurement Act has provided for Medicare coverage for several indications, and many other insurers have followed suit. The challenges for the future include continued recognition of the utility of bone mass measurement, improvements in quality assurance as more instruments are deployed in the community, and the development of advanced methods that ameliorate some of the problems inherent in the methods of measurement. The assessment of bone quality and architecture is a critical area for future research and development in the field of bone densitometry.

## REFERENCES

1. WHO Study Group. Assessment of fracture risk and its application to screening for postmenopausal osteoporosis. Geneva: *WHO Technical Report Series 843*, 1994.
2. Cameron JR, Sorenson G. Measurement of bone mineral in vivo: an improved method. *Science* 1963;142:230–232.
3. Mayor GH, Garn SM, Sanchez TV, et al. Proceedings: The need for differential bone mineral standards for blacks. *Am J Roentgenol* 1976;126:1293–1297.
4. Nord RH. Technical considerations in DPA. In: Genant HK, ed. *Osteoporosis Update 1987*. San Francisco: University of California Printing Services, 1987:203–212.
5. Cann CE, Genant HK. Precise measurement of vertebral mineral content using computed tomography. *J Computed Assist Tomog* 1980;4:493–500.

6. Grampp S, Genant HK, Mathur A., et al. Comparisons of noninvasive bone mineral measurements in assessing age-related loss, fracture discrimination and diagnostic criteria. *J Bone Miner Res* 1997;12:697–711.

7. Yu W, Gluer S, Grampp S, et al. Spinal bone mineral assessment in postmenopausal women: a comparison between DXA and QCT. *Osteoporos Int* 1995;5:433–439.

8. Braillon PM. Quantitative computed tomography precision and accuracy for long-term follow-up of bone mineral density measurements. *J Clin Densitom* 2002;5:259–266.

9. Looker AC, Wahner HW, Dunn WL, et al. Proximal femur bone mineral levels of US adults. *Osteoporos Int* 1995;5:389–409.

10. Lang T, Augat P, Majumdar S. Noninvasive assessment of bone density and structure using computed assisted tomography and magnetic resonance. *Bone* 1998;22:149S–154S.

11. Cann CE, Adams JE, Wood G, et al. CTXA Hip-An extension of classical DXA measurements using QCT. *J Bone Miner Res* 2003;18(Suppl2):S317.

12. Leib ES, Lewiecki EM, Binkley N, et al. Official positions of the International Society for Clinical Densitometry. *J Clin Densitom* 2004;7:1–6.

13. Marshall D, Johnell O, Wedel H. Meta-analysis of how well measures of bone mineral density predict occurrence of osteoporotic fractures. *BMJ* 1996;312:1254–1259.

14. Faulkner KG, von Stetten E, Miller P. Discordance in patient classification using T-scores. *J Clin Densitom* 1999;2:343–350.

15. The Writing Group for the ISCD Position Development Conference. *J Clin Densitom* 2004;7;37–44.

16. Weigert JW, Cann CE. DXA in obese patients: are normal values really normal. *J Women's Imaging* 1999;1:11–17.

17. Sabin MA, Blake GM, MacLaughlin-Black SM, et al. The accuracy of volumetric bone density measurements in dual X-ray absorptiometry. *Calcif Tiss Int* 1995;56:210–214.

18. Gilsanz V. Bone density in children: a review of available techniques and indications. *European J Radiol* 1998;26:177–182.

19. Shiraki M, Ito H, Fujimaki H, Higuchi T. Relation between body size and bone mineral density with special reference to sex hormones and calcium regulating hormones in elderly females. *Endocrinol Jpn* 1991;38:343–349

20. Tothill P, Hannan WJ, Cowen S, et al. Anomalies in the measurement of changes in total-body bone mineral by dual-energy X-ray absorptiometry during weight change. *J Bone Miner Res* 1997;12:1908–1921.

21. Formica C, Loro ML, Gilsanz V, et al. Inhomogeneity in body fat distribution may result in inaccuracy in the measurements of vertebral bone mass. *J Bone Miner Res* 1995;10:1504–1511.

22. Totill P, Avewnell A, Reid OM. Precision and accuracy of measurements of whole body bone mineral: Comparisons between Hologic, Lunar, and Norland dual X-ray absorptiometers. *Br J Radiol* 1994;67:1210–1217.

23. Binkly N. Krueger D, Vallerta-Ast N. An overlying fat panniculus affects femur bone mass measurement. *J Clin Densitom* 2003;6:199–204.

24. DeSimone DP, Steven J, Eduards J, et al. Influence of body habitus and race on bone mineral density of the midradius, hip and spine in aging women. *J Bone Miner Res* 1989;4:827–830.

25. Blake GM, McKeeney DB, Chhaya SC, et al., Dual energy X-ray absorptiometry: The effects of beam hardening on density measurements. *Med Phys* 1992;19:459–465.

26. Grampp S, Lang P, Jergas M, et al. Assessment of skeletal status by peripheral quantitative computed tomography of the forearm: Short-term precision in-vivo and comparison to dual X-ray absorptiometry. *J Bone Miner Res* 1995;10:1566–1576.

27. Boonen S, Cheng XG, Nijs J, et al. Factors associated with cortical and trabecular bone loss as quantified by peripheral computed tomography (pQCT) at the ultradistal radius in aging women. *Calcif Tiss Int* 1997;60:164–170.

28. Nijs J, Westhoven R, Joly J, et al. Diagnostic sensitivity of peripheral quantitative computed tomography measurements at ultradistal and proximal radius in postmenopausal women. *Bone* 1998;22:659–664.

29. Schwahn B, Mokov E, Scheidhaur K, et al, Decreased trabecular bone mineral density in patients with phenylketonuria measured by peripheral quantitative tomography. *Acta Paediatr* 1998;87:61–63.

30. Lettgen B, Neudorf U, Hosse R, et al. Bone density in children and adolescents with rheumatic diseases. Preliminary results of selective measurement of trabecular and cortical bone using peripheral computerized tomography. *Klin Padiatr* 1996;208: 114–117.

31. Lang T, Augat P, Majumdar S. Noninvasive assessment of bone density and structure using computed tomography and magnetic resonance. *Bone* 1998;22:149S–154S.

32. Kalender WA. Effective dose values in bone mineral measurements by photon absorptiometry and computed tomography. *Osteoporos Int* 1992;2:82–87.

33. Lewis MK, Blake GM, Fogelman I. Patient dose in dual X-ray absorptiometry. *Osteoporos Int* 1994;4:11–15.

34. Steel SA, Baker AJ, Sanderson JR, et al. An assessment of the radiation dose to patients and staff from a Lunar-XL Fan Beam Densitometer. *Physiol Meas* 1998;19:17–26.

35. International Commission on Radiation Protection. 1990 Recommendations of the International Commission on Radiological Protection. *Ann ICRP* 1991;21:1–201.

36. Gluer CC, Engelke K, Lang TF, et al. Quantitative computed tomography (QCT) of the lumbar spine and appendicular skeleton. *Eur J Radiol* 1995;20:173–178.

37. Cann CE, Rutt BK, Genant HK, et al. The influence of extraosseous calcification on vertebral mineral density. *Calcif Tiss Int* 1983;35:647.

38. Kleerekoper M, Nelson DA, Flynn MJ, et al. Comparison of radiographic absorptiometry with dual energy X-ray absorptiometry and quantitative computed tomography in older white and black women. *J Bone Miner Res* 1994;9:1745–1749.

39. Guglielmi G. Quantitative computed tomography (QCT) and dual X-ray absorptiometry (DXA) in the diagnosis of osteoporosis. *Eur J Radiol* 1995;20:185–187.

40. Ott SM, Kilcoyne RF, Chesnut CH 3rd. Ability of four different techniques of measuring bone mass to diagnose vertebral fractures in postmenopausal women. *J Bone Miner Res* 1987;2:201–210.

41. Genant HK, Engelke K, Fuerst T, et al. Noninvasive assessment of bone mineral and structure: state of the art. *J Bone Miner Res* 1996;11:707–730.

42. Pacifici R, Rupich R, Griffin M, et al. Dual energy radiography versus quantitative computer tomography for the diagnosis of osteoporosis. *J Clin Endocrinol Metab* 1990;70:705–710.

43. Lang TF, Augat P, Lane NE, et al. Trochanteric hip fractures: strong association with spinal trabecular BMD measured with QCT. *Radiology* 1998;209:525–530.

44. Nelson DA, Kleerekoper M. A practical guide to bone densitometry. In: Kleerekoper M, Siris ES, McClung M, eds. *The Bone and Mineral Manual: A Practical Guide.* San Diego: Academic Press, 1999:3–4.

45. Nelson DA, Kleerekoper M. Indications for bone mass measurement. In: Kleerekoper M, Siris ES, McClung M, eds. *The Bone and Mineral Manual: A Practical Guide.* San Diego: Academic Press, 1999:5–6.

46. Council on Rheumatologic Care. *Bone Density Measurement: Position Statement.* 1997. www.rheumatology.org/publications/position/bonedensity.asp?aud=mem.

47. Carter DR, Bouxsein ML, Marcus R. New approaches for interpreting projected density data. *J Bone Miner Res* 1992;7:137–145.

48. Jergas M, Breitenseher M, Gluer CC, et al. Estimates of volumetric bone density from projectional measurements improve the discriminatory capability of dual X-ray absorptiometry. *J Bone Miner Res* 1995;10:1101–1110.

49. Ebbesen EN, Thomsen JS, Beck-Nielsen H, et al. Age and gender-related differences in vertebral bone mass, density and strength. *J Bone Miner Res* 1999;14:1394–1403.

50. Naganathen V, Sambrook P. Gender differences in volumetric bone density: a study of opposite sex twins. *Osteoporos Int* 2003;14:564–569.

51. Russo CR, Laurentein F, Bandinelli S, et al. Aging bone in men and women: beyond changes in bone mineral density. *Osteoporos Int* 2003;14:531–538.

52. Hayashi T, Saton T, Tanaka D, et al. Evaluation of bone density in newborn infants by computed tomography. *J Pediatr Gastroenterol Nutr* 1996;23:130–134.

53. Lu PW, Cowell CT, LLoyd-Jones SA, et al. Volumetric bone mineral density in normal subjects, aged 5–27 years. *J Clin Endocrinol Metab* 1996;81:1586–1590.

54. Baroncelli GI, Saggese G. Critical ages and stages of puberty in the accumulation of spinal and femoral bone mass: the validity of bone mass measurements. *Horm Res* 2000;54(Suppl 1):2–8.

55. Nelson DA, Koo WK. Interpretation of bone mass measurements in the growing skeleton. *Calc Tiss Int* 1999;65:1–3.

56. Kovanlikaya A, Loro ML, Hangartner TN, et al. Osteopenia in children: CT assessment. *Radiology* 1996;198:781–784.

57. Ott SM, O'Hanlan M, Lipkin EW, et al. Evaluation of vertebral volumetric vs. areal bone mineral density during growth. *Bone* 1997;20:553–556.

58. Kaste SC, Jones-Wallace D, Rose SR, et al. Bone mineral decrements in survivors of childhood acute lymphoblastic leukemias: frequency of occurrence and risk factors for their development. *Leukemia* 2001;15:728–734.

59. Boechat MI, Westra SJ, Van Dop C, et al. Decreased cortical and increased cancellous bone in two children with primary hyperparathyroidism. *Metabolism* 1996;45:76–81.

60. Wasnich RD, Miller PD. Antifracture efficacy of antiresorptive agents are related to changes in bone density. *J Clin Endocrinol Metab* 2000;85:231–236.

61. Miller PD, Siris ES, Barrett-Connor E, et al. Prediction of fracture risk in postmenopausal white women with peripheral bone densitometry: evidence from the National Osteoporosis Risk assessment. *J Bone Miner Res* 2002;17:2222–2230.

62. Department of Health and Human Services. Medicare coverage of and payment for bone mass measurements. *Fed Reg* 1998;63:34320–34328.

63. Lenchik L. Radiologists and bone densitometry. *J Clin Densitom* 1999;2:175–177.

64. Cameron J. Radiation dosimetry, *Environ Health Perspect* 1991;91:45–48.

65. Frank M, Faulkner KG. Automated assessment of exclusion criteria for DXA lumbar spine scans. *J Clin Densitom* 2003;6:401–409.

# Peripheral Bone Densitometry in Rheumatic Diseases

## Paul D. Miller

Bone densitometry is one of the pivotal technological developments that has allowed the quantitative measurement of bone mineral content (BMC). Central dual energy x-ray absorptiometry (DXA) remains the "gold-standard" for the diagnosis of low bone mass, the prediction of fracture risk, and monitoring. Peripheral bone mass measurements have specific clinical utility as well. Peripheral measurements are more affordable and provide access to skeletal health assessment for a large segment of the world population (1).

Peripheral densitometry can be used as a tool to predict both global (all fractures) as well as hip fracture risk in the postmenopausal population (2) (Fig. 5B.1). The National Osteoporosis Risk Assessment (NORA) (3) data has firmly established that fracture risk can be predicted in early postmenopausal women (over 50 years old) using peripheral measurements. This is a shift from the previous concept that peripheral densitometry can only be used for fracture risk prediction in the older postmenopausal population (over 65 years old) (Fig. 5B.2) (3,4).

The International Society of Clinical Densitometry (ISCD) (5) has recently published the results of their Position Development Conference on the utility of peripheral techniques in clinical practice. They state that

- The World Health Organization (WHO) criteria for diagnosis of osteoporosis and osteopenia should not be used with peripheral BMD measurement other than 33% radius.
- Peripheral measurements are useful for assessment of fracture risk.
- Peripheral measurements theoretically can be used to identify patients unlikely to have osteoporosis and to

identify patients who should be treated; however, these cannot be applied in clinical practice until device-specific cutoff points are established.
- Peripheral measurements should not be used for monitoring.

The following discussion embellishes the justification for these position statements.

## WHY PERIPHERAL MEASUREMENTS SHOULD NOT BE USED FOR THE DIAGNOSIS OF OSTEOPOROSIS BY WORLD HEALTH ORGANIZATION CRITERIA

The WHO established the criteria linking BMD of the hip and/or spine and/or forearm to lifetime fracture risk in caucasian postmenopausal women. The forearm region of interest (ROI) is not clearly defined from which the data used to establish the link between prevalence and risk were compiled. The fact that the ROI was not specified should not be taken as a criticism because in 1992 it was not known that different BMD devices used different ROIs (Fig. 5B.3) (6). In addition, the T scores for different BMD devices are calculated from different young-normal reference populations that yield different prevalence numbers (Fig. 5B.4)(7,8). Hence, even if the forearm ROIs were similar, the T score might be different because of inconsistencies in the reference databases used by the different peripheral manufacturers. A standardized, uniform reference population database that could be incorporated by all central and peripheral BMD manufacturers would mitigate T-score discrepancies.

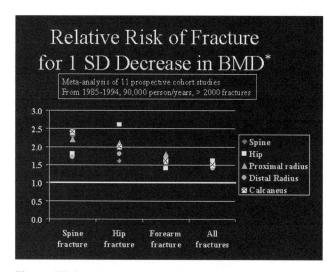

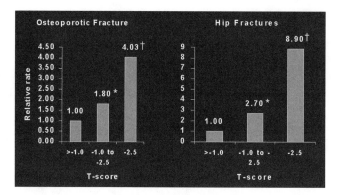

**Figure 5B.2**   One-year fracture rates (all fractures and hip fractures) by T-score classification in the National Osteoporosis Risk Assessment (NORA) (3). T-scores calculated from caucasian female database. All four NORA peripheral devices combined.

**Figure 5B.1**   Fracture risk by skeletal site (both central and peripheral) from a meta-analysis (2).

Until such a project is completed, the differences in T scores between peripheral and central devices bar the use of T scores derived from peripheral devices for the diagnosis of osteopenia and osteoporosis by these technologies.

As discussed in Chapter 5A, the only consistent young-normal reference population database is the National Health and Nutrition Educational Survey III (NHANES III) database for BMD of the hip, which has been incorporated into the three central DXA manufacturer's machines. This consistent database has removed the discordance in T scores at the hip in the central DXA machines. T scores calculated using manufacturer-specific, young-normal reference databases were quite discordant (9). Without a

consistent reference database, the peripheral devices cannot be used for diagnosis using the WHO criteria.

## CAN PERIPHERAL MEASUREMENTS BE USED TO MONITOR THE NATURAL PROGRESSION OF METABOLIC BONE DISEASE OR THE PHARMACOLOGICAL RESPONSE TO TREATMENT?

The ISCD Position Development Conference suggests that peripheral measurements cannot be used to monitor skeletal health. This suggestion is not related to the precision error of the peripheral techniques that are equivalent to central DXA (1%–2%). No one truly understands the

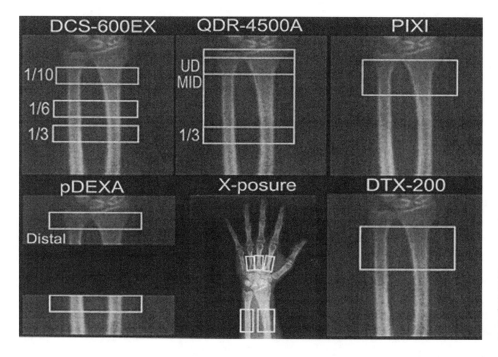

**Figure 5B.3**   Different regions of interest (ROI) measured by different forearm devices (6). In 2004, many forearm BMD technologies exist, all with different ROIs and BMC/BMD volumes.

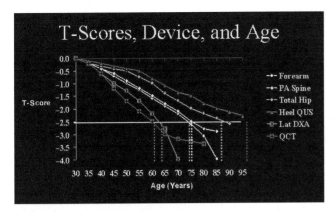

**Figure 5B.4** Discordance between central (DXA and QCT) and peripheral devices in caucasian females (7). T-scores calculated from manufacturer-specific databases.

limitation of peripheral devices to monitor longitudinal change. This limitation might be because of different drug distribution to cortical versus trabecular bone or because of the different structure of peripheral bone versus central skeletal sites. Even the total hip, measured by central DXA, does not show longitudinal change as well as spine DXA. This inability of the hip site to show longitudinal change might be related to the slower response of a skeletal structure with abundant cortical (lower-turnover) bone.

The inability of peripheral techniques to monitor disease or therapy is the most serious limitation of peripheral measurements. Physicians must currently rely on central anterior-posterior (AP)-spine DXA measurements and biochemical markers of bone turnover, which not only have independent value for this intent but also have substantial limitations.

## CAN PERIPHERAL MEASUREMENTS BE USED FOR FRACTURE PREDICTION?

Peripheral BMD measurements can be used for the prediction of the risk for both nonvertebral and vertebral fractures. This is an important appropriate application of peripheral densitometry, especially because the access to peripheral measurements worldwide is increasing. Many nations most likely will never be able to afford population screening strategies using central DXA. Trustworthy fracture risk assessment is an important attribute of all peripheral devices. Peripheral techniques can also be used for hip fracture–risk prediction in postmenopausal women over 50 years of age. Although only limited head-to-head data are available comparing the ability of central to peripheral BMD techniques to predict risk (Fig. 5B.1) (2), data suggest that low peripheral T scores also predict hip fracture risk (8). The challenge is to better define the T-score cut-off that includes the patients at greatest risk for fracture. The T-score cutoff point used for peripheral measurements to define increased fracture risk may be higher than the cutoff point

used for central measurements. Any T score less than –1.0 at a peripheral site predicts an increased risk for fracture (8).

Peripheral T scores of many devices are often at least 0.5 higher than T scores calculated by central techniques (7). Therefore, peripheral T scores are not consistent with central DXA T scores and the prevalence of low bone mass may be underestimated by peripheral devices (Fig. 5B.4) (7). Guidelines have been published suggesting a central DXA measurement may be appropriate if a peripheral T score is more negative than –1.0 (10).

In the NORA dataset (8), the T-score cutoff that best predicted a greater fracture risk by all four peripheral devices was –1.8 (11). In addition, using classification and regression tree analysis (CART) statistical software, 32 non-BMD fracture risk factors were analyzed. The highest risk was seen in women who had a fragility fracture of the ankle, forearm, humerus, or pelvis after the age of 45 years. Combining a preexisting fracture and a peripheral T score of less than or equal to –1.8 captured 75% of all of the 1-year fracture events in NORA. Each peripheral device used in NORA, examined individually, predicted fracture risk with the same power (11). Thus, risk stratification for clinical decisions related to treatment intervention may be enhanced by using a peripheral T-score cutoff of less than or equal to –1.8 in postmenopausal women who have no prior fragility fractures.

There are very limited data regarding the use of peripheral BMD devices for the prediction of fracture risk in patients receiving glucocorticoids, elderly men, or patients with secondary causes of low bone mass. The NORA data does, however, suggest that a low peripheral T score can predict fracture risk in multiethnic, postmenopausal women, in the United States. The NORA study represents the only head-to-head multiethnic fracture data available that included white, Hispanic, Asian, African-American, and Native-American women (12).

In the population receiving glucocorticoids, fractures seem to occur at higher BMD values than observed in normal postmenopausal women (13). Therefore, in this population, it would seem reasonable to select a higher peripheral T score as a threshold for intervention in the glucocorticoid-treated patient, if a central DXA is not available.

However, none of the clinical trials that led to FDA-registration of therapies for the prevention and treatment of postmenopausal osteoporosis, glucocorticoid-induced osteoporosis, or male osteoporosis randomized patients with any peripheral device. It is unknown, therefore, if the approved therapies would show the same degree of fracture risk reduction if patients had been randomized on the basis of a low peripheral BMD value. To the extent that low peripheral values in the postmenopausal population reflect global skeletal fragility, patients treated to improve their bone density based on a low peripheral T score would likely benefit. This, however, has not been proved. Certainly, when available, decisions related to therapeutic intervention should be made on the basis of central BMD measurements.

## REFERENCES

1. Miller PD, Bonnick SL. Clinical application of bone densitometry. In: *Primer on the Metabolic Bone Diseases and Disorders of Mineral Metabolism,* 4th ed. Philadelphia: Lippincott Williams & Wilkins, 1999:152–159.
2. Marshall D, Johnell O, Wedel H. Meta-analysis of how well measurements of bone mineral density predict the occurrence of osteoporotic fractures. *BMJ* 1996;312:1254–1259.
3. Siris ES, Miller PD, Barrett-Conner E, et al. Identification and fracture outcomes of undiagnosed low bone mineral density in postmenopausal women: results from the National Osteoporosis Risk Assessment (NORA). *JAMA* 2001;286:2815–2828.
4. Baran DT, Faulkner KG, Genant HK, et al. Diagnosis and management of osteoporosis: Guidelines for the utilization of bone densitometry. *Calcif Tiss Int* 1997;61:433–440.
5. Leib E, Lewiecki M, Binkley N, et al. Executive summary on the official positions of the International Society for Clinical Densitometry. *J Clin Densitom* 2004;7:1–117.
6. Shepherd J, Cheng XO, Lu Y, et al. Universal standardization of forearm bone densitometry. *J Bone Miner Res* 2002;17:734–745.
7. Faulkner KG, VonStetten E, Miler PD. Discordance in patient classification using T scores. *J Clin Densitom* 1999;2:343–350.
8. Miller PD, Siris ES, Barrett-Conner E, et al. Prediction of fracture risk in post-menopausal Caucasian women with peripheral bone density testing: evidence from the National Osteoporosis Risk Assessment (NORA). *J Bone Miner Res* 2002;17:2222–2230.
9. Faulkner KG, Roberts L, McClung M. Discrepancies in normative data between Lunar and Hologic DXA systems. *Osteoporos Int* 1996;6:432–436.
10. Miller PD, Bonnick SL, Johnston CC Jr, et al. The challenges of peripheral densitometry: which patients need additional central density skeletal measurements? *J Clin Densitom* 1998;1:211–217.
11. Miller PD, Barlas S, Brenneman SK, et al. An approach to identifying osteopenic women at increased short-term risk of fracture. *Arch Int Med* 2004;164:1–8.
12. Barrett-Conner E, Siris E, Wehren LE, et al. Osteoporosis and fracture risk in women of different ethnic groups. *J Bone Miner Res* 2004 (in press).
13. Van Staa TP, Laan RF, Barton IP, et al. Bone density threshold and other predictors of vertebral fracture in patients receiving oral glucocorticoid therapy. *Arthritis Rheum* 2003;11:3224–3229.

# Measurement of Bone Mineral Density-Densitometry in Glucocorticoid-Induced Osteoporosis

*Oscar S. Gluck*    *Michael Maricic*

Bone loss and fractures are the most common adverse effects of glucocorticoids (1) and are among the most common iatrogenic complications of clinical practice. Despite knowledge of the fracture risk associated with glucocorticoids (2) and the availability of effective treatments and published guidelines, physicians, including specialists, don't often measure bone density and prescribe medications to prevent bone loss (3).

## DETECTION OF BONE LOSS CAUSED BY GLUCOCORTICOIDS

Studies examining bone loss caused by low-dose glucocorticoids (GCs) show conflicting results. Some found significant bone loss (4,5) and others did not (6,7). These studies were confounded by their cross-sectional nature, various doses of prednisone studied, and variety of techniques and sites used to measure bone density (central vs. peripheral). In addition, the hormonal state of the patient and the severity of the underlying inflammatory disease were often not controlled.

In studies in which no bone loss was detected, researchers hypothesized that low-dose GC improved the inflammatory disease state and/or mobility status of the patient, thereby preserving bone mass. To separate the bone loss resulting from GCs from the bone loss caused by an underlying inflammatory disease (which is almost always the reason that GCs are given), Pearce (8) examined bone mineral density (BMD) in 9 men who had received 50 mg per day of prednisolone for up to 6 months for antisperm antibodies. BMD decreased 4.6% at the lumbar spine and 2.6% at the trochanter at 6 months. None of these patients had a systemic inflammatory disease. This study supports the concept that glucocorticoids induce bone loss independent of the underlying disease.

A meta-analysis reviewed 66 papers on the effects of GCs on bone density, and found that oral prednisolone (or equivalent) at a dose of 5 mg or greater per day led to significant decreases in bone density (9).

## BMD THRESHOLD FOR FRACTURES IN GLUCOCORTICOID-INDUCED OSTEOPOROSIS

The World Health Organization (WHO) criteria for the densitometric diagnosis of osteoporosis (T score < –2.5) were developed based on approximating the prevalence of fractures in postmenopausal white women to the prevalence of T scores below a certain level in the same population (10). The same type of large epidemiological study does not exist for glucocorticoid-treated patients.

Two early studies suggested that the frequency of vertebral fractures is greater in patients on GCs at the same (11) or even higher BMD (12) than in nonglucocorticoid-treated patients. The study by Peel (11) compared the prevalence of vertebral compression fractures in 76 glucocorticoid-treated rheumatoid females and 347 age-matched controls. The odds ratio (OR) for vertebral compression fracture in glucocorticoid-treated patients was 6.3-fold [confidence interval (CI):3.2–12.3] compared to controls. The lumbar spine BMD in the glucocorticoid-treated patients was decreased only by 0.79 standard deviations (SD) compared to controls: the expected SD difference for an OR of 6.3 would be –2.5, suggesting that there are non-BMD effects of GCs contributing to fracture.

Luengo (12) measured lumbar spine BMD in 32 glucocorticoid-treated and 55 nonglucocorticoid-treated females with vertebral compression fractures. Despite a higher mean lumbar BMD (0.946 gm/cm$^2$ versus 0.830 gm/cm$^2$), the glucocorticoid-treated patients had a higher prevalence of fractures (34% versus 9%). Both of these studies were cross-sectional and had small numbers of patients.

A subsequent report by Selby (13) compared the relationship of BMD and vertebral compression fractures in 82 patients receiving glucocorticoids and 370 not on glucocorticoids from a referral population and plotted the cumulative prevalence of fracture against T scores. He found the relationship between the cumulative frequency of patients of vertebral fractures and bone mass, expressed as T scores, to be identical in the two groups of patients, suggesting that glucocorticoids did not alter the fracture threshold. This was a cross-sectional assessment.

The first prospective study to evaluate the incidence of vertebral fractures in patients taking GCs was reported by van Staa (14) who analyzed the BMD threshold for vertebral fracture in postmenopausal women taking GCs. He compared the incidence of fracture in the placebo groups from the risedronate prevention (15) and treatment (16) trials to the 1-year fracture risk of postmenopausal women not taking GCs in three other trials. In the BMD threshold analysis, even though the women taking glucocorticoids were younger (64.7 vs. 74.1 years old), had higher mean lumbar T scores (–1.8 vs. –2.6) and femoral neck T scores (–0.9 vs. –2.6) and less prevalent fractures (42.9% vs. 58.3%) than the nonglucocorticoid users, the risk of fracture was higher in the GC users than the nonglucocorticoid users [adjusted relative risk (RR) 5.7, CI:2.57–12.54]. Thus, fracture incidence was markedly higher in the glucocorticoid users at any given level of BMD (Fig. 5C.1).

This study supports the concept that factors other than BMD are important to fracture risk in glucocorticoid-treated patients. Whether the increased risk at similar BMD is the result of GCs effects on osteocyte apoptosis, bone turnover, bone microarchitecture, or other factors relating to bone quality is not yet clear. It does appear that a different or higher BMD threshold should be used for estimating fracture risk in patients on glucocorticoids. This has led both

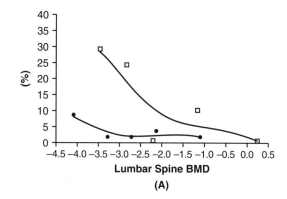

Lumbar Spine BMD

**(A)**

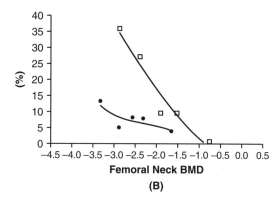

Femoral Neck BMD

**(B)**

**Figure 5C.1**   Incidence of vertebral fracture in patients receiving glucocorticoids (GCs) (*open box*) compared with nonusers of GCs (*), by baseline lumbar spine bone mineral density (BMD) and femoral neck BMD. Individual data points correspond to the incidence in subgroups of the GC user and nonuser populations, based on quintiles of baseline BMD. The solid line is a curve representing smoothing of the individual estimates. (From van Staa TP, Laan RF, Barton P, et al. Bone density threshold and other predictors of vertebral fracture in patients receiving oral glucocorticoids. *Arthritis Rheum* 2003;48:3224–3229, with permission.)

the American College of Rheumatology (17) and the British Bone and Tooth Society (18) to recommend intervention at higher levels of BMD in glucocorticoid-induced osteoporosis (GIOP) as opposed to postmenopausal osteoporosis.

## MONITORING BMD IN GIOP

Dual energy x-ray absorptiometry (DXA) has been demonstrated in prospective, randomized, placebo-controlled trials to be able to monitor response to therapy in glucocorticoid-exposed patients (15,16,19,20). In individual patients, because of the potential rapid loss of bone as a result of GCs and/or rapid increase with bone formation agents, monitoring is recommended every 6 to 12 months (17) compared to the recommendation of every 2 years in nonglucocorticoid patients. The use of peripheral technologies to monitor BMD in GIOP has not been studied and is not recommended.

## NON-DXA TECHNOLOGY IN GIOP

The three major utilities of bone density measurement are to detect low bone mass (to separate abnormal from normal bone mass), to estimate the risk for potential fracture, and to monitor changes in bone density. DXA has been shown to be capable of performing all three of these functions. Alternative technologies for measuring bone density include quantitative ultrasound (QUS) and quantitative computed tomography (QCT) scanning. In nonglucocorticoid-treated patients, these technologies can detect low bone mass in patients. In certain populations, QUS and QCT were able to predict fractures. In GIOP, preliminary studies suggest that they can detect patients with low bone mass and, in the case of QCT, monitor changes in therapy.

## QUANTITATIVE ULTRASOUND

A number of studies have examined the ability of QUS versus DXA to detect low bone density in GC users. A study by Daens (21) compared QUS to DXA in 77 women taking prednisone for inflammatory disease and 100 controls. Those patients on GC had lower values for broadband ultrasound attenuation (BUA), speed of sound (SOS), and lumbar BMD by DXA compared to those not taking GC. Both QUS and DXA were able to discriminate between those taking GC and those not on GC in this study. A study by Martin (22) also demonstrated the ability of calcaneal ultrasound to discriminate low bone density in patients on or not on GCs for rheumatoid arthritis from normals.

Currently, there are no prospective data for assessing fracture risk or for demonstrating the ability to monitor changes in bone density with ultrasound in GIOP; therefore, the utility of QUS in GIOP at the present time is unknown.

## QUANTITATIVE COMPUTED TOMOGRAPHY SCANS

Quantitative computed tomography scanning is the only method currently available for determining the distribution of true volumetric bone density and for separately assessing trabecular and cortical bone. The rate of change of trabecular bone in GIOP and in response to certain medication is greater than the change in combined trabecular and cortical bone measured by DXA. The increased ability of QCT to monitor the effects of bone-forming agents was demonstrated in the study by Lane (23) of parathyroid hormone (PTH) treatment for GIOP. At the end of one year of treatment with PTH, the BMD increase at the lumbar spine measured by DXA was 11%. Volumetric bone density increase in the spine measured by QCT was 33% after the same period of treatment.

---

**TABLE 5C.1**

**RECOMMENDATIONS FOR THE PREVENTION AND TREATMENT OF GLUCOCORTICOID-INDUCED OSTEOPOROSIS**

**Patient beginning therapy with glucocorticoid (prednisone equivalent of ≥5 mg/day) with plans for treatment duration of ≥3 months**
  Modify lifestyle risk factors for osteoporosis
  Smoking cessation or avoidance
  Reduction of alcohol consumption if excessive
  Instruct in weight-bearing physical exercise
  Initiate calcium supplementation
  Initiate supplementation with vitamin D (plain or activated form)
  Prescribe bisphosphonate (use with caution in premenopausal women)

**Patient receiving long-term glucocorticoid therapy (prednisone equivalent of ≥5 mg/day)**
  Modify lifestyle risk factors for osteoporosis
  Smoking cessation or avoidance
  Reduction of alcohol consumption if excessive
  Instruct in weight-bearing physical exercise
  Initiate calcium supplementation
  Initiate supplementation with vitamin D (plain or activated form)
  Prescribe treatment to replace gonadal sex hormones if deficient or otherwise clinically indicated.
  Measure bone mineral density (BMD) at lumbar spine and/or hip
  If BMD is not normal (i.e., T score below −1), then
    Prescribe bisphosphonate (use with caution in premenopausal women)
    Consider calcitonin as second-line agent if patient has contraindication to or does not tolerate alendronate therapy.
  If BMD is normal, follow up and repeat BMD measurement either annually or biannually.

Source: American College of Rheumatology Ad Hoc Committee on Glucocorticoid-Induced Osteoporosis. Recommendations for the prevention and treatment of glucocorticoid-induced osteoporosis. *Arthritis Rheum* 2001;44:1496–1503, with permission.

In nonglucocorticoid-treated patients, several studies have demonstrated that QCT is a valid tool for the detection of low bone mass. QCT has been shown to provide greater discrimination of vertebral fracture subjects from controls than DXA of the spine, likely because of its ability to exclude artifacts such as osteophytes, facet joint degeneration, and aortic calcification (24). However, QCT values tend to be significantly lower than spinal DXA values in the same patient (25) presumably because of differences in the normative data from which the T scores are derived, resulting in a smaller relative SD for QCT compared to DXA. The effect of the smaller QCT SD produces a lower T score for the same BMD. Studies demonstrating the ability of QCT to discriminate controls from patients with low bone density because of GIOP have been limited.

## GUIDELINES FOR BMD MEASUREMENT AND INTERVENTION IN GIOP

When initiating prednisone (≥5 mg/day for ≥3 months) the American College of Rheumatology (ACR) guidelines (17) recommend obtaining a baseline measurement of bone density at the lumbar spine and hip and instituting therapy (Table 5C.1). In patients already receiving long-term prednisone therapy (≥5 mg/day), the ACR guidelines propose pharmacological therapy if the BMD is a T score below –1.0. The British Bone and Tooth Society recommends treatment at a T score below –1.5 (18).

## CONCLUSION

Bone density measurement by DXA is a valuable tool for the assessment of fracture risk and for monitoring patients receiving glucocorticoid therapy. For patients with GIOP fracture at a higher BMD, intervention is recommended at a higher T score than for nonglucocorticoid-exposed patients (Table 5C.1). More research is needed with non-DXA technologies before these devices can be recommended for use in patients with GIOP.

## REFERENCES

1. Saag KG, Koehnke, Caldwell JR, et al. Low dose long-term corticosteroid therapy in rheumatoid arthritis: an analysis of serious adverse events. *Am J Med* 1994;96(2):115–123.
2. van Staa T, Leufkens H, Abenhaim L, et al. Use of oral corticosteroids and risk of fractures. *J Bone Miner Res* 2000;15(6): 993–1000.
3. Solomon DH, Katz JN, Jacobs AM, et al. Management of glucocorticoid-induced osteoporosis in patients with rheumatoid arthritis: rates and predictors of care in an academic rheumatology practice. *Arthritis Rheum* 2002; 46:3136–3142.
4. Laan RF, van Riel PL, van de Putte LB, et al. Low-dose prednisone induces rapid reversible axial bone loss in patients with rheumatoid arthritis. *Ann Intern Med* 1993;119(10):963–968.
5. Hall GM, Spector TD, Griffin AJ, et al. The effect of rheumatoid arthritis and steroid therapy on bone density in postmenopausal women. *Arthritis Rheum* 1993;36:1510–1516.
6. Sambrook PN, Cohen ML, Eisman, et al. Effects of low dose corticosteroids on bone mass in rheumatoid arthritis: a longitudinal study. *Ann Rheum Dis* 1989;48:535–538.
7. Leboff MS, Wade JP, Mackowiak S, et al. Low dose prednisone does not affect calcium homeostasis or bone density in postmenopausal women with rheumatoid arthritis. *J Rheumatol* 1990;18:339–344.
8. Pearce V, Tabensky A, Delmas PD, et al. Corticosteroid-induced bone loss in men. *J Clin Endocrinol Metab* 2000;83:801–805.
9. van Staa TP. Leufkens HG, Cooper C. The epidemiology of corticosteroid-induced osteoporosis: a Meta-analysis. *Osteoporos Int* 2002;13:777–787.
10. World Health Organization. *Assessment of fracture risk and its application to screening for postmenopausal osteoporosis*. Technical report series 843. Geneva: WHO, 1994.
11. Peel NF, Moore DJ, Barrington NA, et al. Risk of vertebral fracture and relationship to bone mineral density in steroid treated rheumatoid arthritis. *Ann Rheum Dis* 1995;54:801–806.
12. Luengo M, Picado C, Del Rio L, et al. Vertebral fractures in steroid dependent asthma and involutional osteoporosis: a comparative study. *Thorax* 1001;46:803.
13. Selby PL, Halsey JP, Adams KRH. Corticosteroids do not alter the threshold for vertebral fracture. *J Bone Miner Res* 2000;15: 952–956.
14. Van Staa TP, Laan RF, Barton IP, et al. Bone density threshold and other predictors of vertebral fracture in patients receiving oral glucocorticoid therapy. *Arthritis Rheum* 2003;11:3224–3229.
15. Cohen S, Levy RM, Keller M, et al. Risedronate therapy prevents corticosteroid-induced bone loss. *Arthritis Rheum* 1999;42: 2309–2318.
16. Reid DM, Hughes RA, Laan RFJM, et al. Efficacy and safety of daily risedronate in the treatment of corticosteroids-induced osteoporosis in men and women: a randomised trial. *J Bone Miner Res* 2000;15:1006–1013.
17. American College of Rheumatology Ad Hoc Committee on Glucocorticoid-Induced Osteoporosis. Recommendation for the prevention and treatment of glucocorticoid-induced osteoporosis. *Arthritis Rheum* 2001;44:1496–1503.
18. Bone and Tooth Society of Great Britain, Royal College of Physicians, and National Osteoporosis Society. *Guidelines on the prevention and treatment of glucocorticoid-induced osteoporosis*. London: Royal College of Physicians, 2003.
19. Saag KG, Emkey R, Schnitzer TJ, et al. Alendronate for the prevention and treatment of glucocorticoid-induced osteoporosis. Glucocorticoid-Induced Osteoporosis Intervention Study Group. *N Engl J Med* 1998;339(5):292–299.
20. Adachi JD, Bensen WG, Brown J, et al. Intermittent cyclical etidronate therapy in the prevention of corticosteroid-induced osteoporosis. *N Engl J Med* 1997;337:382–387.
21. Daens S, Peretz A, de Maertelaer V, et al. Efficiency of quantitative ultrasound measurements as compared with dual-energy x-ray absorptiometry in the assessment of corticosteroid-induced bone impairment. *Osteoporos Int* 1999;10:278–283.
22. Martin JC, Munro R, Campbell MK, Reid DM. Effects of disease and corticosteroids on appendicular bone mass in postmenopausal women with rheumatoid arthritis: comparison with axial measurements. *Br J Rheumatol* 1997;36:43–49.
23. Lane NE, Sanchez S, Modin GW. Parathyroid hormone treatment can reverse corticosteroid-induced osteoporosis. *J Clin Invest* 1998;102:1627–1633.
24. Block JE, Smith R, Gluer CC, et al. Models of spinal trabecular bone loss as determined by quantitative computed tomography. *J Bone Miner Res* 1989;4(2):249–257.
25. Faulkner KG, von Stetten E, Miller P. Discordance in patient classification using T-scores. *J Clin Densitom* 1999;2(3):343–350.

# Radiological Measurements of Periarticular Bone Loss, Erosions, and Joint Space: X-Ray Measurement of Erosions and Joint Space Narrowing

*Désirée van der Heijde*

## AIM OF MEASUREMENT OF RADIOLOGICAL DAMAGE

Measurement of radiological damage can be applied in clinical practice, in cohort studies, and in clinical trials. It can be used to assess the amount of damage at a certain point in time, cross-sectionally, or progression over time, longitudinally. A series of radiographs provides a permanent record for evaluation, in contrast to joint counts, which can be assessed only momentarily.

The information from radiographs is especially useful if it is quantified. Several scoring methods, which are discussed later in this chapter, are available for this purpose. The selection of the most appropriate scoring method is largely dependent on the setting in which it will be applied. For example, in clinical practice and large cohort studies, feasibility is of major importance, while in clinical

trials sensitivity to change is the driving force in the selection of a method. The selection of the scoring method is determined by whether the data are needed to ascertain progression either over a short or long follow-up period or at a single point in time.

Damage assessed on radiographs is a direct consequence of disease activity and other destructive pathophysiological processes (1,2). There is also a close relationship between radiological damage and other outcome measures such as functional capacity and work disability (3). As damage is largely irreversible, structural damage on radiographs is a reflection of cumulative disease activity. More and more reports are becoming available, however, that repair of damage is possible to some extent (4). More information is needed on how frequently this repair occurs, what the meaning of this repair is (i.e., is a joint with repair functioning better than a joint without signs of repair?), how long it takes to see repair, how repair can be assessed best, etc.

Many abnormalities in the joints can be detected on plain films in rheumatoid arthritis (RA). These include soft tissue swelling and proliferation, juxtaarticular and diffuse osteoporosis, marginal bony erosions, subchondral cysts, joint space narrowing as a consequence of cartilage loss, subluxation and malalignment, ankylosis, sclerosis, and osteophytes in severely damaged joints. Both erosions and joint space narrowing are the most specific features in RA, and they can be assessed in a reliable way. Moreover, they give additive information. The focus of this chapter, therefore, is on these features, which are preferably included in a scoring method. Among other features, erosions and joint space narrowing are also important characteristics of psoriatic arthritis (PsA). The presently available scoring methods for PsA are largely based on the scoring methods developed for RA with some modifications. These modifications are in the joints assessed or additional features added to the scoring. An overview of these scoring methods for PsA has been published recently (5).

## JOINTS INCLUDED IN SCORING METHODS IN RA

RA may affect all joints with a synovial membrane; however, the large majority of patients have arthritis in the small joints of the hands, including the wrists, and the feet. Also in early disease, these joints are affected first. Erosions and joint space narrowing on plain films can be detected most easily and reliably in small joints; therefore, the measurement of damage on radiographs is often confined to the joints of hands and wrists and feet. This is valid, as there is a close relationship between the damage in small joints and large joints (6,7). Moreover, in a cohort study with 12 years of follow-up, no patient without damage in the small joints showed damage in the large joints (7); information on the absence or presence of damage on hand and foot radiographs, therefore, could be used as an indication to take films of other joints.

Some of the scoring methods are applied to hand radiographs only. There is, however, an advantage to include radiographs of the feet, as the first erosions are present in the feet and often more damage occurs in the feet (8). The most frequently included joints are the proximal interphalangeal joints (PIPs), the metacarpophalangeal joints (MCPs) of the hands, several joints of the wrist separately or the wrist as a single joint, and the metatarsophalangeal joints (MTPs) of the feet. As RA is a symmetrical polyarthritis, the question exists whether scoring of only one hand and or one foot would provide sufficient information such that both sides would not have to be done. This results in too much loss of information, however, and is, therefore, not advisable.

## SCORING METHODS

In general, scoring methods can be divided into global scoring methods and detailed scoring methods (9). The first type of method gives a score for the entire patient or for the entire joint; the second type of method applies a score for specific features to each joint separately. A completely different group of scoring methods is that which is suitable to assess progression only, such as the carpo:metacarpal index. This latter group does not give an absolute score but a score based on a direct comparison. It is not frequently used and is, therefore, not discussed further.

Table 6A.1 gives an overview of the radiographic scoring systems rank ordered on year of publication. The methods are described below, grouped according to the type of scoring method.

### Global Assessment for the Whole Patient

#### Steinbrocker Index

Steinbrocker, et al. (10) reported in 1949 the first scoring method. This method is based largely on radiographic findings, although information from physical examination and from functional status is also included. It is a four-level staging system, and the joint with the worst stage determines the stage for the entire patient.

#### Kellgren's Method

Kellgren developed a standard set of radiographs to grade joints of hands and wrists on a global scale from 0 to 4 (11,12). The grade is applied to the entire hand and wrist and not to the individual joints.

### Global Assessment per Joint

#### Larsen Score

The Larsen score applies a grade from 0 to 5 to individual joints (13). A standard atlas with reference films is available. Several modifications of the scoring system by the authors have been published (14–16). The method can be applied to both large and small joints. Most frequently, the joints of the hands, wrist, and feet are included in the scoring system. Originally, the wrist is evaluated as a single joint. In one of the modifications, the joint is divided into four quadrants and each quadrant is scored separately (15). Depending on how the wrist is being evaluated, the scoring range for hands and feet is 0–160 or 0–200. The original Larsen scoring method includes soft tissue swelling and juxta-articular osteoporosis in grade 1. Only from grade 2 onwards, definite abnormalities such as erosions are present. The scoring is a combination of erosions and joint space narrowing. Grade 5 represents mutilating

## TABLE 6A.1
### COMPARISON OF RADIOGRAPHIC SCORING SYSTEMS

| Year | Author (reference) | Films | Description of Scoring System | Advantages/Disadvantages |
|------|-------------------|-------|-------------------------------|--------------------------|
| 1949 | Steinbrocker, et al (10) | Hands | Global score based on American Rheumatism Association (ARA) criteria. Ordinal score (range 1–4). | Simple, initial standardization limited by short scale and partiality for severely damaged joints. |
| 1963 | Kellgren and Lawrence (11,12) | Hands and feet | Global score for joint groups including hands, wrists, and feet. Ordinal score (range 0–4). Standard reference films. | Simple semiquantitative scoring system. Lacks sensitivity to progressive damage, and does not grade individual joints of the hands or feet. |
| 1971 | Sharp, et al (23,24) | Hands | Individual score for the joints of the hands and wrists. Erosions (29 joints) and joint space narrowing (27 joints). Ordinal score for erosions (range 0–5, max. 290). Ordinal score for joint space narrowing (range 0–4, max. 216). | Sensitive scoring system but technically demanding. Requires training and is time consuming to apply scoring system accurately and reliably. Later modified and improved by Sharp et al. 1985 (24). |
| 1977 | Larsen, et al (36) | Hands and feet | Global score for all limb joints. Ordinal scale (range 0–5) for erosions and/or joint space narrowing. Standard reference films. | Semiquantitative scoring system for radiographic changes that is easier to learn, but less sensitive to structural change than the Sharp method. Requires compliance with technical recommendations for acquiring x-rays. |
| 1983 | Genant, et al (25) | Hands and feet | Scores erosions (16 joints) and joint space narrowing (11 joints) in the hands and wrist, and scores for erosions (6 joints) and joint space narrowing (6 joints) of the feet. Ordinal scale (range 0–4). | Semiquantitative scoring system. Difficulties assessing changes in grade with progression of structural damage. |
| 1987 | Kaye et al (26) | Hands | Erosions and joint space narrowing scored together for 21 joints of the hands and wrists. Ordinal scale 0, 2, 3, 4. | A simple quantitative scoring system that requires training to efficiently apply. |
| 1989 | van der Heijde et al (20) | Hands and feet | Modified Sharp scoring system, in addition to hands and wrists, includes feet (MTP and IP of big toe). Ordinal score for erosions of hands (range 0–5) and feet (0–10). Ordinal score for joint space narrowing and (sub)luxation (0–4). | Sensitive scoring system for changes in structural damage. Requires training and application of scoring system is time consuming. |
| 1995 | Scott et al (17) | Hands and feet | Modified Larsen scoring system redefines grades of score and adds new reference films. | Modifications enhance sensitivity and increase reliability of scoring system. Less sensitive than Sharp method to changes in structural damage. |
| 1998 | Rau et al (18) | Hands | Modified Larsen scoring system. Osteoporosis and soft tissue swelling are removed from the scoring system. The surface area of the joints damaged by erosions is graded from 0 to 5 in 38 joints of the hands. | Modification improves reliability and sensitivity to change compared to original Larsen method. Relatively easy to apply. |
| 1999 | van der Heijde et al (22) | Hands/feet | Modification of the Sharp/van der Heijde method assigns individual ordinal score (0,1) for erosions (44 joints) and ordinal score for joint space narrowing (42 joints). | Simple, sensitive and reliable scoring method for assessing progression of structural damage. Requires further study to assess performance when applied to patients with longer disease duration. |
| 2000 | Wolfe et al (19) | Hands | Modification of the Larsen scoring system. Three areas in the hands and three in the wrists are graded for erosions. | Simple erosion scale with linear scale. As sensitive and reliable as full Larsen scale. |

Adapted from van der Heijde DM. Radiographic imaging: the "gold standard" for assessment of disease progression in rheumatoid arthritis. *Rheumatology (Oxf)* 2000;39(Suppl 1):9–16, with permission.

abnormality. The modification published in 1995 has modified both the sites to be evaluated as well as the grading (15). Most striking is the deletion of soft tissue swelling and osteoporosis for grade 1. Now erosions less than 1 mm and slight joint space narrowing are graded as 1.

## Scott Modification of Larsen's Method

The grading was redefined by Scott, et al. (17). Moreover, the wrist is scored as a single joint but is weighted by a factor 5 to obtain the total score. The range for hands and feet is 0–200.

## Ratingen Score

This is a modification of the Larsen score, revising the definitions of grade 1 and 2 (18). Osteoporosis and soft tissue swelling are removed from the scoring system. The surface area of the joints destroyed by erosions is graded from 0 to 5 (grade 1 <20%, grade 2 = 21–40%, up to grade 5 >80% destroyed). In total, 38 joints of the hands are scored in a range of 0–190.

## Short Erosion Scale

The short erosion scale (SES) is based on the full Larsen scale as modified in 1995, with erosions starting at grade 1 and no scores being taken for osteoporosis and soft tissue swelling (15,19). By applying statistical techniques, the number of joints was reduced to three in both hands and three in both wrists without loosing sensitivity to change. The data obtained by this method are linear and equally spaced.

## Simple Erosion Narrowing Score

The simple erosion narrowing score (SENS) is based on the van der Heijde modification of Sharp's method for hands and feet (see below) (20–22). It is a simple counting of the number of joints with erosions and the number of joints with joint space narrowing. The same joints as in the van der Heijde–modified Sharp's method are assessed. The scoring range is from 0–86.

## Detailed Scoring Methods

## Sharp's Method

This is the first method describing a detailed scoring system for erosions and joint space narrowing separately for joints in the hands and wrists (23). Originally 27 areas were scored, but in a later modification this was reduced to 17 areas read for erosions and 18 read for joint space narrowing (24). Usually, when the term *Sharp's method* is used, this refers to the modification with the reduced number of areas assessed. Erosions are scored from 0 to 5 per joint.

Erosions are counted when discrete, and surface erosions are scored according to the surface area involved. Joint space narrowing is scored on a 0 to 4 scale, representing focal narrowing (score 1), joint space loss of less than 50% (score 2), joint space loss of more than 50% (score 3), and complete joint space loss or ankylosis (score 4). Subluxation or luxation is not included in the score. In the final analyses, the erosion score, the joint space narrowing score, and the total score (a summation of the erosion and joint space narrowing score) are utilized.

## Genant's Modification of Sharp's Method

Another modification of the Sharp method is described by Genant, which extended the scale for progression from a 6-point scale to an 8-point scale with 0.5 increments from 0 to 3+ for erosions, and from a 5-point scale to a 9-point scale with 0.5 increments from 0 to 4 for joint space narrowing (25).

## Kaye's Modification of Sharp's Method

Kaye, et al. combined the methods described by Genant and Sharp and added a malalignment score to the erosion and joint space narrowing score (26). A main difference is that the score of 1 is not used. Also, the sites scored differ from the original methods. Sites that cannot be evaluated are excluded from analysis. The ultimate score is the absolute score divided by the number of evaluated joints.

## Van Der Heijde's Modification of Sharp's Method

The main modification by van der Heijde was the addition of the joints of the feet to the scoring system (20,21). Moreover, two sites for erosions and two sites for joint space narrowing were deleted from the scoring areas as compared to the Sharp's method (24). The scoring of erosions in the hands remained the same with a range of 0 to 5 per joint. However, for the scoring of erosions in the feet the scoring range was expanded to 10 per joint, with a maximum of 5 for the metatarsal and phalangeal site of the joint. Another major difference is that subluxation and luxation were added to the grading of joint space narrowing.

## Choice of Scoring Method

The setting in which the scoring method is being used is the most important factor in making a choice for a particular scoring method. For clinical practice, feasibility is the major issue. The method should be easily applicable, not time-consuming, easy to learn, and reproducible in hands of usually the same treating physician. For this purpose, the detailed scoring methods are not suitable. A choice could be made between the SENS or one of the Larsen methods. The advantage of the SENS is that it is a simple yes or no phenomenon for erosions and joint space narrowing per joint. The Larsen scale has a grading that is more difficult to apply but has reference films available.

Clinical trials to assess efficacy of treatment are usually not very long in duration. Because of the large costs involved in such studies, and for ethical reasons, the smallest number of patients that can give the answer should be included in a trial. Consequently, a method with the highest sensitivity to change is preferred. Even if the method is (relatively) time-consuming, this is well counterbalanced by the smaller number of patients needed in the trial with a similar power to find a statistically significant difference. The detailed scoring methods are the most sensitive methods, especially when the feet are included (27,28); therefore, these are the methods most used for clinical trials.

For large (observational) cohort studies, there is often a trade-off between feasibility and sensitivity to change. For long-term studies with infrequent time points, sensitivity to change is of lesser importance. On the other hand, if the follow-up periods are short (e.g., 1 year) sensitivity to change could be the most important factor on which to base the choice. For observational cohort studies, therefore, there is no single recommendation for scoring method.

## SCORING PROGRESSION

For the purpose of scoring progression, absolute scores are usually applied to initial and follow-up films, and the scores are subtracted to obtain progression scores. The way the films of the various time points are presented to observers can be done in several ways: single films randomly assigned for time point and patient [single reading], two (or more) time points per patient grouped together without providing information on the correct sequence [paired reading], or two (or more) time points per patient grouped together with information on the correct order of the time points [chronological reading]. The single reading provides the least information to the observer and is, therefore, most prone to reading error. The chronological reading provides the most information and consequently the measurement error is reduced, but expectation bias may be present resulting in overestimation of progression. In comparative studies of the paired and chronological readings, the best signal to noise ratio is obtained by the chronological reading (29). Progression assessed by the chronological reading has been shown to be most closely related to the progression judged by experts as being clinically relevant (30).

Most clinical trials performed to judge efficacy of treatment are scored by paired reading to avoid every possible bias. In addition, it is a better method to judge if repair exists (31).

### Number of Observers

The setting determines how many observers should be used to judge the radiographs. In clinical practice, one observer is sufficient. This is often also the case for observational studies (32). For clinical trials, however, it is advisable to use the scores of two readers for each film and to use the average score of the two readers for the final analysis (32,33).

### Interobserver Reliability

Kappa statistics and intraclass correlation coefficients are appropriate statistics to get information on observer reliability (32). Reliability data on progression scores should be obtained in addition to the status scores. Overall, reliability is good for the published methods.

Additional information on the level of agreement between observers can be obtained by Bland and Altman plots (34), which presents the difference in scores between two observers in relation to the average score. The limits of agreement can be deduced from these data. This results in the smallest detectable difference (SDD) (35), which is the smallest progression that can be detected reliably apart from measurement error. The SDD is a measure of assessing the agreement between readers (32). If progression based on paired or chronological reading is assessed, the smallest detectable change is a more appropriate measure than the SDD (38).

## PRESENTATION OF RADIOGRAPHIC RESULTS OF CLINICAL TRIALS

Experts participating in a roundtable conference published recommendations on how to read, analyze, and report radiographic results from clinical trials (32). Data can be analyzed and reported at either the group level or the individual level. The group level should be the primary analysis. These results should be presented both as means and standard deviations, as well as medians and interquartile ranges. The main reason to present both is that these give additional information as radiographic data of trials are usually not normally distributed. This gives also the best possibility to compare results across trials.

For the presentation of the data on an individual patient level, a cutoff needs to be defined. Ideally, this would be the minimal level of progression that has an impact on the final outcome of the disease. Unfortunately, this is not available for radiographic progression; therefore, surrogate cutoffs are being used. Some authors choose a progression of at least 0 (or at least 0.5 in case the average score of two observers is being used). This does not take into account any type of measurement error. One should, therefore, use the smallest detectable difference (SDD), as described above.

Recently, a new concept has been proposed to present the data from all individual patients as a so-called probability plot (39).

## SUMMARY

Several validated, reliable, and sensitive scoring methods exist for use in clinical practice or in research. Depending on the setting, the optimal scoring method should be selected. To standardize the analysis and interpretation of data, recommendations have been made. Applying these recommendations enhances the interpretability of results of various research efforts.

## REFERENCES

1. Welsing PM, Landewé R, van Riel P, et al. A longitudinal analysis of the cause-effect relationship between disease activity and radiological progression in patients with rheumatoid arthritis. *Arthritis Rheum* 2004;50(7):2082–2093.
2. Landewé R, Geusens P, van der Heijde D, et al. Clinically perceptible arthritis instantaneously influences collagen type-I and type-II degradation in patients with early rheumatoid arthritis. a longitudinal analysis. *Arthritis Rheum* 2004;50(5):1390–1399.
3. van der Heijde D. Radiographic progression in rheumatoid arthritis: does it reflect outcome? Does it reflect treatment? *Ann Rheum Dis* 2001;60[Suppl 3]:47–50.
4. Sharp JT, van der Heijde D, Boers M, et al. Repair of erosions in rheumatoid arthritis does occur. Results from 2 studies by the OMERACT Subcommittee on Healing of Erosions. *J Rheumatol* 2003;30:1102–1107.
5. van der Heijde D, Sharp J, Wassenberg S, Gladman D. Imaging: A review of scoring methods in psoriatic arthritis. *Ann Rheum Dis* 2004 (*in press*).
6. Scott DL, Coulton BL, Popert AJ. Long term progression of joint damage in rheumatoid arthritis. *Ann Rheum Dis* 1986;45(5):373–378.
7. Drossaers-Bakker K, Kroon H, Zwinderman A, et al. Radiographic damage of large joints in long-term rheumatoid arthritis and its relation to function. *Rheumatology* 2000;39:998–1003.
8. van der Heijde DM, van Leeuwen MA, van Riel PL, et al. Biannual radiographic assessments of hands and feet in a three-year prospective follow-up of patients with early rheumatoid arthritis. *Arthritis Rheum* 1992;35(1):26–34.
9. van der Heijde DM. Plain X-rays in rheumatoid arthritis: overview of scoring methods, their reliability and applicability. *Baillieres Clin Rheumatol* 1996;10(3):435–453.
10. Steinbrocker O, Traeger C, Batterman R. Therapeutic criteria in rheumatoid arthritis. *J Am Med Assoc* 1949;140:659–662.
11. Kellgren JH. Radiological signs of rheumatoid arthritis; a study of observer differences in the reading of hand films. *Ann Rheum Dis* 1956;15(1):55–60.
12. Kellgren JH, Lawrence JS. Radiological assessment of rheumatoid arthritis. *Ann Rheum Dis* 1957;16(4):485–493.
13. Larsen A, Dale K, Eek M. Radiographic evaluation of rheumatoid arthritis and related conditions by standard reference films. *Acta Radiol Diagn Stockh* 1977;18:481–491.
14. Larsen A, Thoen J. Hand radiography of 200 patients with rheumatoid arthritis repeated after an interval of one year. *Scand J Rheumatol* 1987;16(6):395–401.
15. Larsen A. How to apply Larsen score in evaluating radiographs of rheumatoid arthritis in long-term studies. *J Rheumatol* 1995;22(10):1974–1975.
16. Larsen A, Horton J, Howland C. The effects of auranofin and parenteral gold in the treatment of rheumatoid arthritis: an X-ray analysis. *Clin Rheumatol* 1984;3[Suppl 1]:97–104.
17. Scott D, Houssien D, Laasonen L. Proposed modification to Larsen's scoring method for hand and wrist radiographs. *Br J Rheumatol* 1995;34:56.
18. Rau R, Wassenberg S, Herborn G, et al. A new method of scoring radiographic change in rheumatoid arthritis. *J Rheumatol* 1998;25(11):2094–2107.
19. Wolfe F, van der Heijde DM, Larsen A. Assessing radiographic status of rheumatoid arthritis: introduction of a short erosion scale. *J Rheumatol* 2000;27(9):2090–2099.
20. van der Heijde DM, van Riel PL, Nuver Zwart IH, et al. Effects of hydroxychloroquine and sulphasalazine on progression of joint damage in rheumatoid arthritis. *Lancet* 1989;1(8646):1036–1038.
21. van der Heijde D. How to read radiographs according to the Sharp/van der Heijde method. *J Rheumatol* 2000;27(1):261–263.
22. van der Heijde D, Dankert T, Nieman F, et al. Reliability and sensitivity to change of a simplification of the Sharp/van der Heijde radiological assessment in rheumatoid arthritis. *Rheumatology* 1999;38(10):941–947.
23. Sharp JT, Lidsky MD, Collins LC, Moreland J. Methods of scoring the progression of radiologic changes in rheumatoid arthritis. Correlation of radiologic, clinical and laboratory abnormalities. *Arthritis Rheum* 1971;14(6):706–720.
24. Sharp JT, Young DY, Bluhm GB, et al. How many joints in the hands and wrists should be included in a score of radiologic abnormalities used to assess rheumatoid arthritis? *Arthritis Rheum* 1985;28(12):1326–1335.
25. Genant HK. Methods of assessing radiographic change in rheumatoid arthritis. *Am J Med* 1983(75):35–47.
26. Kaye JJ, Callahan LF, Nance EP Jr, et al. Bony ankylosis in rheumatoid arthritis. Associations with longer duration and greater severity of disease. *Invest Radiol* 1987;22(4):303–309.
27. Lassere M. Pooled metaanalysis of radiographic progression: comparison of Sharp and Larsen methods. *J Rheumatol* 2000;27(1):269–275.
28. Rau R, Wassenberg S. Bildgebende verfahren in der rheumatologie: Scoring—Methoden bei der rheumatoiden Arthritis. *Z Rheumatol* 2003;62:555–565.
29. van der Heijde D, Boonen A, Boers M, et al. Reading radiographs in chronological order, in pairs or as single films has important implications for the discriminative power of rheumatoid arthritis clinical trials. *Rheumatology* 1999;38(12):1213–1220.
30. Bruynesteyn K, van der Heijde D, Boers M, et al. Detecting radiological changes in rheumatoid arthritis that are considered important by clinical experts: influence of reading with or without known sequence. *J Rheumatol* 2002;29(11):2306–2312.
31. van der Heijde D, Landewé R. Imaging: do erosions heal? *Ann Rheum Dis* 2003;62[Suppl 2]:10–12.
32. van der Heijde D, Simon L, Smolen J, et al. How to report radiographic data in randomized clinical trials in rheumatoid arthritis: guidelines from a roundtable discussion. *Arthritis Rheum* 2002;47(2):215–218.
33. Fries JF, Bloch DA, Sharp JT, et al. Assessment of radiologic progression in rheumatoid arthritis. A randomized, controlled trial. *Arthritis Rheum* 1986;29:1–9.
34. Bland JM, Altman DG. Statistical methods for assessing agreement between two methods of clinical measurement. *Lancet* 1986;1:307–310.
35. Lassere M, Boers M, van der Heijde D, et al. Smallest detectable difference in radiological progression. *J Rheumatol* 1999;26(3):731–739.
36. Larsen A, Dale K. Standardized radiological evaluation of rheumatoid arthritis in therapeutic trials. In: Dumonde DC, Jasani JK, eds. *Recognition of anti-rheumatic drugs*. Lancaster, UK: MTP Press, 1977:285–292.
37. van der Heijde DM. Radiographic imaging: the "gold standard" for assessment of disease progression in rheumatoid arthritis. *Rheumatology (Oxf)* 2000;39[Suppl 1]:9–16
38. Bruynesteyn K, Boers M, Kostense P, et al. Deciding on progression of joint damage in paired films of individual patients: smallest detectable difference or change? *Ann Rheum Dis* 2004;10.1136/ard. 2003.
39. Landewé R, van der Heijde D. Radiographic progression depicted by probability plots: presenting data with optional use of individual values. *Arthritis Rheum* 2004;50(3):699–706.

# Radiological Measurements of Periarticular Bone Loss, Erosions, and Joint Space: The Use of MRI for the Grading of Erosions and Joint Space Narrowing

*Fiona McQueen*

## MAGNETIC RESONANCE IMAGING IN THE ASSESSMENT OF CARTILAGE AND BONY DAMAGE

Magnetic resonance imaging (MRI) is emerging as a powerful tool for rheumatologists interested in quantifying abnormalities of bone in a variety of settings. In rheumatoid arthritis (RA), MRI allows a three-dimensional (3D) view of erosions from an extremely early stage and reveals bone marrow edema, a preerosive lesion associated with an adverse prognosis (1,2). These bony changes can be examined in the context of accompanying soft tissue inflammation, including synovitis and tendonitis, to provide a unique picture of disease activity and progression. Recently, the spondyloarthropathies have begun to be explored with MRI, which has revealed specific features associated with enthesopathy and active spinal lesions (3,4). A considerable literature now exists on MRI of cartilage damage and joint space narrowing in osteoarthritic joints (5–7). Thus, MRI is poised to take its place as an essential part of the rheumatologist's armamentarium, but before that can happen, it is essential that its use moves beyond the descriptive to the quantitative. For this reason, scoring systems have been developed and validated quite rigorously in multicenter studies to expose the strengths and weaknesses of this imaging modality and eventually allow its most effective application in the clinical setting.

### The Physical Basis of MR Imaging

To better understand how MR differs from conventional radiography (CR) in the imaging of erosions and joint space narrowing, one must return to the physical basis of the imaging process itself. The fundamental molecule visualized by MR is the H$^+$ ion, and the feature used to distinguish various tissues and pathological states in the arthritic joint is the water content. This is in stark contrast with CR in which water molecules are not "seen" at all, but rather Ca$^{2+}$ ions define the image produced. An MR image is produced when all the H$^+$ ions within the organ being imaged are exposed to an extremely powerful magnetic field and their own individual polarities become aligned with this. When the external field is withdrawn, each individual proton recovers its own spin and orientation with its attendant longitudinal magnetization (known as T1 relaxation) and this generates an electrical signal, which has a specific spatial location within the tissue and is recorded by a computer. The external field is applied in pulses, and, for example, 256 repetitions may be required to generate an image (8). The density of protons and their relationship with other molecules nearby (such as proteoglycan in cartilage) determines the MR signal. The phenomenon of T2 relaxation is related to the tendency of neighboring spinning protons to fall out of phase with each other. When they are relatively "free" as in synovial fluid, the T2 relaxation time is prolonged and the image appears bright or "high signal," but when constrained as in cartilage, the T2 relaxation time is rapid and the tissue appears dark, or more correctly "low signal"(8).

## MR Scanners, Sequences and Acquisitions

MR scanners are described according to the strength of their magnetic field as 0.2, 1.0, 1.5, and 3.0 Tesla (T) machines. The 0.2 T scanners are generally used in the ambulatory care setting and although image resolution is lower than high-field machines, this can be compensated for by employing specific imaging protocols. Most of the MR data relevant to scoring erosions and joint space narrowing in RA and osteoarthritis (OA) has been obtained using 1.0 and 1.5 T scanners. The other critical piece of equipment is the imaging coil, which receives the alternating current generated by spinning protons and converts it into a signal to make up the image. For a clear image, the signal-to-noise ratio must be high and this is improved with specialized coils available for extremities including dedicated wrist coils (8). In-plane resolution is influenced by the field of view, which should be small enough for good image quality, and the matrix, which optimally should use a large number of units for small pixel size producing a high-density image.

A full discussion of specialist MR sequences available is well beyond the scope of this summary, but some sequences applicable to the imaging of bone are briefly mentioned. As well as T1- and T2-weighted spin-echo sequences described above, fast spin-echo imaging is a technique developed to produce more rapid T2w images with greater resolution. It utilizes 180° radiofrequency pulses followed by phase-encoding gradients to produce echoes from the original signal, which enhance it and provide more contrast in the final image. Short tau inversion recovery (STIR) sequences employ a similar technique, but in this case signal from bone marrow fat is suppressed, allowing bone marrow edema to be well seen. Gradient echo sequences have a 3D capability and include techniques such as fast low-angle shot (FLASH) and spoiled "gradient recalled acquisition in the steady state" (GRASS), which are useful in depicting bone erosions. The paramagnetic contrast agent, gadolinium diethylenetriamine pentaacetic acid (Gd-DTPA) allows MR evaluation of rheumatoid synovitis (8). It can also improve the imaging of bone edema and active erosions, which frequently contain enhancing pannus. The term *acquisitions* applied to MR imaging refers to acquisition of signal from the tissue being scanned. This is affected by the thickness of slices used to make up the final image, and the gap between adjoining slices. Acquisition of signal is increased by a longer time spent under the scanner, which improves image clarity, especially for T2w sequences.

## Distinguishing Erosions Using MR

Erosions are unquestionably of fundamental importance to rheumatologists as they represent (mostly) permanent structural joint damage. They are both a pathological hallmark of RA and a feature that can be used to measure disease progression. Radiographic erosions are recognized by a characteristic breach in the fine "white," or more correctly radio-opaque, bony cortex. Using MR to image the same erosion results in virtually the opposite; an area of altered signal interrupts the "dark" cortical line (low signal as it hardly contains any water) and defines a pocket within the underlying bone. Bone marrow fat is replaced by H$^+$-rich inflammatory tissue that has the following characteristics: it yields an intermediate signal on T1w images and high signal (producing a bright lesion) on post-gadolinium T1w, T2w, or STIR images. MR erosions and bone edema are yet to be compared with their histopathological equivalents. Ostendorf, et al. (9) used miniarthroscopy of metacarpophalangeal (MCP) joints in RA patients to identify bony alterations and chondromalacia, which were frequently recognized as erosions or preerosive lesions on MRI and were correlated with joint space narrowing. However, histological specimens of bone and cartilage could not be taken, and more studies are needed to define the tissue correlates of MR bone lesions.

One must recall that when MR is used to image erosions in RA, it is also likely to reveal surrounding inflammatory change in bone and soft tissues. Thus, erosions often occur adjacent to regions of synovitis and regions associated with edema in the marrow of underlying subcortical bone (1,2). These changes produce high signal on T1w post-Gd and T2w images and the result is a complex pattern of contrasting bright, intermediate, and dark signal, which has the advantage of demonstrating the inflammatory context of the erosion but the disadvantage of (sometimes) making the borders of the lesion hard to define (Fig. 6B.1). To offset this is the multiplanar, tomographic aspect of MR so that areas of potential erosion can be verified in other planes and slices (contrasting with CR where 2D imaging makes some regions such as the wrist very difficult to assess). Importantly, researchers are now investigating whether MR "erosions" can be detected in normal individuals. Ejbjerg, et al. (10) explored this in 28 healthy controls and found precontrast, erosion-like changes at 5/448 MCP and 16/420 carpal sites. Only one of these lesions showed features on T2 fat saturated (FS) and STIR sequences supportive of erosion, and bone marrow edema was not found in any joints. Thus, although erosion-like changes can be seen in some normals, these usually lack evidence of surrounding inflammation and are, therefore, more likely to be associated with degenerative change or previous trauma.

## MRI of Joint Space Narrowing and Cartilage Pathology

MR also has strengths and weaknesses in the imaging of joint space narrowing. On a radiograph, the two cortical borders of adjacent bones can often be clearly seen and the distance between them estimated with a fair degree of accuracy. Of course this space contains many features not seen by CR including cartilage, synovial membrane, and synovial fluid. At a large joint such as a knee or ankle, MR allows direct visualization of cartilage (impossible using CR) by employing, for example, a high-resolution, 3D

gradient, echo fat-suppressed sequence. Cartilage appears as a band of bright signal with adjacent low-signal synovial fluid, intermediate-signal synovial membrane, and on the other side, suppressed bone marrow fat yielding low signal. Furthermore, other sequences can be used to reveal cartilage viability as it becomes waterlogged in the early stages of degeneration with high-signal regions on T2w sequences (11).

Unfortunately, at the small joints of the hand and wrist, MRI is a relatively imprecise method for assessing cartilage thickness and joint space narrowing. Here, the band of cartilage between adjacent carpal bones is very thin with little synovial membrane or fluid intervening and appears on MR as a region of intermediate-low signal between two dark cortical lines. Spatial resolution is lower than that achieved by fine-detail radiographs and CT (Fig. 6B.2) and may be further eroded by partial volume artifacts producing averaging of signal between adjacent areas of different signal intensity. The addition of overlying or adjacent synovitis, tendonitis, bone erosion, and bone edema can further confuse the picture. Advanced MR techniques can be used to overcome these difficulties but are usually only available in specialized units and require longer imaging times (11).

## SCORING JOINT DAMAGE USING MR

### MR Scoring Systems for RA

Despite the fact that MR technology has been available for the last 20 years, quantitative MR scoring systems were not developed until the early 1990s. Recently, the Outcome

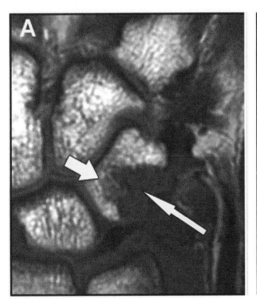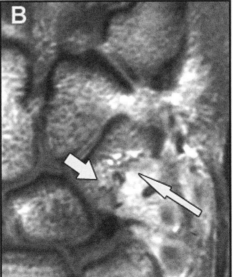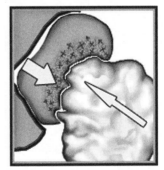

**Figure 6B.1    A:** T1w coronal MR scan of the carpus in a patient with RA shows a large erosion at the triquetrum filled with synovial membrane (*thin arrow*). Adjacent bone edema is low signal (*wide arrow*). (**B**) Post-Gd T1w coronal image shows enhancement within inflamed synovial membrane and in the region of bone edema.

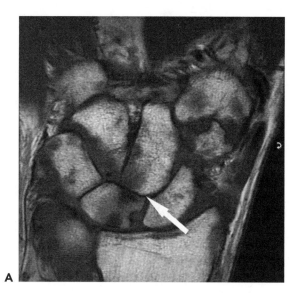 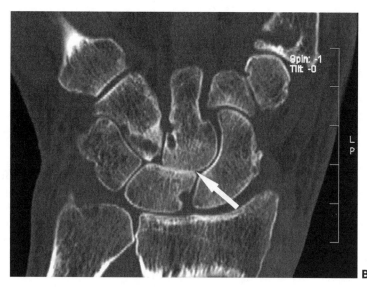

**Figure 6B.2** **A:** T1w coronal MR scan of the wrist in a patient with RA revealing bone edema and erosions at multiple carpal bones. (**B**) Joint space narrowing with "bone-on-bone" apposition of the capitate and lunate (*arrow*) is much better seen on the equivalent high-resolution CT scan.

Measures in Rheumatoid Arthritis Clinical Trials (OMERACT) MRI working party has attempted to create an internationally accepted and validated MRI scoring system, now known as RAMRIS (RA MRI score), for use in RA (12). This is still not comprehensive and does not include an assessment of tendonitis, tenosynovitis, or joint space narrowing, the last one having been abandoned after evidence of poor reliability in a multireader international exercise (13). Other modifications have been made over the 6 years since this system was first proposed, and the score continues to evolve with practical application. Although it was developed for use at the hands and wrists, it is now being applied to other joints such as those in the feet (14).

## Reproducibility of MR Scoring

Many early studies did not address the fundamental issue of scoring reproducibility for MRI erosions. However, in a cohort of early RA patients, McQueen, et al. described MR erosion score data with good interobserver and excellent intraobserver reliability intraclass correlation coefficients [(ICCs) of 0.77–0.84 and 0.92–0.98, respectively] (1). The five-center international exercises conducted by the MRI working party using the RAMRIS revealed interobserver reliability ranging from poor to good with ICCs ranging from 0.15 to 0.85 (15). Training was found to have a significant influence (16) and assessments at the wrist were less reliable than at MCP joints, probably because of the complex anatomy of that area; an observation also described by Østergaard et al (17). Table 6B.1 summarizes these MR reliability results. In comparison, reliability of radiographic scoring for erosions has been shown to be somewhat higher (ICCs for the Sharp score range from 0.40–0.97) (18) with consistent scoring demonstrated by trained readers in the Antitumor Necrosis Factor Trial in Rheumatoid Arthritis with Concomitant Therapy Study

### TABLE 6B.1

**INTRACLASS CORRELATION COEFFICIENTS (ICCs) ESTIMATING RELIABILITY OF MR EROSION SCORES IN RA**

| Study Authors | No. of patients or sites examined | Site | Erosion score ICC |
|---|---|---|---|
| McQueen et al (1) | 42 | Wrist | 0.75–0.84 |
| Conaghan et al (15) | 10 | MCPs | 0.78–0.85 |
| | | Wrist | 0.15–0.45 |
| Østergaard et al (17) | 30 | MCPs | 0.81–0.95 |
| | 10 | Wrist | 0.73–0.74 |
| Bird et al (21) | 5 | MCPs | 0.73–0.87* |

* Semiautomated erosion volume estimation.

Group (ATTRACT) (19) (interobserver ICCs 0.89 at baseline and 54 weeks, personal communication, Professor van der Heijde).

Given the complexity of MR images, which reveal the full range of pathology within the rheumatoid joint including many features that can mimic erosions or blur their borders, these results are not surprising. Nevertheless, the fact that MR scoring of bone erosions is generally less reproducible between observers than radiographic erosion scoring needs to be borne in mind when interpreting the results of clinical trials using MR as an outcome measure. In this situation, a rigorous determination of reliability should to be applied to results before it would be accurate to conclude that, for example, drug X slows the progression of MR erosions more than drug Y. The MRI working party is currently developing an atlas to facilitate the use of the RAMRIS system by rheumatologists, and it is expected that this will improve scoring reliability (20).

## Computerized Systems for Erosion Volume Estimation

Simple observer-based volume estimation has been used in the RAMRIS system to score erosions (1–10; 1 = 10% of bone involvement, and 10 = 100%) but this has also been attempted using computerized systems. Bird, et al. described the outlining of erosion margins to determine volumes, using OSIRIS imaging software (21). The total volume of erosions obtained by this method correlated strongly with the RAMRIS erosion score. Interobserver reliability was found to be good in a separate study (ICCs of 0.73–0.87) (22) (Table 6B.1), but there were large systematic differences in volume estimations by observers, with variation by as much as 100%. This once more draws attention to difficulties in identifying the borders of erosions on MRI; a task that must still be performed by a skilled observer and is not aided by a computer. An NIH group has used another technique employing a "live wire" to delineate MRI erosions before volume computation (3,24). MR erosion volumes were compared with CT estimates and interestingly were higher, suggesting that a rim of bone edema may surround many erosions, blurring boundaries and leading to problems in defining volume. However, interobserver reliability for scoring CT erosions in this study was low and only limited MR sequences were used. In contrast, Perry et al (25) recently found a high degree of concordance between MR and CT erosion scores at the wrist in a group of RA patients, emphasising the importance of using a full range of relevant sequences when defining erosions using MR.

## MR Versus CR for Scoring Bony Change in RA

Although MRI falls short of CR in terms of reproducibility for scoring erosions and joint space narrowing, CR in many situations does not even approach MRI for sensitivity and providing useful information. This has been most clearly illustrated in very early RA when in one study, 45% of patients were erosive on MRI at 4 months from symptom-onset compared with only 12% on CR (26). MR and x-ray (XR) erosion scores then progressed in tandem until at 6 years they had become strongly correlated ($r = 0.79$) (1). Figure 6B-3 shows scans and x-rays from one of these patients and illustrates the early appearance of an MR erosion, which is then recognized on CR the following year. In established disease there is less to distinguish MR from CR as means to monitor erosive progression as has recently been described in the Damage Study (27) where MR scans of the dominant MCPs were slightly less responsive to change over 2 years than CR of both hands.

Østergaard, et al. (28) have shown that MR erosions precede CR erosions by a median of 2 years, and this group recently reported that radiographic lesions were only reliably recognized when MR erosion volumes reached 20%–30% of the metacarpal head (29). To counter the suggestion that small MR erosions are simply in the mind of the imaginative observer, there are several studies comparing MR with ultrasound that show a strong correlation between these modalities, both being more sensitive than CR (30). Several groups have identified MR bone edema, which is undetectable using CR, as a preerosive change (1,2), and in the cohort study referred to above, the bone edema score at presentation was predictive of the total Sharp score 6 years later (1). These findings suggest that distinguishing the borders of an MR erosion from its surrounding zone of bone edema may not be so vitally important if both lesions have adverse prognostic implications.

## Using MR to Score Bone Lesions at the Hands and Feet

One of the criticisms leveled at MR as a way to assess rheumatoid bony damage is that it usually only allows imaging of one body region, such as the dominant hand, contrasting with a more "holistic" picture obtained from CR of both hands and feet. Boutry, et al. (31) recently described MR findings from both hands and both feet in 30 early RA patients. Bone erosions were reported to be bilateral at the hands in 70% and at the feet in 83%, indicating the extent of "data loss" when only one side is examined, but the definition of erosion was less stringent than in previous studies and these figures require confirmation. Ostendorf, et al. (14) used an adapted form of the RAMRIS to score MR scans of MCP joints of the dominant hand and MTP joints of the dominant forefoot in RA patients with an average disease duration of only 2 months (14). Bone edema and erosion were present at MTP joints in 70% and 10%, respectively, of patients whose MCP joints were scored as normal, suggesting that MR of the foot is likely to assume a critical place in the investigation of early disease. Unfortunately, MRI of more than one joint region usually

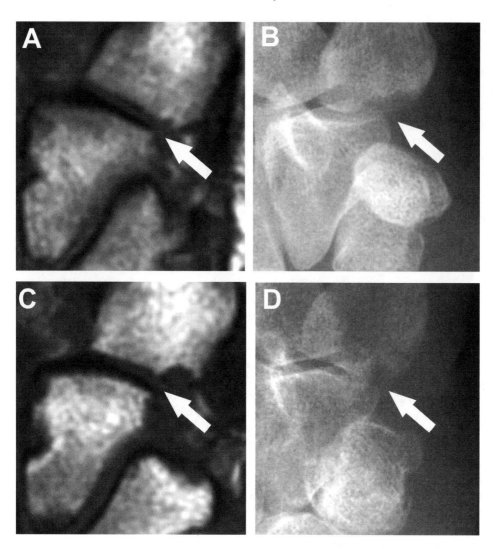

**Figure 6B.3    A:** T1w coronal MR scan of the wrist in an RA patient shows very early erosions at the fifth metacarpal base and the pole of the hamate. (**B**) Radiograph of the same region shows periarticular osteopenia but no erosions. (**C**) MR scan 1 year later reveals progression of erosions at both these sites (and 2 other erosions within the hamate). (**D**) Radiograph 1 year later shows the erosion at the fifth metacarpal base, but hamate lesions remain obscured.

comes at the cost of prolonged scanning time (with associated expense and patient discomfort).

## MRI Scoring of Bony Change in Spondyloarthropathies

Braun, et al. (4) have recently described a new MRI scoring system to determine activity and chronicity of spinal bone lesions in ankylosing spondylitis patients (4). The activity score was determined by the extent of bone edema and erosions adjacent to vertebral margins, which enhanced on STIR and post-Gd T1w turbo spin echo (TSE) sequences, while chronicity required evidence of sclerosis and syndesmophyte formation. Post-Gd T1w sequences were more reliable than STIR sequences for determination of the activity score (interrater variance of 6.8% and 15% of the total variance, respectively) and this demonstrated good sensitivity to change. However, reliability of the chronicity score was low as MRI did not image early syndesmophytes

well, and a study is underway to compare CR with MR in this context.

## MR Bony Change as an Outcome Measure in Clinical Trials

The progression of MR erosions is now being examined as an outcome measure in clinical trials. Østergaard, et al. (32) recently reported MR findings in a small group of RA patients treated with interleukin -1–receptor antagonist (anakinra). Change in the MRI erosion score over 12 weeks correlated with change in the total Sharp score over 36 weeks, suggesting that MR is ideal for early evaluation of treatment efficacy. Braun, et al. (4) used their spondyloarthropathy MR scoring system to determine progression of disease activity at spinal sites in 20 patients and found a 40% improvement in the "active lesion score" in those treated with infliximab. This field is rapidly expanding, and with more reliable MR scoring systems being developed, it is likely that in many settings, MRI will become the imaging method of choice for outcome measurement in clinical trials.

## MR IN OA — SCORING CARTILAGE DEFECTS

Osteoarthritis produces changes in cartilage that appear on MR as surface irregularity, thinning, erosion, and ulceration. The MR signal of cartilage is also altered in early OA as a result of water retention. Broderick, et al. (33) graded the severity of knee OA using MR and arthroscopy on a 0 to 5 scale and found that grades correlated well for severe lesions but poorly for minor cartilage thinning. However, using a different 3D MR sequence to determine the volume of lesions, Raynauld, et al. (6) found excellent interreader agreement for MR cartilage measurements at the knee (ICCs 0.94–0.99).

Data from longitudinal studies in OA are now appearing. Wluka, et al. (7) quantified the decrease in cartilage thickness at the tibia in a cohort of OA patients over 2 years using OSIRIS software and found this to be of the order of 5% per year. Coefficients of variation for MRI measurement of medial and lateral cartilage volumes were 3.4% and 2.0%, respectively, suggesting excellent reproducibility. The authors suggest that the ability of MR to estimate total cartilage volume in this context makes it a much more reliable imaging technique than CR, which relies on joint space narrowing, a two-dimensional assessment of a 3D structure. As in RA, MR also reveals the other features of disease in OA and provides excellent imaging of osteophytes and geodes as well as meniscal degeneration and synovitis. Bone marrow edema is also seen in this disease but is quantitatively less than in RA and has not been associated with prognosis.

## CONCLUSIONS

In summary, the grading of erosions and joint space narrowing using MRI has evolved over the last 10 years to a point where its clinical application is now possible and appropriate. MR differs fundamentally from radiography in its dependence on protons to produce an image, and it is, therefore, capable of revealing the rheumatoid erosion in its inflammatory context, which involves not only neighboring synovium but also frequently cartilage and underlying bone. In some situations, MR should be viewed as complementary to radiographic techniques that may produce more reproducible information about cortical margins and joint space narrowing. Unquestionably MR is the better modality in very early RA when pathological change is frequently subradiographic, and recent studies suggest that imaging regions such as the forefoot and wrist may be particularly fruitful. This application is likely to

become increasingly important in keeping with the current emphasis on early therapeutic intervention in RA, ideally at the preerosive stage. In OA, the development of 3D sequences to accurately measure cartilage volume in large joints means that MR is poised to overtake CR as the method of choice for assessing disease progression. There are downsides to the routine use of MR, however, including a major issue of cost, problems with claustrophobia with some patients, and difficulties in scanning obese individuals or those with surgical hardware stabilizing their joints. More data are still required from clinical trials and observational studies comparing MRI with other imaging modalities before its true potential can be appreciated.

## ACKNOWLEDGMENTS

I would like to acknowledge the assistance of Dr. Neal Stewart for reviewing parts of this manuscript.

## REFERENCES

1. McQueen FM, Benton N, Perry D, et al. Bone oedema scored on magnetic resonance scans of the dominant carpus at presentation predicts radiographic joint damage at the hands and feet six years later in patients with rheumatoid arthritis. *Arthritis Rheum* 2003;48:1814–1827.
2. Savnik A, Malmskov H, Thomsen HS, et al. MRI of the wrist and finger joints in inflammatory joint diseases at 1-yr interval: MRI features to predict bone erosions. *Eur Radiol* 2002;12:1203–1210.
3. McGonagle D, Gibbon W, O'Connor, et al. Characteristic magnetic resonance imaging entheseal changes of knee synovitis in spondyloarthropathy. *Arthritis Rheum* 1998;41:694–700.
4. Braun J, Baraliakos X, Golder W, et al. Magnetic resonance imaging examinations of the spine in patients with ankylosing spondylitis, before and after successful therapy with infliximab. *Arthritis Rheum* 2003;48:1126–1136.
5. Loeuille D, Olivier P, Mainard D, et al. Magnetic resonance imaging of normal and osteoarthritis cartilage. *Arthritis Rheum* 1998;41:963–975.
6. Raynauld JP, Kauffman C, Beaudoin G, et al. Reliability of a quantification imaging system using magnetic resonance images to measure cartilage thickness and volume in human normal and osteoarthritis knees. *Osteoarthritis Cartilage* 2003;11(5):351–360.
7. Wluka AE, Stuckey S, Snaddon J, et al. The determinants of change in tibial cartilage volume in osteoarthritic knees. Arthritis Rheum 2002;46:2065–2072.
8. Peterfy CG. Magnetic resonance imaging of rheumatoid arthritis: the evolution of clinical applications through clinical trials. *Semin Arthritis Rheum* 2001;30:375–396.
9. Ostendorf B, Peters R, Dann P, et al. Magnetic resonance imaging and miniarthroscopy of metacarpophalangeal joints. *Arthritis Rheum* 2001;44:2492–2250.
10. Ejbjerg B, Narvestad E, Rostrup E. Magnetic resonance imaging of wrist and finger joints in healthy subjects occasionally shows changes resembling erosions and synovitis as seen in rheumatoid arthritis. *Arthritis Rheum* 2004;50:1097–1106.
11. Peterfy CG. MR Imaging. *Bailliere's Clin Rheumatol* 1996;10:635–678.
12. Østergaard M, Peterfy C, Conaghan P, et al. OMERACT RA magnetic resonance imaging studies. Core set of MRI acquisitions, joint pathology definitions and the OMERACT RA-MRI scoring system. *J Rheumatol* 2003;30:1385–1386.
13. Østergaard M, Klarlund M, Lassere M, et al. Interreader agreement in the assessment of magnetic resonance images of rheumatoid

arthritis wrist and finger joints- an international multicentre study. *J Rheumatol* 2001;28:1143–1150.

14. Ostendorf B, Scherer A, Modder U, et al. Diagnostic value of magnetic resonance imaging of the forefeet in early rheumatoid arthritis when findings on imaging of the metacarpophalageal joints of the hands remain normal. *Arthritis Rheum* 2004;50:2094–2102.

15. Conaghan P, Lassere M, Østergaard M, et al. OMERACT rheumatoid arthritis magnetic resonance imaging studies. Exercise 4: an international multicentre longitudinal study using the RA-MRI score. *J Rheumatol* 2003;30:1376–1379.

16. McQueen FM, Østergaard M, Conaghan P, et al. OMERACT rheumatoid arthritis magnetic resonance imaging studies. Summary of OMERACT 6 MR imaging module. *J Rheumatol* 2003; 30:1387–1392.

17. Østergaard M, Conaghan P, O'Connor P, et al. Reducing costs, duration and invasiveness of magnetic resonance imaging in rheumatoid arthritis by omitting intravenous gadolinium injection—does it affect assessments of synovitis, bone erosions and bone edema? *Ann Rheum Dis* 2003;62:67.

18. Lassere M, van der Heidje D, Johnson K, et al. The reliability of measures of disease activity and disease damage in rheumatoid arthritis: implications for the smallest detectable difference, the minimal clinically important difference, and the analysis of treatment effects in randomized controlled trials. *J Rheumatol* 2001; 28:892–903.

19. Lipsky PE, van der Heijde DM, St Clair EW, et al. Infliximab and methotrexate in the treatment of rheumatoid arthritis (ATTRACT). *NEJM* 2000;343:1594–1602.

20. Østergaard M, Bird P, McQueen F, et al. The EULAR-OMERACT magnetic resonance imaging in rheumatoid arthritis reference film atlas—a new tool for standardized assessment of rheumatoid joint inflammation and destruction (abstract). *Ann Rheum Dis* 2004;63 (Suppl 1):81–82.

21. Bird P, Lassere M, Shnier R, et al. Computerized measurement of magnetic resonance imaging erosion volumes in patients with rheumatoid arthritis. *Arthritis Rheum* 2003;48:614–624.

22. Bird P, Ejberg B, McQueen F, et al. OMERACT rheumatoid arthritis magnetic resonance imaging studies. Exercise 5: an international multicenter reliability study using computerized erosion volume measurements. *J Rheumatol* 2003;30:1380–1384.

23. Goldbach-Mansky R, Woodburn J, Yao L, et al. Magnetic resonance imaging in the evaluation of bone damage in rheumatoid arthritis: a more precise image or just a more expensive one? *Arthritis Rheum* 2003;48:585–589.

24. Bedair H, Murphy M, Fleming D, et al. A comparison of MRI and CT in detecting carpal bone erosions in early rheumatoid arthritis. *Arthritis Rheum* 2001;45:S222.

25. Perry D, McQueen FM, Stewart N, et al. Detection of erosions in the rheumatoid hand; a comparative study of CT versus MR scanning. *Ann Rheum Dis* 2004; 63 (Suppl 1):OP0081.

26. McQueen FM, Stewart N, Crabbe J, et al. Magnetic resonance imaging of the wrist in early rheumatoid arthritis reveals a high prevalence of erosions at four months after symptom-onset. *Ann Rheum Dis* 1998;57:350–356.

27. Bird P, Kirkham B, Portek I. Documenting damage progression in a two-year longitudinal study of rheumatoid arthritis patients with established disease (the DAMAGE study cohort): Is there an advantage in the use of magnetic resonance imaging as compared with plain radiography? *Arthritis Rheum* 2004;50:1383–1389.

28. Østergaard M, Hansen M, Stoltenberg M, et al. New radiographic bone erosions in the wrists of patients with rheumatoid arthritis are detectable with magnetic resonance imaging a median of two years earlier. *Arthritis Rheum* 2003;48:2128–2131.

29. Ejbjerg B, Narvestad E, Østergaard M. X-ray requires an MRI-estimated bone volume loss of 20-30% to allow certain detection of bone erosions in rheumatoid arthritis metacarpophalangeal joints. *Ann Rheum Dis* 2003;62:163–164.

30. Wakefield R, Gibbon W, Conaghan P, et al. The value of sonography in the detection of bone erosions in patients with rheumatoid arthritis; comparison with conventional radiography. *Arthritis Rheum* 2000;43:2762–2770.

31. Boutry N, Larde A, Lapegue F. Magnetic resonance imaging appearance of the hands and feet in patients with early rheumatoid arthritis. *J Rheumatol* 2003;30:671–679.

32. Østergaard M, Nielsen H, Narvestad E, et al. Radiographic progression during anakinra treatment of rheumatoid arthritis patients is predicted by MRI, but not by conventional markers of disease activity. *Ann Rheum Dis* 2003;62:332.

33. Broderick LS, Turner DA, Renfrew DL, et al. Severity of articular cartilage abnormality in patients with osteoarthritis: evaluation of fast spin-echo MR vs arthroscopy. *Am J Roentgenol* 1994;162:99–103.

# Quality of Life and Its Measurement in Osteoporosis

**Deborah Gold**

Tremendous progress has been made in our understanding and managing the physiologic consequences of osteoporosis in terms of both bone loss and fractures. However, the impact of osteoporosis on patients' quality of life has not yet been fully defined. Quality of life effects of other chronic diseases are viewed as critical to the patients who suffer from them. Multiple articles have been published that focus specifically on how chronic obstructive pulmonary disease (1), chronic pain from stroke (2), diabetes (3), osteoarthritis (4), and rheumatoid arthritis (5) reduce quality of life. This chapter focuses on the psychological and social consequences of osteoporosis and discusses measurement tools that are used to quantify health-related quality of life (HRQOL) in this disorder.

In osteoporosis, we must identify critical components of quality of life that are worsened by bone loss and fractures. Additionally, the worsening of the change in the components of HRQOL should be measured in valid and reproducible ways. Finally, we must design interventions to improve quality of life for patients with osteoporosis.

## PSYCHOLOGICAL IMPACT OF OSTEOPOROSIS

Osteoporosis has a number of important implications that far exceed its physical impact. The consequences of osteoporosis also include financial, psychological, and social effects, which significantly affect the individual as well as the family and community.

Two of the most commonly reported psychological problems associated with osteoporosis are anxiety and depression. Before a symptomatic fracture occurs, patients with osteoporosis are less likely to experience psychological problems from the disease. After a fracture occurs, pain, limited mobility, and feelings of helplessness and hopelessness develop. At that point, few patients have developed coping skills that they can utilize. An initial symptomatic fracture caused by osteoporosis then often generates anxiety. Especially prone to anxiety are women who believe that osteoporosis and fractures are inevitable consequences of aging. Osteoporosis may be viewed as if their lives were "coming to an end." Significant levels of anxiety have been demonstrated in community-dwelling, postmenopausal women recently diagnosed with symptomatic vertebral fracture (6).

Fear of falling, especially for the older woman who may have significant balance challenges, is another concern for many women with osteoporosis. Salkeld, et al. (7) found that fear of hip fracture–related issues was considerable. Nearly all the women questioned would have traded off most of their remaining life expectancy to avoid nursing home placement. Eighty percent of the participants reported that they would rather be dead than have to be placed in a nursing home after a hip fracture. The fear of having a hip fracture and becoming dependent was not a tenable option for these patients.

The second emotional reaction commonly associated with osteoporosis and low bone density is depression. It has been well established that there is an increased prevalence of depression among older patients with chronic illness (8). It should not be surprising that there seems to be a strong relationship between depressive symptoms and osteoporosis. A study by Coelho, et al. (9) measured bone mineral density (BMD) and indices of psychosocial well being in 102 community-dwelling, Portuguese post-menopausal women. Multivariate analyses revealed that women with low BMD and osteoporosis had significantly higher scores on the Beck Depression Inventory than did those women without osteoporosis, even when controlling for other explanatory factors.

## Managing Osteoporosis-Related Anxiety and Depression

Gold and colleagues (10) showed that an osteoporosis education program that included exercise and coping skills reduced anxiety levels of participants compared with a control group that did not receive the intervention. The long-term management of the anxiety associated with osteoporosis should include at least three components: education, empowerment, and exercise, which have been demonstrated to reduce anxiety in this disorder (10). Physical activity seems to play an important role in managing mild to moderate depression as well. Specifically, strength training or aerobic exercise is associated with the significant reduction of depressive symptoms.

One study examined the effects of a multidisciplinary osteoporosis intervention on depression and anxiety (11). Participants included 103 older adults with osteoporosis. Approximately half received instruction in exercise, nutrition, and education in an osteoporosis clinic. No direct psychotherapy or use of psychotherapeutic medications was administered. The other half received usual care in the form of a consultation with an endocrinologist. The two groups did not differ in baseline measurements of depression or anxiety or in the degree of severity of osteoporosis. After participation in the 4-day clinic program, the treatment group showed a significant reduction in degree of depression and anxiety. The control group did not change in these areas. Because this intervention was multidisciplinary, it was impossible to separate out the effects of any specific component such as education, nutrition, or exercise. The results suggest that this type of multidisciplinary intervention successfully decreases depression and anxiety—two primary mental health outcomes of osteoporosis.

## SOCIAL IMPACT OF OSTEOPOROSIS

Patients with osteoporosis can have negative experiences in their interactions with other persons or society. Osteoporosis has two particular social consequences: social role loss and social isolation (12).

Individuals define themselves by the social roles they have, that is, by the positions or functions they have in social units. Each social role is defined by its specific responsibilities and rewards. Our important social roles in modern society typically occur in the family or in the workplace. Women with severe osteoporosis and multiple fractures find it difficult to continue with their social roles. Many of their social roles within their families and at the workplace require physical effort that puts their fragile skeletons at increased risk for fracture.

Social isolation can occur at the same time as or as a result of social role loss. Social interactions throughout life require a certain degree of reciprocity between members of a relationship. This balance or shared effort is that which keeps relationships positive. Osteoporosis often limits the degree to which such reciprocity is possible. Without reciprocity, nonfamilial relationships eventually diminish.

## RESEARCH ON QUALITY OF LIFE AND OSTEOPOROSIS

Peer-reviewed journal articles that included some mention of quality of life associated with osteoporosis did not appear in the medical literature until the late 1980s and early 1990s (13). Many were written in public health, nursing, and geriatric journals. However, searching medical databases for osteoporosis and quality of life captured few of these articles. Instead, these articles can only be found by searching for osteoporosis and coping, social support, or community services.

An attempt was made to identify the coping strategies used by women with osteoporosis and vertebral fractures. This approach was relatively short-lived, perhaps because no pattern of coping had been established as the most effective for osteoporosis. The studies were not randomized clinical trials but evaluated the consequences of osteoporosis on the lives of patients with fragility fractures.

A seminal 1993 editorial in *Calcified Tissue International* highlighted the importance of quality of life as an outcome in osteoporosis clinical trials (14). The ability to conduct such measurement was dependent on the availability of valid and reliable measurement tools. In this editorial, the authors noted that each fracture and each fracture experience is unique and results in a trajectory of social, emotional, and physical challenges based on many factors including family and community support, religious faith, and successful pharmaceutical intervention. Although several generic scales measured global quality of life (e.g., short form (SF)-36, Sickness Impact Profile), none was able to measure the unique constellation of challenges presented by this disease. The 1990s, therefore, became the decade of the development of osteoporosis-specific quality-of-life scales.

## OSTEOPOROSIS-SPECIFIC QUALITY OF LIFE SCALES

The literature on osteoporosis and quality of life includes multiple instruments and their variations. Most of these are self-administered tools. Only a few, such as the

Osteoporosis Assessment Questionnaire (OPAQ) and the Quality of Life Questionnaire of the European Foundation for Osteoporosis (QUALEFFO) have thus far been utilized in large-scale clinical trials (15–17).

The Multiple Outcomes of Raloxifene Endpoints (MORE) study (18) was the first large prospective international clinical trial in which HRQOL data were collected on a large sample of postmenopausal women by use of a validated osteoporosis-targeted questionnaire. In MORE, both the OPAQ and QUALEFFO were utilized. The QUALEFFO includes questions in the domains of pain, physical function, social function, general health perception, and mental function. At baseline, the QUALEFFO was able to discriminate between patients with and without prevalent vertebral fracture and was also sensitive to differences between groups of patients with single versus multiple fractures. The QUALEFFO was also able to detect longitudinal changes in osteoporosis-related quality of life in this trial (19).

The OPAQ was developed by Silverman and Mason and was based on the Arthritis Impact Measurement Scales Questionnaire 2 (4). The OPAQ can be scored by domain or by the four composite dimensions (physical function, symptoms, emotional status, and social interaction) determined through previous factor analysis (20). The physical function dimension includes six domains: walking/bending, standing/sitting, dressing/reaching, household/self-care, transfers, and usual work. The symptoms dimension includes two domains: back pain and fatigue. The emotional status dimension includes four domains: fear of falling, level of tension, body image, and independence. The social interaction dimension includes two domains: social activity and support of family and friends. In MORE, women with a prevalent vertebral fracture at baseline had significantly lower OPAQ scores on physical function, emotional status, clinical symptoms, and overall HRQOL compared with women without a prevalent fracture. HRQOL scores became lower with each subsequent fracture. Incident vertebral fractures significantly decreased OPAQ scores on physical function, emotional status, clinical symptoms, and overall HRQOL.

Similar results were demonstrated in a large study of teriparatide in postmenopausal women with osteoporosis (21). Compared to women without vertebral or nonvertebral incident fractures, women who had fractures reported significant declines in physical functioning, emotional status, and symptoms using the OPAQ (all $p < 0.05$).

## CONCLUSIONS

The morbidity resulting from osteoporotic fractures involves emotional, psychological, and social change as well as physical damage. Only by proper assessment and quantification of the total effects of osteoporosis on quality of life can decisions be made on the categories and aggressiveness of treatment. In most cases, a multidisciplinary approach involving physical therapy, nutrition counseling, and psychosocial support should be considered.

## REFERENCES

1. van Manen JG, Bindels PJ, Dekker FW, et al. The influence of COPD on health-related quality of life independent of the influence of comorbidity. *J Clin Epidemiol* 2003;56(12):1177–1184.
2. Kong KH, Woon VC, Yang SY. Prevalence of chronic pain and its impact on health-related quality of life in stroke survivors. *Arch Phys Med Rehabil* 2004;85(1):35–40.
3. Snoek F, Visser A. Improving quality of life in diabetes: how effective is education? *Patient Educ Couns* 2003;51(1):1–3.
4. Meenan RF, Mason JH, Anderson JJ, et al. AIMS 2—the content and properties of a revised and expanded Arthritis Impact Measurement Scales health-status questionnaire. *Arthritis Rheum* 1992;35(1):1–10.
5. Nichol MB, Harada AS. Measuring the effects of medication use on health-related quality of life in patients with rheumatoid arthritis. A review. *Pharmacoeconomics* 1999;16:433–448.
6. Gold DT, Bales CW, Lyles KW, et al. Treatment of osteoporosis: the psychological impact of a medical education program on older patients. *J Am Geriatr Soc* 1989;37:417–422.
7. Salkeld G, Cameron ID, Cumming RG, et al. Quality of life related to fear of falling and hip fracture in older women: a time trade off study. *BMJ* 2000;320(7231):341–346.
8. Smith Barusch A, Rogers A, Abu-Bader SH. Depressive symptoms in the frail elderly: physical and psychosocial correlates. *Int J Aging Hum Dev* 1999;49:107–125.
9. Coelho R, Silva C, Maia A, et al. Bone mineral density and depression: a community study in women. *J Psychosom Res* 1999;46(1):29–35.
10. Gold DT. Osteoporosis and quality of life psychosocial outcomes and interventions for individual patients. *Clin Geriatr Med* 2003;19(2):271–280.
11. Gold DT, Stegmaier K, Bales CW, et al. Psychosocial functioning and osteoporosis in late life: results of a multidisciplinary intervention. *J Womens Health* 1993;2:149–154.
12. Purser JL, Pieper CF, Branch LG, et al. Spinal deformity and mobility self-confidence among women with osteoporosis and vertebral fractures. *Aging (Milano)* 1999;11(4):235–245.
13. Bowen OR. Osteoporosis: prevention and the quality of life for older Americans. *Public Health Rep* 1989;104[Suppl]:11–13.
14. Greendale GA, Silverman SL, Hays RD, et al. Health-related quality of life in osteoporosis clinical trials. The Osteoporosis Quality of Life Study Group. *Calcif Tiss Int* 1993;53(2):75–77.
15. Silverman SL, Minshall ME, Shen W, et al. The relationship of health-related quality of life to prevalent and incident vertebral fractures in postmenopausal women with osteoporosis results from the multiple outcomes of raloxifene evaluation study. *Arthritis Rheum* 2001;44: 2611–2619.
16. Oglesby AK, Minshall ME, Shen W, et al. The impact of incident vertebral and non-vertebral fragility fractures on health-related quality of life in established postmenopausal osteoporosis: results from the teriparatide randomized, placebo-controlled trial in postmenopausal women. *J Rheumatol* 2003;30:1579–1583.
17. Lips P, Agnusdei D, Caulin F, et al. The development of a European questionnaire for quality of life in patients with vertebral osteoporosis. *Scand J Rheumatol* 1996;103:84–88.
18. Ettinger B, Black DM, Mitlak BH, et al. Reduction of vertebral risk in postmenopausal women with osteoporosis treated with raloxifene. Results from a 3-year randomized clinical trial. *JAMA* 1999; 282:637–645.
19. Oleksik AM, Ewing SK, Duong T, et al. Three years of health related quality of life assessment in postmenopausal women with osteoporosis: impact of incident vertebral fractures, age and severe adverse events. *J Bone Miner Res* 2000;15:1384–1392.
20. Randell AG, Bhalerao N, Nguyen TV, et al. Quality of life in osteoporosis: reliability, consistency and validity of the Osteoporosis Assessment Questionnaire. *J Rheumatol* 1998;25:1171–1179.
21. Neer RM, Arnaud CD, Zanchetta JR, et al. Effect of parathyroid hormone (1–34) on fractures and bone mineral density in postmenopausal women with osteoporosis. *N Engl J Med* 2001;344: 1434–1441.

# Bone Loss and Fragility in the Rheumatic Diseases

# Bone Loss and Fractures in Rheumatoid Arthritis

*Shreyasee Amin*

Rheumatoid arthritis has been reported to adversely affect bone in at least three different ways. It leads to erosion of bone at the joint margins of inflamed joints. There is loss of bone density also at the level of inflamed joints (periarticular osteopenia). Lastly, distant from the involved joints, a more generalized bone loss has been observed. This last problem is of particular concern because of the potential for fragility fractures. The pathophysiologic mechanism for the generalized bone loss observed in rheumatoid arthritis is complex and likely to be multifactorial. Although still a source of some debate, the key factors considered to be involved in this loss of bone density are (a) inflammation, related to active disease; (b) reduced physical function, or mobility; and (c) medication use, particularly glucocorticoids. The relative contribution of these factors to changes in bone density in rheumatoid arthritis remains controversial and are discussed. The scope of the problem of bone loss and fractures in those with rheumatoid arthritis is also reviewed.

## BONE LOSS IN RHEUMATOID ARTHRITIS

Most cross-sectional studies, although not all, have reported that bone density among those with rheumatoid arthritis is lower than healthy controls, or reference populations, at the forearm (1–5), hip (1, 6–12) and spine (1, 6–10, 13–15). The majority of these studies, however, have examined primarily women. In two studies involving a large number of men, one reported lower Z-scores at both the hip and spine (16), while the other observed lower Z-scores for the hip, but not spine, which only achieved statistical significance in men over the age of 60 years (17).

The magnitude of difference in bone density between those with rheumatoid arthritis and healthy control populations is difficult to determine because of the heterogeneity of patients examined in studies with respect to age, gender, menopausal status, disease duration, disease severity, and glucocorticoid use. However, some sense of the difference may be appreciated from a study of 16 sets of monozygotic twins with rheumatoid arthritis (9), in which the majority (n = 14) had only one affected twin with rheumatoid arthritis, and none of whom had significant glucocorticoid use. The rheumatoid arthritis–affected twins had significant mean reductions in bone density at most sites, ranging from 4.6% at the lumbar spine to 9.7% at the femoral neck (9). Others have also suggested that the appendicular skeleton may be more affected than the axial skeleton in those with rheumatoid arthritis (18).

In a longitudinal study examining the changes in bone density among those with early rheumatoid arthritis not treated with glucocorticoids, no differences in bone density changes of the lumbar spine or femoral neck were seen at 12 months when compared with volunteer controls (14). Another longitudinal study demonstrated significantly greater loss at the lumbar spine and femoral neck for women with rheumatoid arthritis when compared with controls who were matched for age and menopausal status (19). Again, these differing results may be related to differences in study populations, especially with respect to disease duration, severity, and glucocorticoid use.

## FRACTURES IN RHEUMATOID ARTHRITIS

There is a paucity of studies examining the risk for fractures among patients with rheumatoid arthritis, and most have examined women, particularly postmenopausal women. And yet, the most clinically important consequence of osteoporosis is a fracture, as it contributes to significant morbidity and mortality among patients, as well as increased health care costs (20).

Michel, et al. (21) studied 395 men and women with rheumatoid arthritis from the American Rheumatism Association Medical Information System (ARAMIS) database who were followed for an average of 6.7 years (22). There were 52 (13%) who sustained at least one fracture, 43 of 304 (14%) women and 9 of 91 (10%) men (21). The most frequent fractures involved the spine (n = 13), foot or ankle (n = 9), and ribs (n = 7) (21). Among those without a diagnosis of known osteoporosis, prednisone use of more than 5 mg/day was most predictive of time to fracture (21).

Hooyman, et al. (23) examined 388 women who had been diagnosed with rheumatoid arthritis over a 25-year period in Rochester, MN and who were subsequently followed for 4,902 person-years. There were 29 patients with proximal femur fractures, 23 with distal forearm, 12 with pelvic, and 12 with proximal forearm fractures (23). The relative risk (RR) was greatest for pelvic fractures [RR = 2.56, 95% confidence interval (CI): 1.32, 4.47] and for proximal femur fractures [RR = 1.51, 95% confidence interval (95% CI): 1.01, 2.17] (23). The relative risks for fracture at the other sites were also increased but did not reach statistical significance. There were 42 women who experienced one or more vertebral fracture, but the relative risk could not be calculated because of the absence of incidence rates in the study population necessary to determine the expected number (23).

Cooper, et al. (24) performed a population-based, case-control study from the United Kingdom (UK), examining 300 men and women over the age of 50 (60 men and 240 women), who were admitted to an orthopaedic unit for proximal femur fracture, and comparing them with 600 age- and sex-matched community controls. There were 14 people (13 women, 1 man) among the cases and 14 among the controls (12 women, 2 men) identified as having rheumatoid arthritis (24). The unadjusted risk (odds ratio, OR) of hip fracture for those with rheumatoid arthritis was 2.1 (95% CI: 1.0, 4.7) (24), and the risk did not change substantially following adjustment for lifestyle factors such as smoking and alcohol intake. However, when functional impairment was included in the model, the excess risk attributable to rheumatoid arthritis was attenuated (OR = 1.3, 95% CI: 0.5, 3.5) (24).

In a cross-sectional cohort study of 5,566 women and 2,187 men, 50 years of age or older, in the population-based Canadian Multicentre Osteoporosis Study (CANMOS), there was no association noted between the presence of rheumatoid arthritis and prevalent vertebral deformity (25). The association with other prevalent fractures was not reported.

In a study from the UK, Spector, et al. (26) studied radiographic vertebral deformity in 149 postmenopausal women with rheumatoid arthritis (age 45–65) and 713 postmenopausal women (age 45–65) from the general population as controls. There were 18 (12.1%) with vertebral fracture among the rheumatoid arthritis group and 44 (2.1%) among controls with an OR of 2.1 (95% CI: 1.2, 3.7) (26). Also from the UK, Peel, et al. (27) studied the prevalence of vertebral deformities in 76 postmenopausal women (ages 50–79 years) with rheumatoid arthritis who had received glucocorticoids for at least 1 month and compared them with 347 population-based, age-matched female controls (ages 50–79 years). Women with rheumatoid arthritis had a prevalence of vertebral deformity of 27.6% compared with 5.8% in the control group. The risk for vertebral deformity among steroid-treated rheumatoid arthritis women was high, with an OR of 6.2 (95% CI: 3.2, 12.3) (27). In a study from Norway, 249 women with rheumatoid arthritis, aged 50 and over, were compared with 249 age- and sex-matched population based controls (28, 29). There were 55 patients (22.1%) among the rheumatoid arthritis group with a vertebral deformity, compared with 38 patients (15.3%) in the control group (OR = 1.74, 95% CI: 1.02, 3.04) (29). The presence of a vertebral deformity was independently associated with the diagnosis of rheumatoid arthritis, bone density, and long-term steroid use (29). There were 53 patients (21.3%) who self-reported a non-vertebral fracture since being diagnosed with rheumatoid arthritis, compared with 50 patients (20.1%) in the control group (28). However, self-reported hip fractures did appear to be higher among those with rheumatoid arthritis (10 vs. 2, OR = 9.0, 95% CI: 1.2, 394.5) (28).

The overall findings do suggest that those with rheumatoid arthritis, particularly women, may be at increased risk for fractures at both axial and appendicular sites. The risk for fractures in men with rheumatoid arthritis has not been well established. Glucocorticoid use and functional impairment may be contributing factors to this increased risk for fractures.

## PATHOGENESIS OF GENERALIZED BONE LOSS AND FRACTURES IN RHEUMATOID ARTHRITIS

The pathophysiological mechanism for the increased risk of generalized osteoporosis and fractures in rheumatoid arthritis patients is complex and felt to be multifactorial. In rheumatoid arthritis, the unique factors that may adversely affect bone metabolism are considered to be (a) inflammation related to active disease; (b) disability with reduced physical function and mobility, and (c) medications, particularly glucocorticoids.

## Disease Activity

Shenstone, et al. (14) reported that among nonsteroid-treated patients with rheumatoid arthritis, those with a disease duration of less than 6 months had the greatest loss in femoral neck bone density over 12 months. Gough, et al. (19) demonstrated that patients with active disease, as measured by mean c-reactive protein (CRP) levels, had significantly greater bone density losses at the hip and spine compared to patients with inactive disease. These studies suggest that the inflammatory process, which is known to contribute to joint damage and bony erosions, may also play a direct role in the pathogenesis of generalized osteoporosis in rheumatoid arthritis.

There is now evidence that the immune system affects bone metabolism (30,31). Osteoclast precursors and mature osteoclasts express a receptor called receptor activator for NF-κB (RANK) (30). Osteoblastic cells induce osteoclastic differentiation and resorptive activity through the expression of a surface membrane protein called osteoprotegrin ligand (OPGL), also called RANKL, which binds to RANK (30). Pro-inflammatory cytokines in rheumatoid arthritis, including tumor necrosis factor-α (TNF-α), interleukin (IL)-I and IL-6, among others, can stimulate bone resorption via an up-regulation of RANKL on fibroblasts and activated T cells (30). Studies have shown that synovial fibroblasts and activated T cells express RANKL and can induce osteoclastogenesis even in the absence of traditional bone resorptive signals (30,31). Osteoprotegrin (OPG) is a soluble decoy receptor for RANKL and regulates bone resorption by blocking RANK to RANKL binding and thereby inhibits osteoclastogenesis. In a mice transgenic model for inflammatory destructive arthritis, blocking RANKL with OPG treatment led to decreased bone and cartilage destruction with no effect on inflammation (32). These studies demonstrate the direct effect of the immune system on bone at the level of inflamed joints. In inflammatory conditions, RANKL is released from cell surfaces by metalloproteases and may be a mechanism for the generalized osteoporosis seen (33).

## Physical Function

Immobility and decreased physical activity are important predictors of bone loss and fractures (34). Among patients with rheumatoid arthritis, pain from active inflammation and damaged joints can lead to decreased physical function, which may play a role in the generalized bone loss seen in rheumatoid arthritis. Several studies have reported an association between low levels of physical activity and low bone density among patients with rheumatoid arthritis (3, 6, 11, 16, 18, 35). In a study of 925 women with rheumatoid arthritis, higher Health Assessment Questionnaire (HAQ) scores were associated with an increased risk not only for osteoporosis (OR = 1.3, 95% CI: 1.07, 1.7) but also for vertebral fractures (OR = 1.7, 95% CI: 1.08, 2.09) (36). Others have also reported that impaired physical function is associated with increased fractures among those with rheumatoid arthritis (23,24,37). In a randomized trial of dynamic strength training in 70 rheumatoid arthritis patients, where there was significant improvement in muscle strength and HAQ scores in the treatment group, the bone density in the femoral neck and spine increased by 0.51 ± 1.64% (mean ± SD) and by 1.17 ± 5.34%, respectively, in the strength-training group, but decreased by 0.70 ± 2.25% and 0.91 ± 4.07%, respectively, in the control group (38). However the bone density changes in the treatment group did not reach statistical significance when compared with the control group (38). The power to detect a significant difference may have been limited. In contrast, when 309 patients with rheumatoid arthritis were assigned to a high-intensity, weight-bearing program for 2 years versus usual care physical therapy, the mean rate of decrease in hip bone density was smaller in the high-intensity group and independently associated with changes in muscle strength and aerobic fitness (39).

## Medications

### Glucocorticoid Medications

Glucocorticoid use is a well-recognized risk factor for osteoporosis and fragility fractures. There is controversy, however, in how much glucocorticoid use contributes to bone loss and fractures in rheumatoid arthritis patients given the fact that they can decrease inflammation and thereby serve to improve physical function, both of which may be beneficial to bones. There have been conflicting reports from cross-sectional and longitudinal studies of rheumatoid arthritis patients with some studies finding no difference in bone density or bone loss between glucocorticoid users and nonusers (15,40–42). Others have reported significantly lower bone density or loss of bone density attributable to glucocorticoid use (18,36,43–45). Again, interpretation of these conflicting results is challenging because patients examined in these studies differ with respect to age, gender, menopausal status, disease duration, and activity, as well as cumulative doses of glucocorticoids used. Still, there are several studies that have suggested that there is an increased risk for fractures, particularly vertebral fractures, among rheumatoid arthritis patients who are glucocorticoid users (29,46–50). However, the reported negative effects of glucocorticoids on bone density or fractures from such studies could also be attributable to confounding by indication, with patients using prescribed glucocorticoids having had more severe disease at onset.

There have been a few randomized, controlled trials with rheumatoid arthritis patients receiving glucocorticoid medication in one treatment arm but not in the other. In 40 rheumatoid arthritis patients on intramuscular gold randomized to prednisone or placebo, trabecular, but not cortical bone density, as measured by quantitative computed tomography (QCT), decreased significantly in the prednisone treated group (51). Bone density did appear to improve with discontinuation of prednisone (51). However, there has been some question as to whether the changes seen in bone density could be, in part, an artifact and related more to changes in marrow fat given the technique used to measure bone density. In another study with 56 rheumatoid arthritis patients randomized to either prednisone or chloroquine, there was a nonsignificant loss of bone density at the hip and spine in the prednisone group (52). In the COBRA study (COmbinatietherapie Bij Reumatoide Artritis), in which 155 rheumatoid arthritis patients were randomized to sulfasalazine alone or to combination of sulfasalazine, methotrexate, and prednisone, there was a slight but not statistically significant greater loss of bone density at the lumbar spine, but not at the hip, at 28 weeks in the combination treatment group (53). Of note, prednisone was discontinued per protocol at 28 weeks, while methotrexate was discontinued at 40 weeks. More recently, van Everdingen, et al. (54) randomized 81 patients with early rheumatoid arthritis to prednisone versus placebo for at least 6 months before sulfasalazine could be added as rescue therapy. There was less radiographic progression in the prednisone-treated group compared to placebo (54). Although there was little difference in bone-density measures between the two groups, there was a nonsignificant increased risk of lumbar vertebral fractures in the prednisone-treated group (54,55). Glucocorticoid medications may affect bone quality and strength not measurable by conventional bone densitometry. Although the power in these studies may have been limited in detecting significant differences between the groups, overall there appeared to be a trend towards lower bone density and possibly increased fractures in those treated with prednisone.

Fortunately, effective therapies are available to prevent and treat glucocorticoid-induced osteoporosis (56,57). In a 2-year longitudinal study of 366 men and women with rheumatoid arthritis, half of whom were current users of glucocorticoid medication, use of antiresorptive agents was associated with decreased risk for bone loss at the hip (OR = 0.43, 95% CI: 0.20, 0.89) and lumbar spine (OR = 0.51, 95% CI: 0.22, 1.18) (58).

### Methotrexate

Methotrexate osteopathy is a recognized complication of high-dose methotrexate used in oncology and is characterized by bone pain, low bone density, and fractures (59). The net effect on bone metabolism of long-term, low-dose methotrexate, as used in rheumatoid arthritis, has been a source of debate. *In vitro* studies suggest that low-dose methotrexate can decrease osteoblast proliferation, although not differentiation (60), as well as decrease osteoblast function (61). On the other hand, in a study of rats with adjuvant-induced arthritis, methotrexate suppressed the arthritis and restored osteogenic activity to normal (62). In human

studies, there are case reports of low-dose methotrexate resulting in stress fractures (63,64). However, both cross-sectional (65,66) and prospective, longitudinal studies (67,68) in rheumatoid arthritis patients have failed to demonstrate lower bone density in methotrexate users compared with nonusers. However, among patients using prednisone doses of 5 mg or more per day, methotrexate users had significantly lower bone density than nonusers (67). In an 18-month, prospective study of 46 premenopausal women with nonsteroid-treated rheumatoid arthritis, randomized to either low-dose methotrexate (7.5 mg per week) or sulfasalazine (2 g per day), there were no significant differences seen in bone density of the lumbar spine or femoral neck between groups (69). In four premenopausal women with rheumatoid arthritis, not on glucocorticoid medications and treated with methotrexate for 1 year, bone histomorphometry results showed no significant differences overall between pre- and posttreatment iliac crest biopsies (70). These studies would suggest that low-dose methotrexate may have no net adverse effects on bone density over short-term follow-up. The effect of methotrexate in combination with glucocorticoid medications on bone density remains unclear.

## SUMMARY

Bone loss and fractures occur with increased frequency in patients with rheumatoid arthritis. The contribution of disease activity, immobility, and medication is difficult to disentangle, but all likely play contributing roles. Controlling disease is essential to decrease inflammation and damage to joints but may also help prevent the generalized loss of bone that can occur. The use of glucocorticoid medications to control disease remains a source of debate, but if used, adjuvant therapy for the prevention and treatment of glucocorticoid-induced osteoporosis is necessary.

## REFERENCES

1. Lane NE, Pressman AR, Star VL, et al. Rheumatoid arthritis and bone mineral density in elderly women. The Study of Osteoporotic Fractures Research Group. *J Bone Miner Res* 1995;10 (2):257–263.
2. Iwamoto J, Takeda T, Ichimura S. Forearm bone mineral density in postmenopausal women with rheumatoid arthritis. *Calcif Tissue Intl* 2002;70(1):1–8.
3. Hansen M, Florescu A, Stoltenberg M, et al. Bone loss in rheumatoid arthritis. Influence of disease activity, duration of the disease, functional capacity, and corticosteroid treatment. *Scand J Rheumatol* 1996;25(6):367–376.
4. Toyoda T, Inokuchi S, Saito S, et al. Bone loss of the radius in rheumatoid arthritis. Comparison between 34 patients and 40 controls. *Acta Orthop Scand* 1996;67(3):269–273.
5. Perez-Edo L, Diez-Perez A, Marinoso L, et al. Bone metabolism and histomorphometric changes in rheumatoid arthritis. *Scand J Rheumatol* 2002;31(5):285–290.
6. Sambrook PN, Eisman JA, Champion GD, et al. Determinants of axial bone loss in rheumatoid arthritis. *Arthritis Rheum* 1987;30(7): 721–728.

7. Kroger H, Honkanen R, Saarikoski S, et al. Decreased axial bone mineral density in perimenopausal women with rheumatoid arthritis—a population based study. *Ann Rheum Dis* 1994;53(1): 18–23.

8. Celiker R, Gokce-Kutsal Y, Cindas A, et al. Osteoporosis in rheumatoid arthritis: effect of disease activity. *Clin Rheumatol* 1995;14(4):429–433.

9. Sambrook PN, Spector TD, Seeman E, et al. Osteoporosis in rheumatoid arthritis. A monozygotic co-twin control study. *Arthritis Rheum* 1995;38(6):806–809.

10. Cortet B, Flipo RM, Blanckaert F, et al. Evaluation of bone mineral density in patients with rheumatoid arthritis. Influence of disease activity and glucocorticoid therapy. *Rev Rhum (Engl Ed)* 1997;64(7-9):451–458.

11. Haugeberg G, Uhlig T, Falch JA, et al. Bone mineral density and frequency of osteoporosis in female patients with rheumatoid arthritis: results from 394 patients in the Oslo County Rheumatoid Arthritis register. *Arthritis Rheum* 2000;43(3):522–530.

12. Gilboe IM, Kvien TK, Haugeberg G, et al. Bone mineral density in systemic lupus erythematosus: comparison with rheumatoid arthritis and healthy controls. *Ann Rheum Dis* 2000;59(2):110–115.

13. Magaro M, Tricerri A, Piane D, et al. Generalized osteoporosis in non-steroid treated rheumatoid arthritis. *Rheumatol Int* 1991;11(2):73–76.

14. Shenstone BD, Mahmoud A, Woodward R, et al. Longitudinal bone mineral density changes in early rheumatoid arthritis. *Br J Rheumatol* 1994;33(6):541–545.

15. Martin JC, Munro R, Campbell MK, et al. Effects of disease and corticosteroids on appendicular bone mass in postmenopausal women with rheumatoid arthritis: comparison with axial measurements. *Br J Rheumatol* 1997;36(1):43–49.

16. Laan RF, Buijs WC, Verbeek AL, et al. Bone mineral density in patients with recent onset rheumatoid arthritis: influence of disease activity and functional capacity. *Ann Rheum Dis* 1993;52(1):21–26.

17. Haugeberg G, Uhlig T, Falch JA, et al. Reduced bone mineral density in male rheumatoid arthritis patients: frequencies and associations with demographic and disease variables in ninety-four patients in the Oslo County Rheumatoid Arthritis Register. *Arthritis Rheum* 2000;43(12):2776–2784.

18. Hall GM, Spector TD, Griffin AJ, et al. The effect of rheumatoid arthritis and steroid therapy on bone density in postmenopausal women. *Arthritis Rheum* 1993;36(11):1510–1516.

19. Gough AK, Lilley J, Eyre S, et al. Generalised bone loss in patients with early rheumatoid arthritis. *Lancet* 1994;344(8914):23–27.

20. Center JR, Nguyen TV, Schneider D, et al. Mortality after all major types of osteoporotic fracture in men and women: an observational study. *Lancet* 1999;353(9156):878–882.

21. Michel BA, Bloch DA, Fries JF. Predictors of fractures in early rheumatoid arthritis. *J Rheumatol* 1991;18(6):804–808.

22. Fries JF, McShane DJ. ARAMIS (the American Rheumatism Association Medical Information System). A prototypical national chronic-disease data bank. *West J Med* 1986;145(6):798–804.

23. Hooyman JR, Melton LJ 3rd, Nelson AM, et al. Fractures after rheumatoid arthritis. A population-based study. *Arthritis Rheum* 1984;27(12):1353–1361.

24. Cooper C, Coupland C, Mitchell M. Rheumatoid arthritis, corticosteroid therapy and hip fracture. *Ann Rheum Dis* 1995;54(1):49–52.

25. Hanley DA, Brown JP, Tenenhouse A, et al. Associations among disease conditions, bone mineral density, and prevalent vertebral deformities in men and women 50 years of age and older: cross-sectional results from the Canadian Multicentre Osteoporosis Study. *J Bone Miner Res* 2003;18(4):784–790.

26. Spector TD, Hall GM, McCloskey EV, et al. Risk of vertebral fracture in women with rheumatoid arthritis. *BMJ* 1993;306(6877):558.

27. Peel NF, Moore DJ, Barrington NA, et al. Risk of vertebral fracture and relationship to bone mineral density in steroid treated rheumatoid arthritis. *Ann Rheum Dis* 1995;54(10):801–806.

28. Orstavik RE, Haugeberg G, Uhlig T, et al. Self reported non-vertebral fractures in rheumatoid arthritis and population based controls: incidence and relationship with bone mineral density and clinical variables. *Ann Rheum Dis* 2004;63(2):177–182.

29. Orstavik RE, Haugeberg G, Mowinckel P, et al. Vertebral deformities in rheumatoid arthritis: a comparison with population-based controls. *Arch Intern Med* 2004;164(4):420–425.

30. Jones DH, Kong YY, Penninger JM. Role of RANKL and RANK in bone loss and arthritis. *Ann Rheum Dis* 2002;61(Suppl 2):32–39.

31. Kong YY, Feige U, Sarosi I, et al. Activated T cells regulate bone loss and joint destruction in adjuvant arthritis through osteoprotegerin ligand. *Nature* 1999;402(6759):304–309.

32. Redlich K, Hayer S, Maier A, et al. Tumor necrosis factor alpha-mediated joint destruction is inhibited by targeting osteoclasts with osteoprotegerin. *Arthritis Rheum* 2002;46(3):785–792.

33. Green MJ, Deodhar AA. Bone changes in early rheumatoid arthritis. *Best Prac Res Clin Rheumatol* 2001;15(1):105–123.

34. Smith EL, Gilligan C. Physical activity effects on bone metabolism. *Calcif Tissue Int* 1991;49[Suppl]:S50–S54.

35. Saario R, Sonninen P, Mottonen T, et al. Bone mineral density of the lumbar spine in patients with advanced rheumatoid arthritis. Influence of functional capacity and corticosteroid use. *Scand J Rheumatol* 1999;28(6):363–367.

36. Sinigaglia L, Nervetti A, Mela Q, et al. A multicenter cross sectional study on bone mineral density in rheumatoid arthritis. Italian Study Group on Bone Mass in Rheumatoid Arthritis.[comment]. *J Rheumatol* 2000;27(11):2582–2589.

37. Michel BA, Bloch DA, Wolfe F, et al. Fractures in rheumatoid arthritis: an evaluation of associated risk factors. *J Rheumatol* 1993;20(10):1666–1669.

38. Hakkinen A, Sokka T, Kotaniemi A, et al. A randomized two-year study of the effects of dynamic strength training on muscle strength, disease activity, functional capacity, and bone mineral density in early rheumatoid arthritis. *Arthritis Rheum* 2001;44(3):515–522.

39. de Jong Z, Munneke M, Lems WF, et al. Slowing of bone loss in patients with rheumatoid arthritis by long-term high-intensity exercise: results of a randomized, controlled trial. *Arthritis Rheum* 2004;50(4):1066–1076.

40. Cortet B, Guyot MH, Solau E, et al. Factors influencing bone loss in rheumatoid arthritis: a longitudinal study. *Clin Exp Rheumatol* 2000;18(6):683–690.

41. Sambrook PN, Cohen ML, Eisman JA, et al. Effects of low dose corticosteroids on bone mass in rheumatoid arthritis: a longitudinal study. *Ann Rheum Dis* 1989;48(7):535–538.

42. Shibuya K, Hagino H, Morio Y, et al. Cross-sectional and longitudinal study of osteoporosis in patients with rheumatoid arthritis. *Clin Rheumatol* 2002;21(2):150–158.

43. Aman S, Hakala M, Silvennoinen J, et al. Low incidence of osteoporosis in a two year follow-up of early community based patients with rheumatoid arthritis. *Scand J Rheumatol* 1998;27(3):188–193.

44. Buckley LM, Leib ES, Cartularo KS, et al. Effects of low dose corticosteroids on the bone mineral density of patients with rheumatoid arthritis. *J Rheumatol* 1995;22(6):1055–1059.

45. Kroot EJ, Nieuwenhuizen MG, de Waal Malefijt MC, et al. Change in bone mineral density in patients with rheumatoid arthritis during the first decade of the disease. *Arthritis Rheum* 2001;44(6):1254–1260.

46. Verstraeten A, Dequeker J. Vertebral and peripheral bone mineral content and fracture incidence in postmenopausal patients with rheumatoid arthritis: effect of low dose corticosteroids. *Ann Rheum Dis* 1986;45(10):852–857.

47. Saag KG, Koehnke R, Caldwell JR, et al. Low dose long-term corticosteroid therapy in rheumatoid arthritis: an analysis of serious adverse events. *Am J Med* 1994;96(2):115–123.

48. McDougall R, Sibley J, Haga M, et al. Outcome in patients with rheumatoid arthritis receiving prednisone compared to matched controls. *J Rheumatol* 1994;21(7):1207–1213.

49. Lems WF, Jahangier ZN, Jacobs JW, et al. Vertebral fractures in patients with rheumatoid arthritis treated with corticosteroids. *Clin Exp Rheumatol* 1995;13(3):293–297.

50. de Nijs RN, Jacobs JW, Bijlsma JW, et al. Prevalence of vertebral deformities and symptomatic vertebral fractures in corticosteroid treated patients with rheumatoid arthritis. *Rheumatology* 2001;40(12):1375–1383.

51. Laan RF, van Riel PL, van de Putte LB, et al. Low-dose prednisone induces rapid reversible axial bone loss in patients with rheumatoid

arthritis. A randomized, controlled study. *Ann Intern Med* 1993;119(10):963–968.

52. van Schaardenburg D, Valkema R, Dijkmans BA, et al. Prednisone treatment of elderly-onset rheumatoid arthritis. Disease activity and bone mass in comparison with chloroquine treatment. *Arthritis Rheum* 1995;38(3):334–342.

53. Verhoeven AC, Boers M, te Koppele JM, et al. Bone turnover, joint damage and bone mineral density in early rheumatoid arthritis treated with combination therapy including high-dose prednisolone. *Rheumatology* 2001;40(11):1231–1237.

54. van Everdingen AA, Jacobs JW, Siewertsz Van Reesema DR, et al. Low-dose prednisone therapy for patients with early active rheumatoid arthritis: clinical efficacy, disease-modifying properties, and side effects: a randomized, double-blind, placebo-controlled clinical trial. *Ann Intern Med* 2002;136(1):1–12.

55. van Everdingen AA, Siewertsz van Reesema DR, Jacobs JW, et al. Low-dose glucocorticoids in early rheumatoid arthritis: discordant effects on bone mineral density and fractures? *Clin Exp Rheumatol* 2003;21(2):155–160.

56. Amin S, Lavalley MP, Simms RW, et al. The comparative efficacy of drug therapies used for the management of corticosteroid-induced osteoporosis: a meta-regression. *J Bone Miner Res* 2002;17(8): 1512–1526.

57. Amin S, LaValley MP, Simms RW, et al. The role of vitamin D in corticosteroid-induced osteoporosis: a meta-analytic approach. *Arthritis Rheum* 1999;42(8):1740–1751.

58. Haugeberg G, Orstavik RE, Uhlig T, et al. Bone loss in patients with rheumatoid arthritis: results from a population-based cohort of 366 patients followed up for two years. *Arthritis Rheum* 2002;46(7): 1720–1728.

59. Ragab AH, Frech RS, Vietti TJ. Osteoporotic fractures secondary to methotrexate therapy of acute leukemia in remission. *Cancer* 1970; 25(3):580–585.

60. van der Veen MJ, Scheven BA, van Roy JL, et al. In vitro effects of methotrexate on human articular cartilage and bone-derived osteoblasts. *Br J Rheumatol* 1996;35(4):342–349.

61. May KP, Mercill D, McDermott MT, et al. The effect of methotrexate on mouse bone cells in culture. *Arthritis Rheum* 1996;39(3): 489–494.

62. Suzuki Y, Nakagawa M, Masuda C, et al. Short-term low dose methotrexate ameliorates abnormal bone metabolism and bone loss in adjuvant induced arthritis. *J Rheumatol* 1997;24(10):1890–1895.

63. Preston SJ, Diamond T, Scott A, et al. Methotrexate osteopathy in rheumatic disease. *Ann Rheum Dis* 1993;52(8):582–585.

64. Zonneveld IM, Bakker WK, Dijkstra PF, et al. Methotrexate osteopathy in long-term, low-dose methotrexate treatment for psoriasis and rheumatoid arthritis. *Arch Dermatol* 1996;132(2): 184–187.

65. Carbone LD, Kaeley G, McKown KM, et al. Effects of long-term administration of methotrexate on bone mineral density in rheumatoid arthritis. *Calcif Tissue Int* 1999;64(2):100–101.

66. Cranney AB, McKendry RJ, Wells GA, et al. The effect of low dose methotrexate on bone density. *J Rheumatol* 2001;28(11):2395–2399.

67. Buckley LM, Leib ES, Cartularo KS, et al. Effects of low dose methotrexate on the bone mineral density of patients |with rheumatoid arthritis. *J Rheumatol* 1997;24(8):1489–1494.

68. Mazzantini M, Di Munno O, Incerti-Vecchi L, et al. Vertebral bone mineral density changes in female rheumatoid arthritis patients treated with low-dose methotrexate. *Clin Exp Rheumatol* 2000; 18(3):327–331.

69. Tascioglu F, Oner C, Armagan O. The effect of low-dose methotrexate on bone mineral density in patients with early rheumatoid arthritis. *Rheumatol Int* 2003;23(5):231–235.

70. Minaur NJ, Kounali D, Vedi S, et al. Methotrexate in the treatment of rheumatoid arthritis. II. In vivo effects on bone mineral density. *Rheumatology* 2002;41(7):741–749.

# Bone Loss and Fractures in Systemic Lupus Erythematosus

*Chin Lee*     *Susan Manzi*     *Rosalind Ramsey-Goldman*

Osteoporosis is an important and preventable condition associated with systemic lupus erythematosus (SLE) (1). Although the incidence of SLE has increased, patient survival has improved over the last several decades (2–4). Accordingly, clinicians have placed a growing emphasis on prevention and treatment of SLE-related comorbidities, such as osteoporosis (5).

Previous cross-sectional and prospective studies offer epidemiologic evidence for reduced bone mineral density (BMD) and increased fracture risk in the SLE population. Bone loss in lupus is likely a multifactorial process, and both traditional and SLE-related risk factors for osteoporosis have been implicated. In this chapter we review the current epidemiologic information on reduced BMD, fracture data, and associated risk factors reported in the SLE population, as well as provide clinically relevant strategies to minimize bone loss and reduce fracture risk in these patients.

## EPIDEMIOLOGY

### Bone Mineral Density in SLE

According to the suggested World Health Organization classification criteria for osteoporosis, SLE patients have lower BMD than do aged-matched controls (6–10). The estimated prevalence of osteoporosis among those with SLE ranges from 4% to 23%, while osteopenia ranges from 25% to 44% (7, 10–17). In SLE patients with disease duration longer than 10 years, the prevalence of osteoporosis is reported to be 15% (18).

The frequency of osteoporosis in SLE varies across different racial groups. The prevalence of osteoporosis among white women with SLE ranges from 12% to 16%. In contrast, among Chinese women with SLE, it is estimated at only 4% to 6% (19). In comparison, the prevalence of osteoporosis in African-American women with SLE is higher than in African-American women without SLE but comparable to that in white women with SLE (20). But African-American women appear to be at greater risk for osteopenia and osteoporosis at the lumbar spine than are white women (21). Variation in the prevalence of osteoporosis among different racial groups may be partially attributable to dissimilarities in inherent calcium metabolism, severity of SLE, as well as the cumulative exposure to specific disease therapies, such as glucocorticoids (19).

The nature of bone loss in SLE is likely heterogeneous (22) involving both trabecular and cortical bone at the hip, spine, and forearm (6,8,11). Although most studies agree that SLE patients have reduced BMD, discrepancies exist with respect to the type of bone (cortical or trabecular) and site (hip, spine, or forearm) affected. Cross-sectional data suggest that BMD at the lumbar spine tends to be lower in SLE patients than in healthy controls, particularly among those with established disease, whereas hip BMD appears somewhat less affected (6–8).

In longitudinal studies, patients with established SLE experience greater bone loss at the spine (14), whereas patients with early, mild disease have no change in BMD at either the spine or hip (17). However, some longitudinal reports have shown no significant bone loss in either the spine or femoral neck in the studied SLE group as a whole, but subgroups of SLE individuals on a higher dose of glucocorticoids experience bone loss at the spine (12, 23,24).

## Fractures in SLE

Fracture data in SLE patients are very limited; however, in addition to findings of reduced BMD, a higher occurrence of fractures in women with SLE has been reported. An early study examining a cohort of SLE patients from two centers reported fractures occurring in 22 of 364 in adulthood. The most common sites of fracture included hip, femur, vertebra, and rib. Low BMD, a predictor of fracture in this study, was strongly associated with both the cumulative and highest prednisone dose used by SLE patients (25).

In a large, population-based cohort of SLE women providing data on self-reported fractures, 12.3% of 702 SLE women reported at least one fracture after being diagnosed with SLE. When compared with a historical, population-based group of women of similar age, women with SLE experienced fractures five times more frequently than expected. Moreover, nearly half of all fractures occurred in SLE women younger than 50 years old or before menopause. This finding is striking given that fractures are the leading cause of morbidity in postmenopausal women over age 55 in the general population (26). Duration of glucocorticoid use was an independent factor related to the time from lupus diagnosis to fracture occurrence (27).

A more recent study found that 9% of 242 patients with SLE experienced nontraumatic fractures from the time of disease onset. Of these individuals, 1 in 5 was osteoporotic, and 1 in 7 was osteopenic, while 1 in 22 had normal BMD at the spine and femoral neck (1). Factors associated with fractures in SLE patients appear to be older age at SLE diagnosis (1) and longer duration of glucocorticoid use (27).

## RISK FACTORS OF SLE-RELATED OSTEOPOROSIS

### Traditional Risk Factors

The traditional risk factors associated with osteoporosis in SLE are those typically associated with osteoporosis in the general population: female sex, women 65 years of age or older, white or Asian race, low body weight (below 127 pounds), a personal or maternal history of fracture, early menopause, and life-style factors, including smoking, a diet low in calcium and vitamin D, and excessive alcohol consumption. Other traditional risk factors include specific medications, such as long-term use of thyroid hormone, and factors increasing the likelihood for falls (28,29)

### SLE-Related Risk Factors

In addition to the traditional risk factors, specific SLE-related risk factors have been identified or suspected to be

associated with lower BMD and increased risk for osteoporosis and fractures among those with SLE. These risk factors may be intrinsic to SLE or may be related to disease treatment. Epidemiologic data, biochemical bone markers, and histomorphometric bone data from murine models point to a relationship between SLE activity and lower BMD; however, the specific pathogenesis of osteoporosis as a result of SLE per se has yet to be elucidated (10,30). In SLE, increased inflammatory mediators and cytokines, such as interleukin (IL)-6, IL-1, tumor necrosis factor (TNF)-α, and receptor activator of NF-κB ligand (RANKL), and reduced osteoprote (OPC) may create a milieu suitable for promoting accelerated bone remodeling and reducing BMD (31). Data supporting SLE per se as a risk factor for bone loss come from studies demonstrating lower BMD in SLE women without prior glucocorticoid exposure than in healthy controls (6,8). Furthermore, an association between disease activity and lower BMD, not attributable to glucocorticoid use alone, has been reported (10).

Active SLE has been associated with ovarian dysfunction, including transient and premature menopause, which may account for low BMD observed in some young SLE women of reproductive age that appears to be independent of glucocorticoid exposure (8,32,33). One must recognize such patients because these women are at increased risk for development of osteoporosis later in life (7).

Although a less direct cause of bone loss, reduced physical activity because of fatigue and musculoskeletal symptoms such as arthritis experienced by SLE patients can also contribute to the development of osteoporosis. Prospective data suggest regular exercise, defined as a minimum of 40 minutes of aerobic exercise three times per week, may be a protective factor for bone loss at the femoral neck in SLE patients taking glucocorticoids (34).

Avoiding sunlight and using a topical sunscreen is commonly recommended as a means to avoid SLE flares or disease symptoms; but this practice can result in vitamin-D deficiency and is yet another risk factor for bone loss. Exposure to ultraviolet light allows dermal conversion of 7-dehydrocholesterol to an inert form of vitamin D, an important regulator of serum calcium levels. Subsequent hydroxylation in the liver and kidney leads to the production of the biologically active 1, 25-dihydroxyvitamin D, which in turn aids in both the intestinal absorption of dietary calcium and the maturation of osteoclasts that mobilize calcium from bone. Additionally, renal disease in SLE may disrupt production of active vitamin D and, consequently, lead to bone loss (35).

Specific therapies to manage SLE can affect bone mass via different mechanisms. As previously mentioned, glucocorticoids have been associated with reduced BMD and bone loss in SLE. The ability of glucocorticoids to induce bone loss and increase fracture risk is not unique to SLE and occurs through both direct and indirect means. Glucocorticoids can inhibit osteoblastogenesis and promote apoptosis of osteoblasts and osteocytes, key cells in bone formation (36). Glucocorticoids can also reduce intestinal calcium absorption and increase urinary calcium excretion resulting in secondary hyperparathyroidism and suppress the action or synthesis of sex hormones, thereby promoting further bone loss.

Previous studies have documented reduced BMD either at the spine or hip among those with SLE previously treated with glucocorticoids compared with healthy controls (12,19,24) in trabecular or cortical bone (10). Cumulative glucocorticoid dose has been associated with lower spine BMD in individuals with SLE when compared with those without glucocorticoid use (8). Furthermore, the duration of steroid use, peak steroid dose, and current use of steroids have all been linked to reduced BMD at the spine and hip in SLE patients (12). However, not all studies have shown a similar relationship between glucocorticoid use in SLE, including dose or duration of use, and lower BMD at the lumbar spine or femoral neck (7,11). Absence of a relationship in some reports may be partially attributable to a relatively small number of SLE subjects studied (37).

Immunosuppressive therapies can also lead to ovarian dysfunction and indirectly reduce BMD. Cyclophosphamide, an important immunosuppressive agent used to treat organ-or life-threatening SLE, is capable of inducing premature menopause (38,39) and is a disease-related risk factor for bone loss. Cyclosporine has been associated with osteoclast activation, osteoblast suppression, and retardation of bone formation. Low BMD seen with cyclosporine use has been reported primarily in posttransplant patients (40). Nevertheless, cyclosporine remains a therapeutic option in SLE, and its use should be viewed as a potential risk factor for bone loss. High-dose methotrexate administration in the treatment of oncology patients has been associated with bone loss and fractures, but long-term administration and dosages used to treat SLE have no reported adverse effects on BMD (41).

Bone loss can also be promoted by prolonged use of the anticoagulant therapy heparin. In some SLE patients, anticoagulants are required to manage hypercoagulable states, such as antiphospholipid antibody syndrome (APS). Although oral anticoagulants such as warfarin or coumadin are usually the treatment of choice, they are contraindicated in pregnancy because of their associated risk for teratogenicity. Pregnant women with SLE who also have secondary APS are often treated with heparin to minimize their risk for miscarriage. Unfractionated heparin can reduce cancellous bone by promoting osteoclastic bone destruction and reducing osteoblastic activity. Patients on long-term unfractionated heparin may have up to a 30% reduction in BMD, and 2% to 3% may experience symptomatic vertebral fractures (42). On the other hand, low-molecular-weight heparin seems to have a less deleterious effect on bone than unfractionated heparin when used in SLE women during pregnancy (43).

Anticonvulsant therapy may be required for symptomatic treatment of seizures in patients with neuropsychiatric SLE (44). Chronic administration of anticonvulsants is an independent risk factor for lower BMD and has been associated with increased fractures. Although the mechanism by which anticonvulsants lead to these abnormalities is unclear, they may accelerate vitamin-D metabolism, resulting in decreased calcium absorption, cause secondary hyperparathyroidism, and decreased BMD. Although no study has specifically assessed the potential bone loss with anticonvulsant use in SLE, chronic use of such drugs in SLE patients remains another factor that may contribute to bone loss (45).

## EVALUATION OF OSTEOPOROSIS IN SLE

Many of the current strategies for monitoring and diagnosing osteoporosis in the general population also apply to those with SLE (Fig. 9.1). Loss of height and spinal kyphosis are late physical findings consistent with underlying osteoporosis, and the former has been a predictor of future fractures. Despite the potential for technical limitations, osteopenia identified on thoracic lumbar spine films can occur when there is loss of approximately 20% to 40% of bone mass (46). SLE patients presenting with either physical and/or radiographic finding(s) suggestive of underlying bone loss should prompt further investigation.

Early detection of bone loss can be achieved by performing a BMD test. Because of the heterogeneity of bone loss in SLE, BMD measurement at both the spine and hip should be performed, and assessment of the distal forearm can provide further information. BMD measurements should be obtained at approximately 2-year intervals as this should allow for determination of a significant change. A difference of 2% to 3% at the lumbar spine and 4% to 6% at the hip are viewed as significant (46). However, those at higher risk for new or recurrent fractures, such as individuals on glucocorticoid therapy or those with prior fragility fractures, can have a significant change in BMD over a shorter time interval in these patients. Obtaining BMD measurements as frequently as every 6 to 12 months may be warranted.

Initial laboratory evaluations should include a complete blood count with differential, serum chemistries, including calcium, alkaline phosphatase, creatinine, and thyroid-stimulating-hormone and parathyroid-hormone levels. Additional tests, such as bone specific alkaline phosphatase, serum hormone levels (e.g., testosterone, follicular stimulating hormone), and urinary electrolytes can be assessed if clinically appropriate (46). With respect to biochemical bone parameters, lower levels of osteocalcin, a marker associated with bone formation, and elevated serum carboxyterminal cross-linked telopeptide of type-I collagen, indicative of bone resorption, have been observed in SLE patients suggesting bone loss because of disease (47,48). Yet, other studies have found no appreciable correlation between biochemical bone markers with bone loss

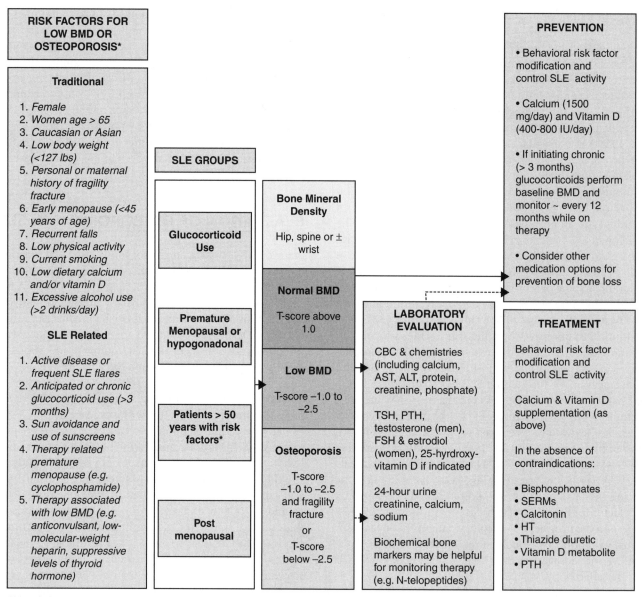

**Abbreviations**

BMD (bone mineral density), CBC (complete blood count), AST (alkaline phosphatase), ALT (aminotransferase), TSH (thyroid-stimulating hormone), PTH (parathyroid hormone), FSH (follicular-stimulating hormone), APL (antiphospholipid antibodies), SERMs (selective estrogen receptor modulators), HT (hormone therapy).

**Figure 9.1** Evaluation and management of bone health in SLE patients.

in SLE (12,49). Inconsistency in the predictive value of biochemical bone markers for bone loss in SLE patients may be due to the relatively small numbers of patients evaluated in some prior studies. Because biochemical bone markers reflect the dynamic nature of bone turnover, multiple measurements over time may better predict future changes in BMD and may indeed be useful in monitoring SLE patients. Further study will help define the clinical utility of biochemical bone markers in management of bone health in SLE. Similarly, active investigation of the potential role of cytokines and inflammatory mediators likely

involved in the pathogenesis of osteoporosis in SLE is ongoing, and at present, their clinical applicability is yet undefined.

## PREVENTION AND TREATMENT OF OSTEOPOROSIS IN SLE

Initial preventive measures consist of behavioral modification of both traditional and SLE-related risk factors when possible (Fig. 9.1). Minimizing frequency and severity of

SLE disease activity is in itself a treatment goal, but it may also have long-term benefit on bone health. Beyond modification of risk factors, specific therapeutic agents available for prevention and treatment of bone loss in SLE patients are discussed below and in greater detail in subsequent chapters.

## Calcium and Vitamin D

Calcium supplementation alone has been shown to have a modest, but statistically significant positive effect on BMD at one or more skeletal sites in both perimenopausal and postmenopausal women (50). In a double-blinded, randomized, placebo-controlled study investigating the prevention of glucocorticoid-induced osteoporosis in a group of patients with a variety of inflammatory diseases, including SLE, there was no significant difference in percent change in BMD at 36 months between vitamin D plus 1000 mg/day of calcium versus placebo (51). Recent meta-analyses, however, have found a benefit of calcium supplementation for prevention of bone loss and a trend toward reduction of vertebral fractures, but it is unclear whether calcium intake reduces the incidence of nonvertebral fractures (52,53). In another meta-analysis, vitamin D plus calcium was superior to no therapy or calcium alone in the management of glucocorticoid-induced osteoporosis (54). Because of low toxicity and cost, all patients starting on glucocorticoids should receive prophylactic therapy with calcium and vitamin D in the absence of any contraindications, including nephrolithiasis, hypercalciuria, or hypocalcemia. Adult SLE patients on glucocorticoid therapy should receive 1500 mg per day of oral calcium supplementation. Vitamin D at the generally recommended amount of 400 to 800 IU can aid in absorption of dietary calcium and may assist in maintaining BMD and reduce risk of fractures and, therefore, should be taken with calcium supplementation (52,55). Currently, there is insufficient information on any protective benefits of calcium with or without vitamin-D supplementation in SLE patients who are premenopausal and/or not receiving glucocorticoids.

## Hormone Therapy

Hormone therapy (HT) has proven benefits for increasing BMD both in younger perimenopausal and older postmenopausal non-SLE women (52). A conjugated estrogen (0.625 mg)-progesterone combination with 1 gram of calcium carbonate prevented bone loss at the lumbar spine in hypogonadal premenopausal SLE women receiving chronic steroid therapy compared with SLE women given calcitriol with the same amount of calcium carbonate (56). Similarly, results of a 1-year, randomized, double-blind, placebo-controlled trial suggested that transdermal estradiol may prevent bone loss in postmenopausal SLE women at the lumbar spine and femur without increasing disease activity (49). The use of hormones in SLE is controversial despite its likely benefits on bone. In addition to SLE being a disease of young women of reproductive age, estrogen exposure causes worsening of disease in murine models of lupus, and there have been case reports of disease flares in SLE patients receiving hormones (57). However, a population-based, case-control study failed to find an increased risk of SLE with estrogen exposure (58).

Exogenous estrogen can increase hypercoagulability; therefore, HT and oral contraceptive use is contraindicated in SLE patients with APS (59). Additionally, data from the Women's Health Initiative indicated HT reduced hip and vertebral fractures, but the study was prematurely halted because of adverse events in cardiovascular-related mortality and breast cancer endpoints (60). Because there is accumulating information for increased cardiovascular risk in SLE, there is concern for the added cardiovascular risk posed by using hormone therapy in SLE patients. Nevertheless, the bone benefits of hormones may be gained by SLE patients who require HT for menopausal symptoms severe enough to interfere with their quality of life and by those individuals who cannot take other bone protective agents. Any plans to initiate hormone therapy in SLE patients should be done only after the risks and benefits of HT have been thoroughly discussed between patient and physician.

## Selective Estrogen Receptor Modulators

Selective estrogen receptor modulators (SERMs), such as raloxifene, toremifene, and tamoxifen, interact with the estrogen receptor to induce selective agonist or antagonist action in estrogen-responsive target tissues. Raloxifene (60 mg/day) has been shown to increase BMD in the spine and femoral neck and decrease vertebral but not nonvertebral fractures and is currently approved for the prevention and treatment of postmenopausal osteoporosis. Similar to HT, women receiving raloxifene had increased risk of venous thromboembolus compared with women taking placebo [relative risk (RR) = 3.1; 95% confidence interval (CI): 1.5–6.2] (61). Unlike HT, raloxifene has not been associated with any increased risk for cardiovascular events (62). Physicians should consider bone protective agents other than SERMs for SLE patients with APS or underlying hypercoagulopathy. Raloxifene, however, may be an alternative option for SLE patients requiring bone protective agents who are not ideal candidates for HT and have no risk factors for hypercoagulopathy as it modestly improves BMD in non-SLE patients.

## Bisphosphonates

Bisphosphonates, which include alendronate, risedronate, etidronate, and pamidronate, possess a high affinity for bone hydroxyapatite and are potent inhibitors of osteoclastic bone resorption (46). Multiple well-designed, randomized, controlled trials have demonstrated the efficacy of bisphosphonates to increase BMD and reduce vertebral and nonvertebral fractures. Bisphosphonates can also preserve BMD in patients receiving long-term glucocorticoid therapy (63). In the absence of contraindications, bisphosphonates should be considered for use in SLE patients with osteoporosis and/or prior fragility fractures and for prevention of glucocorticoid-induced osteoporosis because of their proven efficacy for reducing fractures.

## Calcitonin

Calcitonin, an endogenous peptide that inhibits osteoclast activity, is available in nasal, subcutaneous, and intramuscular form and may be offered as an alternative for SLE patients unable to take HT, raloxifene, or bisphosphonates. It has been shown to increase BMD in the spine and femoral neck (64) and to decrease vertebral fractures, but convincing data for nonvertebral fractures are lacking. In light of the limited information on fracture prevention, calcitonin should be regarded as second-line therapy in managing osteoporosis in SLE patients. Additionally, calcitonin may relieve acute pain resulting from vertebral fractures (63) and, therefore, may be of benefit in pain reduction in SLE patients sustaining vertebral fractures.

## Parathyroid Hormone

Parathyroid hormone (PTH) is an endogenous, 84-amino-acid peptide with anabolic properties that can promote bone formation. Although primary hyperparathyroidism or conditions of endogenous, sustained excess PTH have been known to contribute to cortical bone loss, intermittent administration of PTH can increase BMD to a greater extent than can other available agents, restore the microarchitecture, and increase bone size. PTH given at the 20 μg dose has been shown to reduce both vertebral fractures (RR = 0.35; 95% CI: 0.22–0.55) and nonvertebral fragility fractures (RR = 0.47; 95% CI: 0.25–0.88). PTH is being evaluated as a potential therapeutic agent for glucocorticoid-induced osteoporosis, but at present, no data exist to recommend its use for prevention or treatment of glucocorticoid-induced osteoporosis in the setting of SLE. Among its contraindications, PTH is not approved for use in children and young adults with open epiphyses or women during pregnancy. Notably, long-term PTH at high doses has been associated with an increased risk of osteosarcoma in rats, but no cases of osteosarcoma have been reported in human trials (63). PTH should be viewed as second line therapy and reserved for SLE patients at greatest risk for fractures or with prior or current fragility fractures in whom bisphosphonate therapy is poorly tolerated or contraindicated. Because of limited data on the long-term effects, PTH administration should be limited to no more than 1 to 2 years.

## Combination Therapies and Potential Future Treatments

HT combined with alendronate appears to improve BMD to a greater extent than either agent used alone. Risedronate and estrogen used together have demonstrated small increases in BMD at the spine, hip, and wrist after 1 year. There is rapid bone loss, however, upon withdrawal of HT. Similarly, raloxifene combined with alendronate appears to modestly improve BMD at the spine, hip (femoral neck), and wrist compared with either agent used alone. Studies have suggested that gains in BMD achieved with PTH treatment can be preserved when followed by alendronate or estrogen therapy (63). On the other hand, there is no evidence of synergy between PTH and alendronate, and concurrent use of alendronate may reduce the anabolic effects of PTH (65). Similarly, the use of alendronate has been shown to impair the ability of PTH to increase BMD at the lumbar spine and the femoral neck in men (66).

The benefits of hydroxychloroquine in SLE are well-recognized, but there is minimal data on bone health. Hydroxychloroquine use has been associated with higher BMD of the hip and spine in women with SLE (15), but additional studies are needed to validate these findings and to determine whether any benefit exists for lowering fracture occurrence. Thiazide diuretics have been shown to improve gastrointestinal absorption and decrease urinary excretion of calcium, which can help minimize hypercalciuria associated with glucocorticoid use. In the setting of low urinary calcium, SLE patients receiving glucocorticoid therapy may benefit from thiazide diuretics as a means of preventing bone loss (35). Dehydroepiandrosterone (DHEA) or prasterone, a weak androgen used to control lupus activity, may be useful in preserving BMD in SLE patients receiving glucocorticoids (67,68), but further study is ongoing. Other agents including fluoride, insulin growth factor type 1 (IGF-I), and statins may have some benefit in improving BMD in SLE patients, but results of active clinical trials will shed greater light on their clinical utility. Finally, other potential therapies for reducing bone loss in SLE may include biologic agents involving monoclonal antibodies directed against specific cytokine targets, such as IL-1, IL-6, and RANK-L.

## SUMMARY

Bone loss and fractures are emerging as important lupus-related conditions paralleling increased SLE incidence and survival. Bone loss in SLE is likely a multifactorial process involving both traditional and SLE-related risk factors for osteoporosis. Improved recognition of these risk factors is essential for early identification and prompt initiation of preventive measures to minimize further bone loss and fracture risk. Currently available knowledge on agents used in the prevention and treatment of osteoporosis in SLE are largely derived from studies performed in the non-SLE population. Therefore, awareness of specific caveats in the use of bone protective agents germane to SLE is important to optimize bone health and minimize therapeutic toxicity in the SLE patient.

## ACKNOWLEDGMENT

This work was supported by grants from the National Institutes of Health (K24 AR 02138, K24 AR 02213, K12 P60 AR48098, T32 AR 07611, P60 AR 30692, P60 AR 30692), the Arthritis Foundation Clinical Science Grant, Lupus Foundation of Illinois, and Arthritis Foundation Greater Chicago Chapter and by unrestricted educational grants from Proctor & Gamble Pharmaceuticals and Merck & Co., Inc.

We are indebted to Janice M. Sabatine, Ph.D. for her technical and editorial assistance in the preparation of this manuscript.

## REFERENCES

1. Gordon C. Long-term complications of systemic lupus erythematosus. *Rheumatology (Oxf)* 2002;41(10):1095–1100.
2. Urowitz MB, Gladman DD, Abu-Shakra M, Farewell VT. Mortality studies in systemic lupus erythematosus. Results from a single center. III. Improved survival over 24 years. *J Rheumatol* 1997;24(6):1061–1065.
3. Uramoto KM, Michet CJ Jr, Thumboo J, et al. Trends in the incidence and mortality of systemic lupus erythematosus, 1950–1992. *Arthritis Rheum* 1999;42(1):46–50.
4. Trager J, Ward MM. Mortality and causes of death in systemic lupus erythematosus. *Curr Opin Rheumatol* 2001;13(5):345–351.
5. Cervera R, Khamashta MA, Font J, et al. European Working Party on Systemic Lupus Erythematosus. Morbidity and mortality in systemic lupus erythematosus during a 10-year period: a comparison of early and late manifestations in a cohort of 1,000 patients. *Medicine (Baltimore)* 2003;82(5):299–308.
6. Kalla AA, Fataar AB, Jessop SJ, Bewerunge L. Loss of trabecular bone mineral density in systemic lupus erythematosus. *Arthritis Rheum* 1993; 36: 1726–1734.
7. Formiga F, Moga I, Nolla JM, et al. Loss of bone mineral density in premenopausal women with systemic lupus erythematosus. *Ann Rheum Dis* 1995; 54(4): 274–276.
8. Houssiau FA, Lefebvre C, Depresseux G, et al. Trabecular and cortical bone loss in systemic lupus erythematosus. *Br J Rheumatol* 1996;35:244–247.
9. Trapani S, Civinini R, Ermini M, et al. Osteoporosis in juvenile systemic lupus erythematosus: a longitudinal study on the effect of steroids on bone mineral density. *Rheumatol Int* 1998;18:45–49.
10. Sinigaglia L, Varenna M, Binelli L, et al. Determinants of bone mass in systemic lupus erythematosus: a cross sectional study on premenopausal women. *J Rheumatol* 1999; 26(6): 1280–1284.
11. Kalla AA, Kotze TJvW, Meyers OL. Metacarpal bone mass in systemic lupus erythematosus. *Clin Rheumatol* 1992;11:1–8.
12. Kipen Y, Buchbinder R, Forbes A, et al. Prevalence of reduced bone mineral density in systemic lupus erythematosus and the role of steroids. *J Rheumatol* 1997;24(10):1922–1929.
13. Gilboe I, Kvien TK, Haugeberg G, Husby G. Bone mineral density in systemic lupus erythematosus: comparison with rheumatoid arthritis and healthy controls. *Ann Rheum Dis* 2000;59:110–115.
14. Jardinet D, Lefebvre, Depresseux G, et al. Longitudinal analysis of bone mineral density in premenopausal female systemic lupus erythematosus patients: deleterious role of glucocorticoid therapy at the lumbar spine. *Rheumatol* 2002;39:389–392.
15. Lakshminarayanan S, Walsh S, Mohanraj M, Rothfield N. Factors associated with low bone mineral density in female patients with systemic lupus erythematosus. *J Rheumatol* 2001;28(1):102–108.
16. Becker A, Fischer R, Scherbaum WA, Schneider M. Osteoporosis screening in systemic lupus erythematosus: impact of disease duration and organ damage. *Lupus* 2001;10(11):809–814.
17. Leong NM, Shamiyeh E, Chung AH, et al. Longitudinal analysis of bone mineral density in women with recent onset systemic lupus erythematosus. *J Bone Miner Res* 2003;18(2):S398.
18. Swaak AJ, van den Brink HG, Smeenk RJ, et al. Systemic lupus erythematosus: clinical features in patients with a disease duration of over 10 years, first evaluation. *Rheumatology (Oxf)* 1999;38(10):953–958.
19. Li EK, Tam LS, Young RP, et al. Loss of bone mineral density in Chinese pre-menopausal women with systemic lupus erythematosus treated with corticosteroids. *Br J Rheumatol* 1998;37:405–410.
20. Cummings S, Melton III LJ. Epidemiology and outcomes of osteoporotic fractures. *Lancet* 2002;359:1761–1767.
21. Chadha A, Shamiyeh E, Manzi S, et al. Race may not protect against low bone mineral density in women with lupus. *J Bone Miner Res* 2003;18(2):S154.
22. Boyanov M, Robeva R, Popivanov P. Bone mineral density changes in women with systemic lupus erythematosus. *Clin Rheumatol* 2003;22:318–323.
23. Kalla AA, Meyers OL, Parkyn ND, Kotze TJ. Osteoporosis screening-radiogrammetry revisited. *Br J Rheumatol* 1989;28(6):511–517.
24. Pons F, Peris P, Guanabens N, et al. The effect of systemic lupus erythematosus and long-term steroid therapy on bone mass in pre-menopausal women. *Br J Rheumatol* 1995;34742–746.
25. Petri M. Musculoskeletal complications of systemic lupus erythematosus in the Hopkins Lupus Cohort: an update. *Arthritis Care Res* 1995;8(3):137–145.
26. Melton LJ III, Thamer M, Ray NF, et al. Fractures attributable to osteoporosis: report form the National Osteoporosis Foundation. *J Bone Miner Res* 1997;12:16–23.
27. Ramsey-Goldman R, Dunn JE, Huang CF, et al. Frequency of fractures in women with systemic lupus erythematosus: comparison with United States population data. *Arthritis Rheum* 1999;42(5):882–890.
28. Lunt M, Masaryk P, Scheidt-Nave C, et al. The effects of lifestyle, dietary dairy intake and diabetes on bone density and vertebral deformity prevalence: the EVOS study. *Osteoporos Int* 2001;12(8):688–698.
29. Albrand G, Munoz G, Sornay-Rendu E, et al. Independent predictors of all osteoporosis-related fractures in healthy post-menopausal women: the OFELY study. *Bone* 2003;32:78–85.
30. Schapira D, Kabala A, Raz B, Israeli E. Osteoporosis in murine systemic lupus erythematosus—a laboratory model. *Lupus* 2001;10:431–438.
31. Linker-Israeli M, Deans RJ, Wallace DJ, et al. Elevated levels of endogenous IL-6 in systemic lupus erythematosus. A putative role in pathogenesis. *J Immunol* 1991;147(1):117–123.
32. Pasoto SG, Mendonca BB, Bonfa E. Menstrual disturbances in patients with systemic lupus erythematosus without alkylating therapy: clinical, hormonal and therapeutic associations. *Lupus* 2002;11(3):175–180.
33. Medeiros MC, Silveira VL, Menezes AT, Carvalho RC. Risk factors for ovarian failure in patients with systemic lupus erythematosus. *Braz J Med Biol Res* 2001;34(12):1561–1568.
34. Kipen Y, Briganti E, Strauss B, et al. Three year followup of bone mineral density change in premenopausal women with systemic lupus erythematosus. *J Rheumatol* 1999;26:310–317.
35. Sen D, Keen RW. Osteoporosis in systemic lupus erythematosus: prevention and treatment. *Lupus* 2001;10:227–232.
36. Weinstein RS, Jilka RL, Parfitt AM, Manolagas SC. Inhibition of osteoblastogenesis and promotion of apoptosis of osteoblasts and osteocytes by glucocorticoids. Potential mechanisms of their deleterious effects on bone. *J Clin Invest* 1998;27:465–483.
37. Dhillon VB, Davies MC, Hall ML, et al. Assessment of the effect of oral corticosteroids on bone mineral density in systemic lupus erythematosus: a preliminary study with dual energy x-ray absorptiometry. *Ann Rheum Dis* 1990;49:624–626.

38. Boumpas DT, Austin HA, Vaughan EM, et al. Risk for sustained amenorrhea in patients with systemic lupus erythematosus receiving intermittent pulse cyclophosphamide therapy. *Ann Intern Med* 1993;119:366–369.

39. Huong du L, Amoura Z, Duhaut P, et al. Risk of ovarian failure and fertility after intravenous cyclophosphamide. A study in 84 patients. *J Rheumatol* 2002;29(12):2571–2576.

40. Cueto-Manzano AM, Konel S, Crowley V, et al. Bone histopathology and densitometry comparison between cyclosporine a monotherapy and prednisolone plus azathioprine dual immunosuppression in renal transplant patients. *Transplantation* 2003;75(12):2053–2058.

41. Cranney AB, McKendry RJ, Wells GA, et al. The effect of low dose methotrexate on bone density. *J Rheumatol* 2001;28(11):2395–2399.

42. Ruiz-Irastorza G, Khamashta MA, Nelson-Piercy C, Hughes GR. Lupus pregnancy: is heparin a risk factor for osteoporosis? *Lupus* 2001;10(9):597–600.

43. Pettila V, Leinonen P, Markkola A, et al. Postpartum bone mineral density in women treated for thromboprophylaxis with unfractionated heparin or LMW heparin. *Thromb Haemost* 2002;11:680–682.

44. Brey RL, Escalante A. Neurological manifestations of antiphospholipid antibody syndrome. *Lupus* 1998;7[Suppl 2]:S67–74 (Review).

45. Farhat G, Yamout B, Mikati MA, et al. Effect of antiepileptic drugs on bone density in ambulatory patients. *Neurology* 2002;58(9):1348–1353.

46. Marcus R, Feldman D, Kelsey J. *Osteoporosis: Imaging of osteoporosis*, 2nd ed. Academic Press: Harcourt Science and Technology, 2001:411–431.

47. Redlich K, Ziegler S, Kiener HP, et al. Bone mineral density and biochemical parameters of bone metabolism in female patients with systemic lupus erythematosus. *Ann Rheum Dis* 2000;59(4):308–310.

48. Hansen M, Halberg P, Kollerup G, et al. Bone metabolism in patients with systemic lupus erythematosus. Effect of disease activity and glucocorticoid treatment. *Scand J Rheumatol* 1998;27(3):197–206.

49. Bhattoa HP, Kiss E, Bettembuk P, Balogh A. Bone mineral density, biochemical markers of bone turnover, and hormonal status in men with systemic lupus erythematosus. *Rheumatol Int* 2001;21(3):97–102.

50. Nordin BE. Calcium and osteoporosis. *Nutrition* 1997;13(7–8):664–686.

51. Adachi JD, Bensen WG, Bianchi F, et al. Vitamin D and calcium in the prevention of corticosteroid induced osteoporosis: a 3 year follow-up. *J Rheumatol* 1996;23(6):995–1000.

52. Shea B, Wells G, Cranney A, et al. Meta-analyses of therapies for postmenopausal osteoporosisVII: Meta-analysis of calcium supplementation for the prevention of postmenopausal osteoporosis. *Endocr Rev* 2002;23:552–559.

53. Homik J, Suarez-Almazor ME, Shea B, et al. Calcium and vitamin D for corticosteroid-induced osteoporosis. *Cochrane Database Syst Rev* 2000;(2):CD000952.

54. Amin S, LaValley MP, Simms RW, Felson DT. The role of vitamin D in corticosteroid-induced osteoporosis: a meta-analytic approach. *Arthritis Rheum* 1999;42(8):1740–1751.

55. Sambrook P, Birmingham J, Kelly P, et al. Prevention of corticosteroid osteoporosis. A comparison of calcium, calcitriol, and calcitonin. *N Engl J Med* 1993;328(24):1747–1752.

56. Kung AW, Chan TM, Lau CS, et al. Osteopenia in young hypogonadal women with systemic lupus erythematosus receiving chronic steroid therapy: a randomized controlled trial comparing calcitriol and hormonal replacement therapy. *Rheumatology (Oxf)* 1999;38(12):1239–1244.

57. Lakasing L, Khamashta M. Contraceptive practices in women with systemic lupus erythematosus and/or antiphospholipid syndrome: what advice should we be giving? *J Fam Plann Reprod Health Care* 2001; 27(1): 7–12.

58. Askanase AD, Buyon JP. Reproductive health in SLE. *Best Pract Res Clin Rheumatol* 2002;16(2):265–280.

59. Cooper GS, Dooley MA, Treadwell EL, et al. Hormonal and reproductive risk factors for development of systemic lupus erythematosus: results of a population-based, case-control study. *Arthritis Rheum* 2002;46(7):1830–1839.

60. Rossouw JE, Anderson GL, Prentice RL, et al. Writing Group for the Women's Health Initiative Investigators. Risks and benefits of estrogen plus progestin in healthy postmenopausal women: principal results from the Women's Health Initiative randomized controlled trial. *JAMA* 2002;288(3):321–333.

61. Ettinger B, Black DM, Mitlak BH, et al. Reduction of vertebral fracture risk in postmenopausal women with osteoporosis treated with raloxifene: results from a 3-year randomized clinical trial. Multiple Outcomes of Raloxifene Evaluation (MORE) Investigators. *JAMA* 1999;282(7):637–645.

62. Barrett-Connor E, Grady D, Sashegyi A, et al; MORE Investigators (Multiple Outcomes of Raloxifene Evaluation). Raloxifene and cardiovascular events in osteoporotic postmenopausal women: four-year results from the MORE (Multiple Outcomes of Raloxifene Evaluation) randomized trial. *JAMA* 2002;287(7):847–857.

63. Brown SA, Rosen CJ. Osteoporosis. *Med Clin North Am* 2003;87(5):1039–1063.

64. Cardona JM, Pastor E. Calcitonin versus etidronate for the treatment of postmenopausal osteoporosis: a meta-analysis of published clinical trials. *Osteoporos Int* 1997;7(3):165–174.

65. Black DM, Greenspan SL, Ensrud KE, et al; PaTH Study Investigators. The effects of parathyroid hormone and alendronate alone or in combination in postmenopausal osteoporosis. *N Engl J Med* 2003;349(13):1207–1215.

66. Finkelstein JS, Hayes A, Hunzelman JL, et al. The effects of parathyroid hormone, alendronate, or both in men with osteoporosis. *N Engl J Med* 2003;349(13):1216–1226.

67. Van Vollenhoven RF, Park JL, Genovese MC, et al. A double-blind, placebo-controlled, clinical trial of dehydroepiandrosterone in severe systemic lupus erythematosus. *Lupus* 1999;8:181.

68. Nishimura J, Ikuyama S. Glucocorticoid-induced osteoporosis: pathogenesis and management. *J Bone Miner Metab* 2000;18(6):350–352.

# Bone Disease in Ankylosing Spondylitis and Psoriatic Arthritis

**10**

*Atul Deodhar*

The bone changes in ankylosing spondylitis (AS) and psoriatic arthritis (PsA) are unique among inflammatory arthritides. The underlying inflammatory process leads to simultaneous opposing effects on bone such as bone loss as well as new bone formation. At one extreme, severe localized bone erosions and acrolysis (extensive resorption of the distal phalanges) can occur, leading to arthritis mutilans in PsA. In AS, axial bone loss can lead to spinal osteoporosis and vertebral fractures. At the other extreme, the underlying pathological process results in new bone formation with bridging syndesmophytes and calcification of paraspinal ligaments.

Peripheral extraarticular enthesitis, a clinical hallmark of the seronegative spondyloarthropathies, demonstrates both erosions (bone loss) and spurs (new bone formation) in advanced phases. The presence of bone resorption plus new bone formation, often in the same joint, suggests a disordered pattern of bone remodeling in PsA and AS (1).

## BONE DISEASE IN ANKYLOSING SPONDYLITIS

### Generalized Bone Loss

The cause of systemic osteoporosis in AS is multifactorial. Spinal immobility caused by inflammatory back pain may cause disuse osteoporosis (2). Increased plasma levels of proinflammatory cytokines such as tumor necrosis factor (TNF)-$\alpha$ and interleukin (IL)-6 that stimulate osteoclastic bone resorption have been found in AS patients (3). Levels of plasma, insulin-like growth factor-1 (IGF-1), a bone-promoting peptide, have been found to decrease with

an inverse correlation to TNF-$\alpha$ levels. Also, levels of IGF-1–binding protein-3 (IGFBP-3), an important cofactor that modulates the bioavailability and activity of IGF-1, were significantly lower in AS patients than in healthy subjects (4).

Markers of disease activity such as erythrocyte sedimentation rate (ESR), C-reactive protein (CRP), and Bath ankylosing spondylitis disease activity index (BASDAI) have shown a significant positive correlation with urinary pyridinium cross-link excretion, a biochemical marker of bone resorption (3,5). In a study of 66 women with AS, markers of bone formation (osteocalcin and bone specific alkaline phosphatase, BSAP) were significantly lower and markers of bone resorption (deoxypyridinoline) were higher than controls (6). Taken together, these data suggest that osteoblastic cell function is impaired in AS (in part because of low IGF-1 levels) and osteoclastic activity is increased (because of high TNF-$\alpha$ levels). Persistent inflammation plays an important role in the pathogenesis of osteoporosis in AS.

The importance of TNF-$\alpha$ in the pathogenesis of bone loss in AS has been demonstrated by a study of 29 patients with AS who received infliximab (a chimeric monoclonal anti-TNF antibody) and had a statistically significant increase in BMD at the spine and total hip (7).

### Bone Mineral Density in AS

Posteroanterior (PA) bone density studies of the lumbar spine in AS are generally fraught with technical challenges. Calcification of paraspinal ligaments as well as development of syndesmophytes in late AS can lead to difficulties in the assessment of true lumbar bone mineral density (BMD) using dual energy x-ray absorptiometry (DXA).

The new bone formation may obscure osteoporotic verte-brae and may give spuriously normal results. Under these circumstances, more accurate assessment of BMD may be obtained by measurement of hip BMD. Quantitative CT scanning or lateral DXA scanning may be alternative meth-ods to assess the true extent of low bone density (8). It is, therefore, of utmost importance that one consider the site and method of bone density measurement when consider-ing results of studies on osteoporosis in AS.

Vertebral osteoporosis (T score worse than or equal to −2.5) is a common complication of AS, with a prevalence between 18% and 62% in various series (9). The preva-lence of low bone mass is greater in males, with increasing age, and in patients with syndesmophytes, cervical fusion, and peripheral joint involvement. However, these variables may be indicators of advanced disease and/or disease dura-tion and are not necessarily independent predictors of sys-temic bone loss.

A study of 66 men with "mild AS" (as defined by a mobile lumbar spine with absent or incipient syndesmo-phytes) showed the presence of osteopenia (T score between −1 to −2.5) in most patients, with a mean T score at the lumbar spine and femoral neck of −1.1 and −1.4, respectively. Disease duration had no effect on the bone density (2). Another study of 73 patients with mild or advanced AS measured BMD at the PA lumbar spine and at the total hip (10). The BMD at both sites was reduced com-pared to age-matched normal controls. There was no dif-ference in lumbar spine BMD between patients with mild or advanced AS. In contrast, at the total hip, there was an increased frequency of osteoporosis in patients with advanced AS compared to those with mild AS. This obser-vation may be related to the new bone formation in the spines of patients with more severe AS.

In a 2-year longitudinal study in 54 patients with AS, the PA lumbar spine BMD did not show significant change, whereas BMD at the femoral neck fell by 1.6% (11). The 24-month change in femoral neck BMD was related to per-sistent systemic inflammation defined as an elevated ESR. The mean percentage change was 4.1% ± 5.7% in those with a high ESR compared to 1.2% ± 3.9% in patients with a low ESR; $p = 0.007$. These results suggest that persistent inflammation is an etiologic factor of bone loss in AS.

### Fractures in AS

Vertebral fractures in AS are common with an odds ratio of 6 to 1 (2). In AS, the risk of a vertebral fracture over a 30-year period is 14% compared to 3.4% for a control population (9). In a cohort study in Rochester, Minnesota (12), there was no increase in the risk of limb fractures; however, there was a large increase in the risk of thoracolumbar compression frac-tures with standardized morbidity ratio equal to 7.6 [95% confidence interval (CI): 4.3–12.6] among patients with AS.

Patients with spinal fusion resulting from AS, may frac-ture through both the anterior and posterior elements of

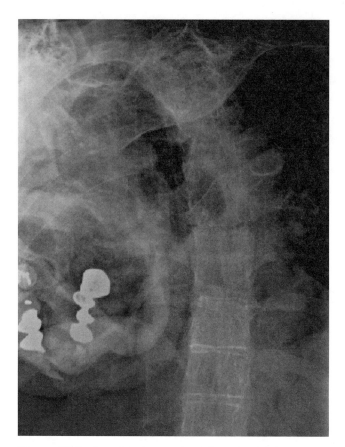

**Figure 10.1**  Pseudoarthrosis T4–5 following a fall in a patient with longstanding ankylosing spondylitis.

the spinal column. This results in a pseudoarthrosis at the discovertebral junction (Fig. 10.1). Pseudoarthrosis may occur after minimal trauma and may be difficult to visual-ize on plain radiographs (13). Diagnosis may require com-puted tomography (CT) or magnetic resonance imaging (MRI) (14). Because of segmental instability above and below the pseudoarthrosis, cord compression may devel-op. The resulting neurological deficit can range from mild sensory loss to complete paraplegia (15).

### Focal Bone Disease in AS

Characteristic focal bony changes specific to AS are Romanus and Andersson lesions. Romanus lesions are focal destructive areas along the anterior margin of the dis-covertebral junction (16). Concomitant bone erosion and bone formation creates a squared contour, with reactive sclerosis leading to a "shiny corner." Andersson lesions are foci of bone destruction occurring throughout the dis-covertebral junction.

## NEW BONE FORMATION IN AS

The molecular mechanisms of new bone formation in spondyloarthropathies are not well elucidated. In an immunohistologic study on biopsy specimens of the sacroil-iac (SI) joints from 5 patients with active AS, a high amount of TNF-α mRNA was found (17). However, near the site of new bone formation, transforming growth factor β (TGF-β) mRNA was detected. The authors concluded that TGF-β might be involved in new bone formation in AS (18).

## BONE DISEASE IN PSORIATIC ARTHRITIS

### Generalized Bone Loss

Very few studies have examined bone mass measurements in patients with psoriatic arthritis (PsA). In a study of 20 patients with cutaneous plaque psoriasis, no significant differences in BMD were found between patients and controls. Patients with psoriatic arthritis, however, had a significantly lower mean lumbar spine Z-score compared to those without arthritis (19). In a large study on 186 patients with nonaxial PsA, BMD at lumbar spine, femoral neck, and total body was significantly lower in patients than in the healthy subjects matched for sex, menopausal status, and age (17).

Grisar and colleagues (20) studied biochemical markers of bone metabolism in patients with PsA, AS, and reactive arthritis. Bone resorption markers (urinary deoxypyridino-line and cross-linked telopeptide of collagen-I) were significantly increased in all groups of patients and in PsA correlated with the acute phase response (C-reactive protein and ESR). This indicated that bone loss in PsA is related to underlying inflammation.

### Fractures in PsA

There are few studies specifically looking at the prevalence of fractures in patients with PsA. The only published series include reports of insufficiency (stress) fractures in PsA (21).

### Focal Bone Loss in PA

In a study comparing patients with rheumatoid arthritis (RA) and PsA, periarticular bone loss occurred in both diseases (22). Periarticular osteoporosis was related to measures of joint inflammation in RA but not in PsA.

Ritchlin and colleagues found a marked increase in osteoclast precursors in blood samples from PsA patients with radiographic erosions (1). Peripheral blood mononu-clear cells (precursors of osteoclasts) from PsA patients readily formed osteoclasts in vitro without exogenous stimulation from receptor activator of NF-κB ligand (RANKL) or macrophage colony stimulating factor (MCSF). Osteoprotegerin (a decoy receptor for RANKL) and anti-TNF antibodies inhibited osteoclast formation.

Osteoclasts were found to be prominently situated at the bone-pannus junction. RANKL expression was dramatically upregulated in the synovial lining. Based on these results, the authors suggested a model for understanding the pathogenesis of aggressive bone erosions in PsA. According to this model, osteoclast precursors arise from TNF-α–activated peripheral blood mononuclear cells that migrate to the inflamed synovium and subchondral bone, where they are exposed to unopposed RANKL and TNF-α. This leads to development of osteoclasts at the erosion front and within the subchondral bone, resulting in a bidi-rectional assault on psoriatic bone (1).

## TREATMENT OF BONE DISEASE IN AS AND PsA

In a community survey of 449 British rheumatologists, only one-third of the respondents indicated that assessment of osteoporosis formed part of their routine management of AS (23). Twelve percent stated that they would not treat osteoporosis in AS. There is a need, therefore, for increased awareness of bone disease in AS.

Pulse intravenous (IV) pamidronate has been used as a therapy for AS. In a study with 84 patients with AS refractory to nonsteroid antiinflammatory drugs (NSAID), IV pamidronate (60 mg monthly for 6 months) was associated with significant reduction in clinical markers of disease activity (BASDAI) compared to patients receiving pamidronate 10 mg IV monthly (24). The mechanism of action remains unclear.

In a study of 29 patients with spondylarthropathy treated with infliximab for 6 months, there was a statistically significant increase in BMD both at the spine and total hip (7).

Currently bisphosphonates are the most commonly used medications for the treatment of osteoporosis in AS (9).

## REFERENCES

1. Ritchlin CT, Haas-Smith SA, Li P, et al. Mechanisms of TNF-alpha- and RANKL-mediated osteoclastogenesis and bone resorption in psoriatic arthritis. *J Clin Invest* 2003;111(6):821–831.
2. Mitra D, Elvins DM, Speden DJ, Collins AJ. The prevalence of verte-bral fractures in mild ankylosing spondylitis and their relationship to bone mineral density. *Rheumatology (Oxf)* 2000;39(1):85–89.
3. Lange U, Teichmann J, Stracke H. Correlation between plasma TNF-alpha, IGF-1, biochemical markers of bone metabolism, markers of inflammation/disease activity, and clinical manifestations in anky-losing spondylitis. *Eur J Med Res* 2000;5(12): 507–511.
4. Toussirot E, Nguyen NU, Dumoulin G, et al. Insulin-like growth fac-tor-I and insulin-like growth factor binding protein-3 serum levels in ankylosing spondylitis. *Br J Rheumatol* 1998;37(11): 1172–1176.
5. Lange U, Jung O, Teichmann J, Neeck G. Relationship between disease activity and serum levels of vitamin D metabolites and parathyroid hormone in ankylosing spondylitis. *Osteoporos Int* 2001;12(12):1031–1035.
6. Speden DJ, Calin AI, Ring FJ, Bhalla AK. Bone mineral density, cal-caneal ultrasound, and bone turnover markers in women with ankylosing spondylitis. *J Rheumatol* 2002; 29(3):516–521.
7. Demis E, Roux C, Breban M, Dougados M. Infliximab in spondy-larthropathy—influence on bone density. *Clin Exp Rheumatol* 2002;20[6Suppl28]:S185–S186.

8. Bronson WD, Walker SE, Hillman LS, et al. Bone mineral density and biochemical markers of bone metabolism in ankylosing spondylitis. *J Rheumatol* 1998;25(5):929–935.

9. Bessant R, Keat A. How should clinicians manage osteoporosis in ankylosing spondylitis? *J Rheumatol* 2002;29(7):1511–1519.

10. Capaci K, Hepguler S, Argin M, Tas I. Bone mineral density in mild and advanced ankylosing spondylitis. *Yonsei Med J* 2003;44(3):379–384.

13. Maillefert JF, Aho LS, El Maghraoui A, et al. Changes in bone density in patients with ankylosing spondylitis: a two-year follow-up study. *Osteoporos Int* 2001;12(7):605–609.

12. Cooper C, Carbone L, Michet CJ, et al. Fracture risk in patients with ankylosing spondylitis: a population based study. *J Rheumatol* 1994;21(10):1877–1882.

13. Goldberg AL, Keaton NL, Rothfus WE, Daffner RH. Ankylosing spondylitis complicated by trauma: MR findings correlated with plain radiographs and CT. *Skeletal Radiol* 1993;22(5):333–336.

14. Shih RR, Chen PQ, Li YW, Hsu CY. Spinal fractures and pseudoarthrosis complicating ankylosing spondylitis: MRI manifestation and clinical significance. *J Comput Assist Tomogr* 2001; 25(2):164–170.

15. Taggard DA, Traynelis VC. Management of cervical spinal fractures in ankylosing spondylitis with posterior fixation. *Spine* 2000;25(16):2035–2039.

16. Jevtic V, Kos-Golja M, Rozman B, McCall I. Marginal erosive discovertebral "Romanus" lesions in ankylosing spondylitis demonstrated by contrast enhanced Gd-DTPA magnetic resonance imaging. *Skeletal Radiol* 2000;29(1):27–33.

17. Frediani B, Allegri A, Falsetti P, et al. Bone mineral density in patients with psoriatic arthritis. *J Rheumatol* 2001;28(1):138–143.

18. Braun J, Bollow M, Neure L, et al. Use of immunohistologic and in situ hybridization techniques in the examination of sacroiliac joint biopsy specimens from patients with ankylosing spondylitis. *Arthritis Rheum* 1995;38(4):499–505.

19. Millard TP, Antoniades L, Evans AV, et al. Bone mineral density of patients with chronic plaque psoriasis. *Clin Exp Dermatol* 2001;26(5):446–448.

20. Grisar J, Bernecker PM, Aringer M, et al. Ankylosing spondylitis, psoriatic arthritis, and reactive arthritis show increased bone resorption, but differ with regard to bone formation. *J Rheumatol* 2002;29(7):1430–1436.

21. Maenpaa HM, Soini I, Lehto MU, Belt EA. Insufficiency fractures in patients with chronic inflammatory joint diseases. *Clin Exp Rheumatol* 2002;20(1):77–79.

22. Harrison BJ, Hutchinson CE, Adams J, et al. Assessing periarticular bone mineral density in patients with early psoriatic arthritis or rheumatoid arthritis. *Ann Rheum Dis* 2002;61(11):1007–1011.

23. Bessant R, Harris C, Keat A. Audit of the diagnosis, assessment, and treatment of osteoporosis in patients with ankylosing spondylitis. *J Rheumatol* 2003;30(4):779–782.

24. Maksymowych WP, Jhangri GS, Fitzgerald AA, et al. A six-month randomized, controlled, double-blind, dose-response comparison of intravenous pamidronate (60 mg versus 10 mg) in the treatment of nonsteroidal anti-inflammatory drug-refractory ankylosing spondylitis. *Arthritis Rheum* 2002;46(3):766–773.

# Osteoarthritis

## 11

*Marc C. Hochberg    Joan M. Meyer*

Osteoarthritis (OA) is the most common form of arthritis (1). OA, when it involves the hip and/or knee, accounts for more functional limitation and physical disability than any other chronic disease among adults and is the most common indication for total hip and total knee replacement. It is estimated that the costs associated with OA exceed 2% of the gross national product in developed countries (2).

OA is now recognized to be a disorder that affects all the tissues of the diarthrodial joint including the articular cartilage, subchondral bone, synovium, and periarticular soft tissues (3). While the pathogenesis of OA has long been characterized primarily by degradation of the articular cartilage with secondary changes occurring in the subchondral bone, recent work has refocused attention on the role of the subchondral bone as an important component of the disease process. Indeed, remodeling of subchondral trabecular bone and calcified cartilage with increased bone turnover and reduced subchondral bone mineral density may be a primary phenomenon in not only the development but also the progression of OA (4,5). This hypothesis is supported by the positive results of trials of antiresorptive agents, including calcitonin and bisphosphonates, in preclinical models of osteoarthritis (6–11).

This chapter focuses on the clinical epidemiologic data demonstrating a relationship between both systemic and local changes in bone mass and turnover and the development and progression of lower limb OA. Early studies of this relationship were of the cross-sectional or case-control design and were unable to establish a cause-and-effect relationship. Furthermore, interpretation of results of these studies was influenced by heterogeneity in the measurement of bone mass and bone mineral density using different techniques at multiple sites and by variation in the definition of osteoarthritis, clinical or radiographic, and specific joint groups affected by OA, among other factors. More recent studies, however, have been of the cohort design, both retrospective and prospective, and provide insight into a causal relationship. Finally, the effects of osteoarthritis and longitudinal changes in bone mineral density and fracture risk are examined.

## OSTEOARTHRITIS OF THE HIP

Foss and Byers were the first to examine the relationship between bone mass and osteoarthritis of the hip (12). They found that the distribution of bone mass, estimated using the percent cortical area of the second metacarpal, differed between 140 patients who had undergone surgical treatment of hip fracture (mean age 81 years, 121 women) and 100 patients who had undergone surgical treatment of hip osteoarthritis (mean age 63 years, 68 women). The majority of patients with hip osteoarthritis had bone mass above the nintieth percentile, while 45% of the hip fracture cases had bone mass below the tenth percentile. The authors suggested that differences in body weight and physical activity between the groups might have contributed to the development and maintenance of higher bone density in the subjects with hip osteoarthritis. Since then numerous cross-sectional studies have examined the relationship between bone mass, measured by various techniques, and osteoarthritis of the hip, and this topic has been the subject of several reviews (13,14). In general, subjects with clinical or radiographic hip osteoarthritis have higher levels of bone mineral density than patients with osteoporosis and normal controls, although results differ somewhat by site of bone measurement.

Both cross-sectional and prospective data on the relationship between bone mineral density and hip osteoarthritis are available from the Study of Osteoporotic Fractures (SOF), a landmark cohort study of risk factors for hip fracture in 9,704 elderly white women begun in 1986 (15–20). Using data from the baseline examination and first follow-up visit, Nevitt and colleagues (15) showed that women with radiographic evidence of moderate to severe hip osteoarthritis had significantly higher age-adjusted bone mineral density at both appendicular (distal and proximal radius and calcaneus) and axial (lumbar spine and hip) sites than women without hip osteoarthritis. Further adjustment for anthropometric variables associated with bone mineral density had very little effect on this relationship. In contrast, while women with mild hip osteoarthritis had significantly higher age-adjusted bone mineral density at all sites except for the radius, after adjustment for anthropometric variables, only the differences at the femoral neck and lumbar spine remained statistically significant.

Radiographs of the pelvis were taken in women who attended the fourth follow-up visit a mean of 8 years after their baseline visit to allow the study of factors associated with the development and progression of radiographic hip osteoarthritis (16,18–20). Among 5,242 women with normal hip radiographs at their baseline visit, higher bone mineral density was associated with a significantly greater risk of developing radiographic hip osteoarthritis characterized by the presence of moderate or larger osteophytes; adjusted odds ratios were 1.5 and 1.9 for the third and highest quartiles compared with the lowest quartile for bone mineral density measured at either the femoral neck or distal radius (Fig. 11.1) (16). Similar results were found when calcaneus bone mineral density was used as the predictor variable. However, when the outcome was incidence of radiographic hip osteoarthritis characterized by marked joint space narrowing (minimal joint space of 1.5 mm or less), there was no relationship between baseline bone mineral density and incidence of radiographic hip osteoarthritis.

Few data are available on the longitudinal changes in bone mineral density in subjects with radiographic hip osteoarthritis. Arden and colleagues analyzed longitudinal data from 5,552 participants in the SOF followed for a mean of 7.4 years and reported that older women with

radiographic hip osteoarthritis had a slower adjusted rate of loss of bone mineral density at the femoral neck than women without hip osteoarthritis (17). The mean rate of decline in women with radiographic hip osteoarthritis was 0.29% per year compared with 0.51% per year in those without hip osteoarthritis. There was no significant difference in the mean rate of decline in bone mineral density at either the lumbar spine or calcaneus between women with and without radiographic hip osteoarthritis. The results reported by Burger and colleagues (21) from the Rotterdam Study contrast with those noted above. Among 714 men and 1,009 women aged 55 and over with serial bone mineral density measurements a mean of only 2.2 years apart, the rate of decline in femoral neck bone mineral density was significantly higher in those with radiographic hip osteoarthritis than in those without radiographic osteoarthritis at either the hip or knee in both sexes. These differences persisted even after adjustment for age, body mass index, and level of physical disability. The reasons for the discrepancy in findings between these two studies are not clear.

## OSTEOARTHRITIS OF THE KNEE

Several cross-sectional studies have reported the association between higher adjusted mean levels of bone mineral density measured at the lumbar spine and/or hip and the presence of radiographic osteoarthritis at the knee, characterized by the presence of osteophytes (21–26). Higher levels of bone mineral density at the lumbar spine and/or femoral neck are associated as well with an increased risk of developing radiographic osteoarthritis of the knee, characterized by the presence of osteophytes (27–30). Data from 473 elderly women (mean age 70 years) enrolled in the Framingham Study showed that women in the second through fourth quartiles of femoral neck bone mineral density had a two-fold greater multiple variable adjusted odds of developing incident radiographic knee osteoarthritis over 8 years of follow-up compared to women in the lowest quartile of bone mineral density (28).

Similar results were noted in analyses of data from both the Chingford Study and Baltimore Longitudinal Study of Aging. Among 715 middle-aged women (mean age 54 years) enrolled in the Chingford Study who were free of radiographic knee osteoarthritis at baseline and followed for 4 years, those who developed radiographic knee osteoarthritis defined by new osteophytes had significantly higher baseline bone mineral density at both the lumbar spine and femoral neck than women who did not develop incident osteophytes (29). Similarly, among a cohort of 289 men and women aged 20 and above (mean age 61 years) followed for a mean of 10 years between radiographs, the odds of developing incident radiographic knee osteoarthritis was significantly greater among

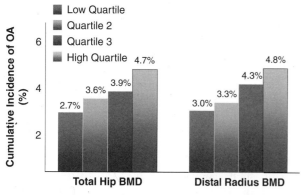

**Figure 11.1** Cumulative incidence of radiographic hip osteoarthritis characterized by moderate or larger osteophytes by quartile of bone mineral density measured either at the femoral neck or distal radius, Study of Osteoporotic Fractures. Data from Nevitt M, et al. High BMD increases the risk of new hip OA in elderly women, but osteoporosis is not protective. *Osteoporosis Int* 2000;11[Suppl 2]:S101(abst).

those with higher baseline lumbar spine but not femoral neck bone mineral density, even after adjusting for potential confounding variables (30).

In contrast to higher femoral neck bone mineral density being a risk factor for the development of incident radiographic knee osteoarthritis, higher femoral neck bone mineral density was protective against progression of radiographic knee osteoarthritis, characterized by joint space narrowing (28). Women in the third and fourth quartiles of femoral neck bone mineral density had significantly multiple variable adjusted odds of having progressive radiographic knee osteoarthritis over 8 years of follow-up compared to women in the lowest quartile of bone mineral density. Similar trends not reaching statistical significance were noted among women in the Chingford Study (29).

As with hip osteoarthritis, results of analyses of the longitudinal changes in bone mineral density in subjects with radiographic knee osteoarthritis compared with subjects with normal knee radiographs are conflicting (21,27,30). Burger and colleagues noted that women but not men with radiographic knee osteoarthritis had a greater rate of decline in femoral neck bone mineral density than subjects with neither radiographic hip or knee osteoarthritis (21). In women, the rate of decline increased with greater baseline severity as defined by Kellgren-Lawrence grade and was independent of level of physical disability. In contrast, Sowers and colleagues found that pre- and perimenopausal women (mean age 37 years) with radiographic knee osteoarthritis did not have a decline in their age-adjusted bone mineral density over 3 years while women without knee osteoarthritis did (27). Furthermore, the differences in change in lumbar spine but not femoral neck bone mineral density were statistically significant between these groups. Hochberg and colleagues studied the rate of decline in bone mineral density at the distal radius in 296 white male and 138 white female participants aged 20 and above (mean age 61 years) in the Baltimore Longitudinal Study of Aging (30). The mean interval between first and last bone mineral density measurements was $12 \pm 4$ years in men and $6 \pm 2$ years in women.

The adjusted rate of decline in bone mineral density was significantly greater than zero in both men and women with and without radiographic knee OA; these rates did not significantly differ from one another.

## RELATIONSHIP BETWEEN RADIOGRAPHIC OSTEOARTHRITIS AND RISK OF FRACTURES

While patients with radiographic hip and/or knee osteoarthritis have higher adjusted levels of bone mineral density, they do not appear to be protected from the complications of low bone mineral density as there appears to be no difference in the rate of fractures. Among older women in the Study of Osteoporotic Fractures with radiographic hip osteoarthritis, there was no difference in the risk of osteoporotic fractures, including both hip and vertebral fractures, over a mean follow-up of 7.4 years (17). A lack of association between radiographic osteoarthritis and subsequent osteoporotic fractures was also noted in data from the Chingford Study population (31). Possible explanations for this absence of fracture risk reduction despite the higher adjusted bone mineral density may include differences in muscle strength and body sway, which might contribute to the risk of falling (32). Bergink and colleagues adjusted for potential confounding variables, including both bone mineral density and parameters of postural stability, and found that subjects with radiographic knee osteoarthritis had significantly higher incidence of both vertebral and nonvertebral fractures than persons without radiographic knee osteoarthritis (33).

## MECHANISMS FOR THE ASSOCIATION BETWEEN HIGHER SYSTEMIC BONE MINERAL DENSITY AND RADIOGRAPHIC OSTEOARTHRITIS

Several sources of data suggest that the relationship between higher bone mineral density and radiographic osteoarthritis may be because of shared genetic factors between these conditions (34). Daughters of women with radiographic hand osteoarthritis have higher adjusted bone mineral density at the hip than daughters of women with normal hand radiographs, even after adjustment for daughter's body mass index and mother's body mass index and bone mineral density (35). On the other hand, mothers of patients with osteoarthritis of the hip had a reduced rate of hip fractures than expected based on rates in the general population (36). Data from the St. Thomas Adult Twin Register confirmed the presence of a genetic contribution as well as supported a role for local factors specifically in subjects with hip osteoarthritis (37). These investigators studied 160 monozygotic and 414 dizygotic white female twin pairs, aged 40 and above, and found that the adjusted odds of having radiographic features of hip osteoarthritis, characterized by osteophytes, was 1.80 per unit difference in bone mineral density of the ipsilateral femoral neck. There was no association when radiographic hip osteoarthritis was defined solely on the basis of joint space narrowing. There was also no significant association between radiographic hip osteoarthritis and bone mineral density at the contralateral hip, lumbar spine, or total body.

A number of studies have examined the association between specific candidate genes known to be associated with bone mineral density with osteoarthritis (reviewed in 38). Most but not all studies have found an association between polymorphisms of the vitamin D receptor gene and radiographic osteoarthritis (39–45). Similarly, the majority of the studies of the estrogen receptor alpha gene and osteoarthritis have shown an association between polymorphisms in this gene with radiographic changes, particularly osteophytosis (43,46,47).

Another factor that might explain the relationship between higher bone mineral density and radiographic hip and/or knee osteoarthritis is effects on prostaglandin metabolism related to the use of nonsteroidal antiinflammatory drugs for symptomatic management of osteoarthritis (48–50).

## BONE TURNOVER IN OSTEOARTHRITIS

Cross-sectional studies have produced conflicting results on differences in bone turnover in persons with radiographic osteoarthritis and controls (reviewed in 51). Stewart and colleagues (52) reported that bone turnover, as measured by urinary excretion of pyridinium crosslinks, was increased in patients with radiographic osteoarthritis compared to age-matched controls; no differences were noted, however, in serum osteocalcin levels between the groups. Garnero and colleagues, on the other hand, found that three measures of bone turnover, serum osteocalcin and the serum and urinary C-telopeptide of type I collagen (CTX-I), were all significantly lower in 67 patients with knee osteoarthritis compared with age-matched healthy controls (53). Similarly, Sowers and colleagues (27) also found lower serum osteocalcin levels among younger women with knee osteoarthritis compared to controls.

A retrospective cohort study to examine the relationship between bone-turnover markers in patients with osteoarthritis was reported by Battica and colleagues (54). They compared urinary excretion of two markers of bone resorption, CTX and N-telopeptide of type I collagen (NTX), in 71 postmenopausal women with either incident or progressive knee osteoarthritis, 36 women with stable nonprogressive knee osteoarthritis, and 50 controls with normal radiographs and bone mineral density. Urinary excretion of NTX was significantly greater in women with incident or progressive knee osteoarthritis compared with both controls and women with nonprogressive osteoarthritis; urinary excretion of CTX was significantly greater in women with incident or progressive knee osteoarthritis than controls but did not differ from that in women with nonprogressive osteoarthritis (Fig. 11.2). These data suggest that elevated bone turnover is associated with development and/or progression of radiographic knee osteoarthritis and extend older observations of Dieppe and colleagues (55) based on scintigraphy.

## SUBCHONDRAL TRABECULAR BONE IN OSTEOARTHRITIS

Subchondral trabecular bone volume in the femoral head of patients with hip osteoarthritis has been reported to be increased largely due to an increase in trabecular number

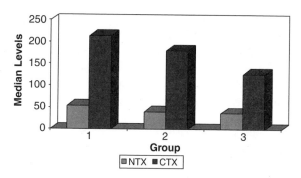

**Figure 11.2** Median average values for urinary excretion of type I collagen N-terminal telopeptides (NTX, nanomoles of bone collagen equivalent per millimoles of creatinine) and C-terminal telopeptides (CTX, milligrams per moles of creatinine) by presence of incident and/or progressive radiographic knee osteoarthritis *(Group 1)*, nonprogressive radiographic knee osteoarthritis *(Group 2)*, or controls without radiographic knee osteoarthritis or osteoporosis *(Group 3)*. (Data from Battica P, Cline G, Hart DJ, et al. Evidence for increased bone resorption in patients with progressive knee osteoarthritis. *Arthritis Rheum* 2002;46:3178–3184.)

and reduced separation between trabeculae (56). Despite the increase in trabecular volume, the individual trabeculae are less mineralized resulting in reduced material density (57). This reduced mineralization is the result of increased turnover in the subchondral trabecular bone (58). Similar changes in subchondral trabecular bone have been identified in the knee using the technique of macroradiography combined with Fractal Signature Analysis (59). Patients with early knee osteoarthritis have thickening of the horizontal subchondral trabeculae; in later stages of disease, the vertical trabeculae become thinner and perforated resulting in less dense, more porous, and mechanically weaker bone. These findings were confirmed in recent studies that measured bone mineral density in the tibial plateau in patients with knee osteoarthritis. Karvonen and colleagues (60) found significantly decreased periarticular subchondral tibial bone mineral density in women with radiographic knee osteoarthritis compared to controls with normal knee radiographs. In a 1-year longitudinal study of 56 patients with symptomatic knee osteoarthritis, those subjects in the highest quartile of tibial subchondral bone mineral density had significantly greater loss of joint space in the medial compartment than subjects in the lowest quartile (61). This relationship may be explained by inclusion of both subchondral cortical as well as trabecular bone in the region of interest resulting in measurement of areas of subchondral sclerosis, where the apparent density differs from the actual material density (5).

## SUMMARY

Clinical epidemiologic studies generally demonstrate a consistent causal association between bone mineral density and radiographic changes of osteoarthritis at the hip and/or knee, characterized by osteophytosis. This association probably reflects the role of shared genetic factors contributing to both the development of higher peak bone mineral density and greater endochondral ossification of calcified cartilage. Localized changes in the subchondral trabecular bone in patients with osteoarthritis of the hip and/or knee suggest, however, that the material density of subchondral bone is reduced. This is probably related to increased local bone turnover. The findings that antiresorptive agents inhibit the development and/or progression of cartilage lesions in preclinical models of osteoarthritis suggest a potential role for these agents in the treatment of patients with early osteoarthritis (62). Preliminary data from a randomized, placebo-controlled trial of risedronate in patients with knee osteoarthritis provide limited support for this hypothesis (63). Future studies in this area are warranted and eagerly anticipated.

# REFERENCES

1. Lawrence RC, Helmick CG, Arnett FC, et al. Estimates of the prevalence of arthritis and selected musculoskeletal disorders in the United States. *Arthritis Rheum* 1998;41:778–789.
2. Yelin E, Callahan LF. The economic cost and social and psychological impact of musculoskeletal conditions. National Arthritis Data Work Group. *Arthritis Rheum* 1995;38:1351–1362.
3. Felson DT. Osteoarthritis: new insights. Part I: The disease and its risk factors. *Ann Intern Med* 2000;133:635–646.
4. Burr DB, Radin EL. Microfractures and microcracks in subchondral bone: are they relevant to osteoarthrosis? *Rheum Dis Clin North Am* 2003;29:675–685.
5. Burr DB. Anatomy and physiology of mineralized tissues: role in the pathogenesis of osteoarthritis. *Osteoarthritis Cart* 2004;12[Suppl A]:S20–S30.
6. Manicourt DH, Altman RD, Williams JM, et al. Treatment with calcitonin suppresses the responses of bone, cartilage, and synovium in the early stages of canine experimental osteoarthritis and significantly reduces the severity of the cartilage lesions. *Arthritis Rheum* 1999;42:1159–1167.
7. Myers SL, Brandt KD, Burr DB, et al. Effects of a bisphosphonate on bone histomorphometry and dynamics in the canine cruciate deficiency model of osteoarthritis. *J Rheumatol* 1999;26:2645–2653.
8. Muehleman C, Green J, Williams JM, et al. The effect of bone remodeling inhibition by zoledronic acid in an animal model of cartilage matrix damage. *Osteoarthritis Cart* 2002;10:226–233.
9. Meyer JM, Farmer RW, Prenger MC. Risedronate but not alendronate slows disease progression in the guinea pig model of primary osteoarthritis. *J Bone Miner Res* 2001;16[Suppl 1]:S305(abst).
10. Meyer JM, Dansereau SM, Farmer RW, et al. Bisphosphonates structurally similar to risedronate slow disease progression in the guinea pig model of primary osteoarthritis. *Arthritis Rheum* 2001;44[9 Suppl]:S307 (abst).
11. Hayemi T, Pickareski M, Wesolowski GAA, et al. Alendronate inhibits osteophyte formation and partially protects cartilage deterioration in the rat anterior cruciate ligament transection model of osteoarthritis. *Ann Rheum Dis* 2003;62[Suppl 1]:110 (abst).
12. Foss MVL, Byers PD. Bone density, osteoarthritis of the hip, and fracture of the upper end of the femur. *Ann Rheum Dis* 1972;31:259–264.
13. Star VL, Hochberg MC. Osteoporosis in patients with rheumatic diseases. *Rheum Dis Clinic North Am* 1994;20:561–576.
14. Stewart A, Black AJ. Bone mineral density in osteoarthritis. *Curr Opin Rheumatol* 2000;12:464–467.
15. Nevitt MC, Lane NE, Scott JC, et al. Radiographic osteoarthritis of the hip and bone mineral density. *Arthritis Rheum* 1995;38:907–916.
16. Nevitt M, Lane N, Hochberg M, Williams E, for the SOF Research Group. High BMD increases the risk of new hip OA in elderly women, but osteoporosis is not protective. *Osteoporosis Int* 2000;11[Suppl 2]:S101(abst).
17. Arden NK, Nevitt MC, Lane NE, et al. Osteoarthritis and risk of falls, rates of bone loss, and osteoporotic fractures. Study of Osteoporotic Fractures Research Group. *Arthritis Rheum* 1999;42:1378–1385.
18. Lane NE, Williams EN, Hung Y-Y, et al. Association of nitrate use with risk of new radiographic features of hip osteoarthritis in elderly white women: the Study of Osteoporotic Fractures. *Arthritis Rheum (Arthritis Care Res)* 2003;49:752–758.
19. Lane NE, Nevitt MC, Hochberg MC, et al. Progression of radiographic hip osteoarthritis over 8 years in a community sample of elderly white women. *Arthritis Rheum* 2004;50: 1477–1486.
20. Hochberg MC. Do risk factors for incident hip osteoarthritis (OA) differ from those for progression of hip OA? *J Rheumatol* 2004;31[Suppl 70]: 6–9.
21. Burger H, van Daele PL, Odding E, et al. Association of radiographically evident osteoarthritis with higher bone mineral density and increased bone loss with age. The Rotterdam Study. *Arthritis Rheum* 1996;39:81–86.
22. Hannan MT, Anderson JJ, Zhang Y, et al. Bone mineral density and knee osteoarthritis in elderly men and women. The Framingham Study. *Arthritis Rheum* 1993;36:1671–1680.
23. Hart DJ, Mootoosamy I, Doyle DV, Spector TD. The relationship between osteoarthritis and osteoporosis in the general population: the Chingford Study. *Ann Rheum Dis* 1994;53:158–162.
24. Hochberg MC, Lethbridge-Cejku M, Scott WW Jr, et al. Upper extremity bone mass and osteoarthritis of the knees: data from the Baltimore Longitudinal Study of Aging. *J Bone Miner Res* 1995;11:432–438.
25. Lethbridge-Cejku M, Tobin JD, Scott WW Jr, et al. Axial and hip bone mineral density and radiographic changes of osteoarthritis of the knee: data from the Baltimore Longitudinal Study of Aging. *J Rheumatol* 1996;23:1943–1948.
26. Sowers MF, Hochberg M, Crabbe JP, et al. Association of bone mineral density and sex hormone levels with osteoarthritis of the hand and knee in premenopausal women. *Am J Epidemiol* 1996; 143:38–47.
27. Sowers M, Lachance L, Jamadar D, et al. The associations of bone mineral density and bone turnover markers with osteoarthritis of the hand and knee in pre-and perimenopausal women. *Arthritis Rheum* 1999;42:483–489.
28. Zhang Y, Hannan MT, Chaisson CE, et al. Bone mineral density and risk of incident and progressive radiographic knee osteoarthritis in women. *J Rheumatol* 2000;27:1032–1037.
29. Hart DJ, Cronin C, Daniels M, et al. The relationship of bone density and fracture to incident and progressive radiographic osteoarthritis of the knee. The Chingford Study. *Arthritis Rheum* 2002;46:92–99.
30. Hochberg MC, Lethbridge-Cejku M, Tobin JD. Bone mineral density and osteoarthritis: data from the Baltimore Longitudinal Study of Aging. *Osteoarthritis Cart* 2004;12[Suppl A]:S45–S48.
31. Arden NK, Griffiths GO, Hart DJ, et al. The association between osteoarthritis and osteoporotic fracture: the Chingford Study. *Br J Rheumatol* 1996;35:1299–1304.
32. Jones G, Nguyen T, Sambrook PN, et al. Osteoarthritis, bone density, postural stability, and osteoporotic fractures: a population based study. *J Rheumatol* 1995;22:921–925.
33. Bergink AP, van der Klift M, Hofman A, et al. Osteoarthritis of the knee is associated with vertebral and nonvertebral fractures in the elderly: the Rotterdam Study. *Arthritis Rheum (Arthritis Care Res)* 2003;49:648–657.
34. Dequeker J, Aerssens J, Luyten FP. Osteoarthritis and osteoporosis: clinical and research evidence of inverse relationship. *Aging Clin Exp Res* 2003;15:426–439.
35. Naganathan V, Zochling J, March L, Sambrook PN. Peak bone mass is increased in the hip in daughters of women with osteoarthritis. *Bone* 2002;30:287–292.
36. Astrom J, Beertema J. Reduced risk of hip fracture in the mothers of patients with osteoarthritis of the hip. *J Bone Jt Surg* 1992;74B:270–271.

37. Antoniades L, MacGregor AJ, Matson M, Spector TD. A cotwin control study of the relationship between hip osteoarthritis and bone mineral density. *Arthritis Rheum* 2000;43:1450–1455.

38. Jordan JM, Kraus VB, Hochberg MC. Genetics of osteoarthritis. *Curr Rheum Rep* 2004;6(1):7–13.

39. Uitterlinden AG, Burger H, Huang Q, et al. Vitamin D receptor genotype is associated with radiographic osteoarthritis at the knee. *J Clin Invest* 1997;100:259–263.

40. Keen RW, Hart DJ, Lanchbury JS, Spector TD. Association of early osteoarthritis of the knee with a Taq I polymorphism of the vitamin D receptor gene. *Arthritis Rheum* 1997;40:1444–1449.

41. Aerssens J, Dequeker J, Peeters J, et al. Lack of association between osteoarthritis of the hip and gene polymorphisms of VDR, COL1A1 and COL2A1 in postmenopausal women. *Arthritis Rheum* 1998;41:1946–1950.

42. Huang J, Ushiyama T, Inoue K, et al. Vitamin D receptor gene polymorphisms and osteoarthritis of the hand, hip, and knee: a case-control study in Japan. *Rheumatology* 2000;39:79–84.

43. Loughlin J, Sinsheimer JS, Mustafa Z, et al. Association analysis of the vitamin D receptor gene, the type I collagen gene COL1A1, and the estrogen receptor gene in idiopathic osteoarthritis. *J Rheumatol* 2000;27:779–784.

44. Uitterlinden AG, Burger H, van Duijn CM, et al. Adjacent genes, for COL2A1 and the vitamin D receptor, are associated with separate features of radiographic osteoarthritis of the knee. *Arthritis Rheum* 2000;43:1456–1464.

45. Baldwin CT, Cupples LA, Joost O, et al. Absence of linkage or association for osteoarthritis with the vitamin D receptor/type II collagen locus: the Framingham Osteoarthritis Study. *J Rheumatol* 2002;29:161–165.

46. Ushiyama T, Ueyama H, Inoue K, et al. Estrogen receptor gene polymorphism and generalized osteoarthritis. *J Rheumatol* 1998;25:134–137.

47. Bergink AP, van Meurs JB, Loughlin J, et al. Estrogen receptor alpha gene haplotype is associated with radiographic osteoarthritis of the knee in elderly men and women. *Arthritis Rheum* 2003;48:1913–1922.

48. Bauer DC, Orwoll ES, Fox KM, et al. Aspirin and NSAID use in older women: effect on bone mineral density and fracture risk, Study of Osteoporotic Fractures Research Group. *J Bone Miner Res* 1996;11:29–35.

49. Morton DJ, Barrett-Connor EL, Schneider DL. Nonsteroidal anti-inflammatory drugs and bone mineral density in older women. *J Bone Miner Res* 1998;13:1924–1931.

50. Carbone LD, Tylavsky FA, Cauley JA, et al. Association between bone mineral density and the use of nonsteroidal anti-inflammatory drugs and aspirin: impact of cyclooxygenase selectivity. *J Bone Miner Res* 2003;18:1795–1802.

51. Hunter DJ, Spector TD. The role of bone metabolism in osteoarthritis. *Curr Rheum Rep* 2003;5:15–19.

52. Stewart A, Black A, Robins SP, Reid DM. Bone density and bone turnover in patients with osteoarthritis and osteoporosis. *J Rheumatol* 1999;26:622–626.

53. Garnero P, Piperno M, Gineyts E, et al. Cross sectional evaluation of biochemical markers of bone, cartilage, and synovial tissue metabolism in patients with knee osteoarthritis: relations with disease activity and joint damage. *Ann Rheum Dis* 2001;60:619–626.

54. Battica P, Cline G, Hart DJ, et al. Evidence for increased bone resorption in patients with progressive knee osteoarthritis. *Arthritis Rheum* 2002;46:3178–3184.

55. Dieppe P, Cushnaghan J, Young P, Kirwan J. Prediction of the progression of joint space narrowing in osteoarthritis of the knee by bone scintigraphy. *Ann Rheum Dis* 1993;53:557–563.

56. Fazzalari NL, Parkinson IH. Fractal properties of subchondral cancellous bone in severe osteoarthritis of the hip. *J Bone Miner Res* 1997;12:632–640.

57. Li B, Aspden RM. Composition and mechanical properties of cancellous bone from the femoral head of patients with osteoporosis and osteoarthritis. *J Bone Miner Res* 1997;12:641–651.

58. Mansell JP, Bailey AJ. Abnormal cancellous bone metabolism in osteoarthritis. *J Clin Invest* 1998;101:1596–1603.

59. Buckland-Wright C. Subchondral bone changes in hand and knee osteoarthritis detected by radiography. *Osteoarthritis Cart* 2004;12[Suppl A]:S10–S19.

60. Karvonen RL, Miller PR, Nelson DA, et al. Periarticular osteoporosis in osteoarthritis of the knee. *J Rheumatol* 1998;25:2187–2194.

61. Bruyere OO, Dardenne C, Lejeune E, et al. Subchondral tibial bone mineral density predicts future joint space narrowing at the medial femoro-tibial compartment in patients with knee osteoarthritis. *Bone* 2003;32:541–545.

62. Spector TD. Bisphosphonates: potential therapeutic agents for disease modification in osteoarthritis. *Aging Clin Exp Res* 2003;15:413–418.

63. Spector TD, Conaghan P, Buckland-Wright JC, et al. Risedronate produces disease modification and symptomatic benefit in the treatment of knee osteoarthritis: results from the BRISK Study. *Arthritis Rheum* 2003;48:3650 (abst).

# Bone Loss Due to Medications

# Glucocorticoid-Induced Osteoporosis: Epidemiology

*Lenore M. Buckley*

In 1932, Harvey Cushing described Cushing's disease and the association between excess endogenous glucocorticoids (GCs) and fractures—occurring in up to 50% of Cushing's disease patients (1). Fractures caused by excess GCs remained a rare event until 1948 when substance E (cortisol) was first used to treat a patient with rheumatoid arthritis (RA). By 1950, fractures were described as an adverse event in RA patients who received exogenous GCs (2), and in 1994 Saag and colleagues (3) reported that fractures were the most common serious adverse event associated with long-term GC use in patients with RA.

Over the last 20 years, there have been significant advances in the accuracy, reproducibility, and reliability of the technology available to assess bone mass using bone densitometry. Because of these advances, the relationship between GC use and fractures has slowly unfolded revealing risk factors, dose and timing relationships, and the potential for recovery of bone mass when GC treatment is discontinued. In addition, the mechanisms of the detrimental effects of GC on bone are better understood, and there have been significant pharmacologic advances in treatments to prevent bone loss during GC treatment and to treat GC-induced osteoporosis. This chapter will review the epidemiology of GC-induced osteoporosis.

## GLUCOCORTICOID USE AND BONE DENSITY: EFFECTS OF DOSE AND TIMING OF TREATMENT

In 1987, Sambrook and colleagues (4) reported the results of one of the first studies examining the relationship between low-dose GCs and bone mineral density (BMD). Using dual photon absorptiometry, they assessed bone density in 111 patients with RA and found an association between low-dose prednisone use (average dosage 10 mg/d) and lower hip BMD in men but not in women (who were taking a lower mean dosage of prednisone of 8 mg/d). In 1993, Hall and colleagues (5) reported an association between even lower doses of GCs and bone mass (5). In a study of BMD using dual energy x-ray absorptiometry (DXA) in 195 women with RA, current GC use at an average dose of 6.9 mg was associated with a reduction in BMD of 6.9% at the lumbar spine (LS) and 7.4% at the hip after adjustment for potential confounding variables. In addition, Hall reported that past users of GCs had BMD similar to those who had never used GCs, suggesting that bone mass can increase after GC treatment is terminated. In 1995, Buckley and colleagues (6) reported lower lumbar spine BMD in GC-treated RA patients taking as little as 5 to 9 mg per day of prednisone but no effect of this lower dose of GCs on femoral neck BMD (6). This is consistent with the clinical observation that vertebral and rib fractures are more common than hip fractures in GC users.

The pattern and timing of bone loss was unclear from these retrospective cross-sectional studies. In 1993, Laan and colleagues (7) reported the effects of low-dose GCs on BMD in a prospective study of RA patients starting treatment with prednisone at a dosage of 10 mg per day. Patients were treated with prednisone for 12 weeks, and the treatment was discontinued by week 20. Using quantitative computed tomography (QCT), a sensitive measure of trabecular bone density, they reported an 8.2% decline in the BMD of the trabecular bone of the LS but little change in the cortical bone of the vertebral body. After withdrawal of GCs, the trabecular lumbar spine BMD increased 5.2%. This study demonstrated that bone loss occurs very quickly after the initiation of GC treatment and that trabecular bone is more sensitive to the detrimental effect of GCs and confirmed that bone density increases after GC treatment is discontinued.

Later clinical trials have given a similar picture of rapid onset of bone loss at the initiation of GC treatment. In a study of the effects of calcitonin and calcitriol in new users of prednisone, patients receiving calcium supplementation alone had a change of −4.3% in LS BMD in year one (average prednisone dosage of 13.5 mg/d) and −2.35% in year two (average prednisone dosage of 7.5 mg/d) and a change of −2.9% and −1.35% at the femoral neck at year one and two, respectively (8). Among long-term GC users, bone loss is slow and restricted primarily to the LS. Buckley and colleagues (9) reported a 2% decrease in LS BMD and no significant change in femoral neck BMD in patients with RA taking an average dosage of prednisone of 5.6 mg/d. Saag and colleagues (10) reported a 1% to 2% decrease in lumbar spine bone mass in new and chronic users of GCs receiving only calcium and vitamin D supplements.

A number of studies have demonstrated that the amount of bone loss from GC treatment is similar in men and women, both premenopausal and postmenopausal (10,11). However, fractures are more likely to occur in those with the lowest bone mass; therefore, most studies find the highest fracture rates in postmenopausal women.

## GLUCOCORTICOID USE AND FRACTURES

In 1984, in a retrospective cohort study of 388 patients with RA followed at the Mayo Clinic, Hooyman and colleagues (12) found an increased risk of all fractures (RR = 1.5) in patients with RA compared to healthy controls (12). Patients with RA who were not treated with GCs had a relative risk (RR) of hip fracture of 1.4 compared to a RR of 2.15 in RA patients who were GC users, and the risk of vertebral fractures was four times greater in GC users, than nonusers. The risk of pelvic fractures was also elevated. In this study, estrogen use appeared to be protective. The small number of patients did not allow a more detailed study of the timing and dosage of GC use on fracture risk. In a similar retrospective study, De Nijs and colleagues (13) studied the incidence of vertebral fractures in 205 RA patients treated with GCs and 205 RA controls. They reported that 25% of GC treated patients had a vertebral deformity and 8% had a symptomatic vertebral fracture compared to 13% and 1.5%, respectively in non-GC-treated RA patients. For every 1 mg increase in prednisone dose there was an increase in the RR of fracture of 1.05.

There are few *prospective* studies of fracture in GC users. Saag and colleagues (10) reported a vertebral fracture rate of 3.7% at 1 year in new and chronic users of GCs who received calcium and vitamin D in a clinical trial and that postmenopausal women had the highest fracture rate (7.6%). Van Staa and colleagues (14) reviewed prospective data from the risedronate trials in GC-treated patients. They examined new and long-term GC users who received placebo treatment during these trials and found a vertebral fracture rate of 16.5% at 1 year in patients who received only calcium supplementation (with or without vitamin D). Fracture rates were similar in new and long-term users of GCs. In this study, the risk factors associated with incident fracture risk were baseline BMD [RR = 1.85, 95% confidence interval (CI):1.06–3.21] and daily GC dose (RR = 1.62, 95% CI:1.11–2.36). New fractures occurred in 12.3% of patients with a daily prednisone dose of ≤ 15 mg and 25% of those taking prednisone at a daily dose of more than 15 mg.

None of these studies were large enough to address the relationship between GC use and femoral fractures. In 2000, van Staa and colleagues (15) reported the results of a large retrospective cohort study from the UK General Practice Data Base (GPDB) comparing the relative rates of fracture in 244,235 patients receiving oral GC matched to patients of similar age and sex receiving nonsystemic GC prescriptions (topical, aural, ophthalmic, and nasal). The GC-treated patients were followed for an average of 1.3 years, received a mean of 6.8 oral GC prescriptions per year, and were most likely to be taking oral GCs for a respiratory condition (40%). Of the users and nonusers of oral GCs, 1.6% and 1.3%, respectively, had sustained a vertebral fracture in the year before the study. Over the study period, the incidence of nonvertebral fracture was 2.0 per 100 patient years in the oral GC users compared to 1.3 in the non-GC-treated group (Fig. 12A.1). After adjustment for possible confounders, the RR of nonvertebral fractures was 1.33 (95% CI:1.29–1.38). The RR of hip fracture was increased in GC users to 1.61 (95% CI:1.47–1.76), and the RR of vertebral fractures was even higher at 2.6 (95% CI:2.31–2.92).

A number of studies have suggested a relationship between GC dose and fracture risk. In a study of RA patients in the Arthritis, Rheumatism and Aging Medical Information (ARAMIS) database, only history of osteoporosis and prednisone use predicted time to fracture with a RR of fracture of 6.3 in patients with known osteoporosis and 1.9 for prednisone users (16). Fracture rates were highest in those taking prednisone at a dosage over 5 mg/day. The study by van Staa and colleagues (15) confirmed a relationship between GC dose and fracture risk. In their study, patients were divided into three groups by average daily prednisolone dose—low dose (<2.5 mg), moderate dose (2.5–7.5 mg), and high dose (>7.5 mg). Vertebral fracture rates increased in the low-dose group and femoral fractures increased in the moderate dose group (Fig. 12A.2). This study confirmed three important aspects of the relationship between GCs and fractures:

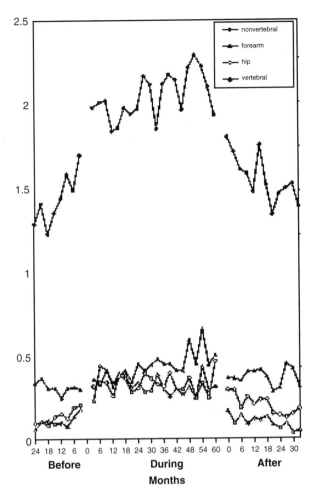

**Figure 12A.1** Incidence of nonvertebral, forearm, hip, and vertebral fractures before, during, and after corticosteroid treatment. (From van Staa TP, Leukens HGM, Abenhaim L, et al. Use of oral corticosteroids and risk of fractures. *J Bone Miner Res* 2000;15:993–1002, with permission.)

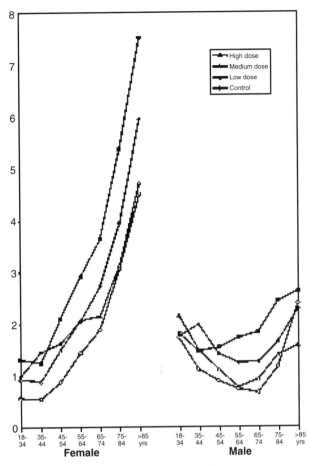

**Figure 12A.2** Incidence of nonvertebral fractures stratified by daily corticosteroid dose, age, and gender. (From van Staa TP, Leukens HGM, Abenhaim L, et al. Use of oral corticosteroids and risk of fractures. *J Bone Miner Res* 2000;15:993–1002, with permission.)

- GCs effects on fracture are dose dependent.
- Even low dosages of GCs (≤2.5 mg/d) increase vertebral fracture risk.
- Slightly higher dosages of GCs (≥5.0 mg/d) are needed to increase hip fracture risk.

In addition, van Staa and colleagues (15) confirmed that fracture risk increases with age in both men and women and that fracture rates are highest in postmenopausal women. Fracture risk increases rapidly after the initiation of GC treatment rising to a relative risk of 2 during the first 3 months, and that rate remained stable over 5 years of follow-up.

A number of studies have suggested that the effects of GCs on bone are at least partly reversible. Studies of BMD in patients with endogenous Cushing's disease showed rapid improvement in bone mass after surgery (17,18). Van Staa and colleagues (15) also reported a rapid decline in fracture risk in the first year after the cessation of GC treatment (Fig. 12A.1). In a subgroup of 7095 GC-treated patients in the GPDB who stopped oral GCs after at least 6 months of use, the nonvertebral fracture rate was 2.4 per 100 person years (100 cases) in the first year and 1.8 in the second year (41 cases). It is not clear from this data if the higher risk of fracture resulting from GC treatment is entirely reversible.

Interestingly, the increased risk of fractures in the patients in the GPDB may not solely be the result of the effects of GCs on bone. GCs can cause myopathy, increasing the tendency to fall. Van Staa and colleagues (15) found that the rate of falls in the GPDB cohort rose rapidly after GC treatment was initiated (1.6 per 100 person years in the year before the study and 2.8 in the first 3 months of GC treatment.)

## Do Fracture Rates Occur at a Higher Bone Density in GC-Treated Patients?

There is debate about whether fractures occur at higher BMD in GC-treated patients than in non-GC-treated patients. It has been hypothesized that GCs could affect fractures in ways other than through their effects on bone density, such as changes in bone architecture, bone resorption, or muscle strength and balance. Two studies of patients with prevalent vertebral fractures have shown similar BMD levels in GC- and non-GC-treated patients (19,20). Selby and colleagues (19) looked at the BMD and x-rays of patients referred to participating centers for osteoporosis. They compared vertebral fracture rates in patients who were currently taking prednisone at a daily dose of 5 mg (n = 82) and those who were not receiving GC treatment (n = 370). Vertebral fractures were more common in the GC-treated patients (53% versus 35%) and were more likely to be multiple (37% versus 15%). Among patients with vertebral fractures, the median lumbar spine T score was slightly lower in GC-treated patients (−2.74 versus −2.65), but the difference was not statistically significant.

To address this question, van Staa and colleagues (14) collected data prospectively from osteoporosis clinical trials assessing the efficacy of risedronate (14). Using data from the placebo-treated patients, they compared vertebral fracture rates in the 59 GC-treated postmenopasual (PMP) women in two risedronate GC trials (new and long-term GC users) with 1,899 PMP women who were not taking GCs. The GC users were younger (64.7 years versus 74.1 years), had higher baseline BMD, (T score at the lumbar spine was −1.8 versus −2.6), and had fewer prevalent fractures (49.2% versus 58.3%) at the initiation of the studies. Over the year of follow-up, however, the GC-treated patients had a higher incidence of new vertebral fractures (16% versus 7%) at lower mean BMD (Fig. 12A.3). The adjusted relative risk of fracture was 5.67 in GC users (95% CI:2.57–12.54). The authors concluded, at similar levels of BMD, postmenopausal women taking GCs, compared to nonusers of GCs, had a considerably higher risk of fracture. However, the BMD used in the analysis was taken at the start of the study (when some patients had just initiated GC treatment) rather than at the time of fracture or at the end of the year. So, it is unclear whether the fractures occurred at higher BMD in GC users or if the BMD had dropped during GC treatment and fractures were occurring at similar BMD to that of non-GC users who had fractures. The authors commented that another limitation of the study was the small number of GC users and inability to control for disease severity in users and nonusers of GCs.

## BONE MASS AND FRACTURES IN GLUCOCORTICOID-TREATED CHILDREN

### Growth

The effects of GC treatment on bone are more complex in children because GCs have detrimental effects on both bone growth (and, therefore, total bone volume) and bone density. Childhood growth rate and final adult height are important determinants of fractures. People with a

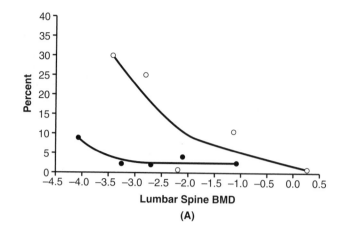

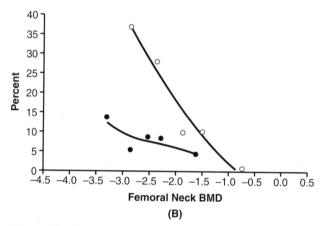

**Figure 12A.3** Incidence of vertebral fracture in patients receiving glucocorticoids (GCs) *(open box)* compared with nonusers of GCs *(*)*, by baseline lumbar spine bone mineral density (BMD) and femoral neck BMD. Individual data points correspond to the incidence in subgroups of the GC user and nonuser populations, based on quintiles of baseline BMD. The solid line is a curve representing smoothing of the individual estimates. (From van Staa TP, Laan RF, Barton P, et al. Bone density threshold and other predictors of vertebral fracture in patients receiving oral glucocorticoids. *Arthritis Rheum* 2003;48:3224–3229, with permission.)

childhood growth rate more than one standard deviation below the mean have a four-fold increase in risk of fracture (21). GCs impede skeletal growth leading to short stature in some children, but the extent of this effect and the potential for recovery of growth velocity is not well understood. In a study of 362 children with asthma, children on continuous GC treatment had a lower mean height than non-GC-treated children and those who received intermittent GC treatment (22). Foote and colleagues (23) described a similar relationship between growth and GC use in children with nephrotic syndrome, but most children recovered linear growth after GC treatment was discontinued. Kotaniemi (24) studied BMD and growth in children with juvenile chronic arthritis and found that the 43 patients with polyarticular arthritis who received GC treatment were significantly shorter than non-GC-treated children (height 143.0 cm versus 150.6 cm, respectively) and that GC treated children had lower BMD and volumetric BMD at both the lumbar spine and femoral neck ($p < 0.01$). Chesney and colleagues (25) found that GC use had concomitant effects on growth and bone density, but when GC treatment was stopped there was improvement in height and bone density.

## Bone Density and Fractures

BMD is more difficult to measure in children. Changes in bone size, which occur in three dimensions, can falsely increase bone density as measured by DXA, which is a two-dimensional measurement. Z scores rather than T scores are generally used when assessing bone density with DXA in children, and measurements have to be corrected for volumetric changes of growth. Given these limitations, Falcini and colleagues (26) reported that the lumbar spine BMD of GC-treated children with juvenile chronic arthritis (JCA) was lower than that of JCA children who never received GCs. Ansell and colleagues (27) described a relationship between GC use and poor growth and fractures in children with JCA and that there was a linear relationship between GC dose and fractures. In a study of fracture rates in GC-treated children with JCA, children with vertebral fractures had received a daily dose of prednisone 2.3 times higher than that given to children who had not had a fracture and all those with a fracture had received at least 5 g of prednisone.

In a study of children from the UK GPDB who had received GC treatment for any reason, the odds ratio of fracture was increased to 1.32 (95% CI:1.02-1.69) in children who had received four or more courses of oral GCs, with an OR of 2.17 for a fracture of the humerus (28). Higher GC doses are associated with shorter height and greater fracture risk, but the effects were very variable suggesting that not only the dose of GCs but also the time in sexual maturation when they are given may be very important in determining their long-term effects.

## PREVENTION AND TREATMENT OF GLUCOCORTICOID OSTEOPOROSIS IN THE COMMUNITY

Although there is now a clearly proven relationship between GC treatment and bone loss and medications are available to prevent GC-induced bone loss, the majority of GC-treated patients never receive preventive treatment. A survey of GC-treated patients in 1999 found low usage of medications to prevent bone loss and that only 45% of postmenopausal women were taking a preventive treatment (29). Using a large HMO administrative database, Mudano and colleagues found that only 40% of GC-treated postmenopausal women were being treated with an antiresorptive agent (30). Yood and colleagues (31) studied 224 health-plan employees receiving GC treatment and found that 62% were receiving some intervention (medication or

lifestyle change) to prevent GC osteoporosis. The factors that were associated with greater likelihood of intervention were female sex, age, prednisone dose, and physician specialty.

GCs are prescribed by primary care physicians and a number of different specialists. Studies show significant practice variations between physicians of different specialties in the use of agents to prevent and treat GC osteoporosis (32,33). Solomon and colleagues (33) examined the use of medications to prevent bone loss in 236 GC-treated patients with RA followed in an academic rheumatology practice and found that approximately one-third of the patients were not receiving treatments to prevent bone loss and only 23% had bone density testing.

## CONCLUSIONS

Studies of the natural history of GC-induced osteoporosis and fracture have revealed

- GC treatment leads to rapid declines in bone mass.
- GC-induced bone loss is dose related. Current daily dose rather than cumulative dose is the best predictor of bone mass and fracture.
- GCs have the greatest detrimental effect on trabecular bone mass leading to a higher rate of vertebral fractures. Prednisone dosages of less than 2.5 mg per day are associated with an increase in vertebral fracture risk.
- GCs also have a detrimental effect on cortical bone and cause an increase femoral fracture risk at dosages of prednisone of more than 2.5 mg per day.
- Pelvic fractures are common in GC-treated patients.
- Fracture rates increase quickly with GC treatment (within 3 months).
- Some of the increase in fracture rates is likely the result of extraskeletal factors such as an increase in falls.
- Bone loss from GC use is at least partially reversible, and fracture rates decline when GC treatment is discontinued.
- Men and women have similar amounts of bone loss resulting from GC use.
- Fractures are more frequent in patients with baseline low bone mass such as postmenopausal women.
- Fractures from GC treatment can occur in patients who do not have osteoporosis at the initiation of GC treatment and may occur at higher bone density than in non-GC-treated patients.
- Children are also at risk for fractures from GC use because of its effects on bone density and bone growth.
- Epidemiology studies suggest that GC-induced osteoporosis is greatly underdiagnosed and undertreated.

## REFERENCES

1. Cushing H. The basophil adenomas of the pituitary and their clinical manifestations. *Bull Johns Hopkins Hosp* 1932;50:137–195.

2. Boland EW, Headley NE. Management of rheumatoid arthritis with smaller (maintenance) doses of cortisone acetate. *JAMA* 1950;144:365–367.

3. Saag KG, Koehnke R, Caldwell J, et al. Low dose long-term corticosteroid therapy in rheumatoid arthritis: an analysis of serious adverse events. *Am J Med* 1994;96:115–123.

4. Sambrook P, Eisman J, Champion D, et al. Determinants of axial bone loss in rheumatoid arthritis. *Arthritis Rheum* 1987;30:721–728.

5. Hall GM, Spector TD, Griffin AJ, et al. The effect of rheumatoid arthritis and steroid therapy on bone density in postmenopausal women. *Arthritis Rheum* 1993;36:1510–1516.

6. Buckley LM, Leib ES, Cartularo K, et al. The effects of corticosteroids on the bone mineral density of patients with rheumatoid arthritis. *J Rheumatol* 1995;22:1055–1059.

7. Laan RF, van Riel PL, van de Putte LB, et al. Low-dose prednisone induced rapid reversible bone loss in patients with rheumatoid arthritis. *Ann Intern Med* 1993;119:963–968.

8. Sambrook P, Birmingham J, Kelly P, et al. Prevention of GC osteoporosis: a comparison of calcium, calcitriol, and calcitonin. *N Engl J Med* 1993;328:1747–1752.

9. Buckley LM, Leib ES, Cartularo KS, et al. Calcium and vitamin D supplementation prevents bone loss in the spine secondary to low-dose corticosteroids in patients with rheumatoid arthritis. *Ann Intern Med* 1996;125:961–968.

10. Saag K, Emkey R, Schnitzer TJ, et al. Alendronate for the prevention and treatment of glucocorticoid osteoporosis. *N Engl J Med* 1998;339:292–299.

11. Adachi J, Cranney A, Goldsmith CH, et al. Intermittent cyclic therapy with etidronate in the prevention of corticosteroid induced bone loss. *J Rheumatol* 1994;21:1922–1926.

12. Hooyman JR, Melton LJ, Nelson AM, et al. Fractures after rheumatoid arthritis. *Arthritis Rheum* 1984;27:1353–1361.

13. De Nijs RN, Jacobs JW, Bijlsma JW, et al. Prevalence of vertebral deformities and symptomatic vertebral fractures in corticosteroid treated patients with rheumatoid arthritis. *Rheumatology* 2001;40:1375–1383.

14. van Staa TP, Laan RF, Barton P, et al. Bone density threshold and other predictors of vertebral fracture in patients receiving oral glucocorticoids. *Arthritis Rheum* 2003;48:3224–3229.

15. van Staa TP, Leukens HGM, Abenhaim L, et al. Use of oral corticosteroids and risk of fractures. *J Bone Miner Res* 2000;15:993–1002.

16. Michel BA, Bloch DA, Wolfe F, Fries JF. Fractures in rheumatoid arthritis: an evaluation of associated risk factors. *J Rheumatol* 1993;20:1666–1669.

17. Rizzato, Montemurro L. Reversibility of exogenous corticosteroid-induced bone loss. *Eur Respir J* 1993;6:116–119.

18. Hermus AR, Huysman DA, Smals AG, et al. Remarkable improvement of osteopenia after cure of Cushing's syndrome. *Horm Metab Res* 1994;26:209–210.

19. Selby PL, Halsey JP, Adams KRH, et al. Corticosteroids do not alter the threshold for vertebral fracture. *J Bone Miner Res* 2000;15:952–956.

20. Naganathan V, Jones G, Nash P, et al. Vertebral fracture risk with long-term corticosteroid therapy. *Arch Intern Med* 2000;160:2917–2922.

21. Cooper C, Eriksson JG, Forsen T, et al. Maternal height, childhood growth, and risk of hip fracture in later life: a longitudinal study. *Osteoporosis Int* 2001:12:623–629.

22. Falliers CJ, Tan LS, Szentivanyi J, et al. Childhood asthma and steroid therapy as influences on growth. *Amer J Dis Child*.1963;105:127–137.

23. Foote KD, Brocklebank JT, Meadow SR. Height attainment in children with steroid-dependent nephrotic syndrome. *Lancet* 1985;2:917–919.

24. Kotaniemi A, Savolainen A, Kroger H, et al. Development of bone mineral density at the lumbar spine and femoral neck in juvenile chronic arthritis—a prospective one year followup study. *J Rheumatol* 1998;25:2450–2455.

25. Chesney RW, Mazess RB, Rose P, Jax DK. Effect of prednisone on growth and bone mineral content in childhood glomerular disease. *Am J Dis Child* 1978;132:768–772.

26. Falcini F, Trapani S, Civinini R, et al. The primary role of steroids on the osteoporosis in juvenile rheumatoid arthritis patients evaluated by dual x-ray absorptiometry. *J Endocrinol Invest* 1996;19:165–169.

27. Voronos S, Ansell B, Reeve. Vertebral collapse in juvenile arthritis: its relationship with glucocorticoid therapy. *Calcif Tissue Int* 1987;41:75–78.

28. van Staa TP, Cooper C, Leufkens HG, Bishop N. Children and the risk of fracture caused by oral corticosteroids. *J Bone Miner Res* 2003;18:913–918.

29. Buckley LM, Marquez, M, Feezor R, et al. Prevention of corticosteroid induced osteoporosis: results of a patient survey. *Arthritis Rheum* 1999;42:1736–1739.

30. Mudano A, Allison J, Hill J, et al. Variations in glucocorticoid prevention in a managed care cohort. *J Rheum* 2001;28:1298–1305.

31. Yood RA, Harrold LR, Fish L, et al. Prevention of glucocorticoid-induced osteoporosis: experience in a managed care setting. *Arch Intern Med* 2001;161:1322–1327.

32. Buckley LM, Marquez M, Hudson J, et al. Variations in physicians judgments about corticosteroid osteoporosis by physician specialty. *J Rheumatol* 1998;25:2195–2202.

33. Solomon DH, Katz JN, Jacobs AM, et al. Management of glucocorticoid-induced osteoporosis in patients with rheumatoid arthritis: rates and predictors of care in an academic rheumatology practice. *Arthritis Rheum* 2002;46:3136–3142.

# Glucocorticoid-Induced Osteoporosis: Pathophysiology

*Ernesto Canalis*

Glucocorticoid-induced osteoporosis (GIOP) is the most common form of secondary osteoporosis, and it is a frequent complication of the use of systemic glucocorticoids. These steroids have marked effects on mineral and skeletal metabolism leading to bone loss and eventually to osteoporotic fractures (1). Often there are concomitant factors playing a role in the osteoporosis following the therapeutic use of glucocorticoids, including the hormonal state of the patient, individual differences in sensitivity to glucocorticoids and the underlying disease (2). This by itself carries a significant risk of osteoporosis, and patients with rheumatic disorders, such as rheumatoid arthritis and systemic lupus erythematosus, as well as patients with chronic obstructive pulmonary disease, chronic inflammatory bowel disease, and organ transplants are at a higher risk of osteoporosis than the general population (2). This is the result of disease chronicity and excessive exposure of skeletal tissue to systemic cytokines and a variety of therapeutic agents with detrimental effects on the skeleton. This chapter focuses on the direct and indirect effects of glucocorticoids on the skeleton and mechanisms leading to bone loss (Fig. 12B.1).

Although the direct effects of glucocorticoids on skeletal cells are the most significant determinants of their impact on skeletal metabolism, some of the effects observed in GIOP are indirect and mediated by changes in the synthesis or activity of systemic hormones and of growth factors present in the bone microenvironment (Table 12B.1). Recent research has centered on the effects of glucocorticoids on the fate, life span, and function of cells of the osteoblast and osteoclast lineages and their consequences on bone formation and bone resorption. Analysis of biopsies obtained from patients receiving therapy with glucocorticoids reveal increased bone resorption and decreased bone formation (3); however, patients eventually reach a state of decreased bone formation and remodeling. The observed bone resorption appears to occur in the initial phases of skeletal exposure to glucocorticoids and may be responsible for the rapid bone loss that follows the initiation of therapy with these steroids. The decreased bone remodeling is secondary to the loss of skeletal cells and is responsible for a continued loss of bone occurring at an apparent slower rate. These phases are reflected, clinically, by a rapid loss of bone mineral density occurring in the first 3 to 6 months after exposure to glucocorticoids, followed by a modest steady decline or even an apparent stabilization of bone mineral density as the disease progresses. Despite this, the detrimental effects of glucocorticoids on the skeleton continue and the risk of fractures increases, as these are related to the dose and duration of treatment with glucocorticoids.

## EFFECTS OF GLUCOCORTICOIDS ON BONE RESORBING CELLS

Glucocorticoids have direct and indirect effects on cells of the osteoclast lineage leading to increased bone resorption (Table 12B.2). Glucocorticoids cause a decrease in the intestinal absorption of calcium and an increase in the urinary excretion of calcium. The exact mechanisms are not known, but changes in intestinal calcium transport appear secondary to a resistance to the effects of vitamin D, because vitamin D levels are not altered (4). The decrease

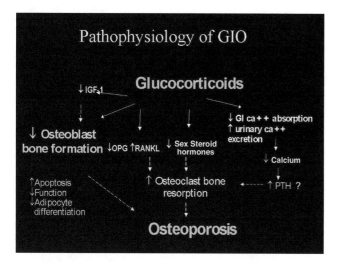

**Figure 12B.1** Direct and indirect effects of glucocorticoids on bone formation and resorption.

in calcium absorption and increased urinary excretion of calcium cause modest elevations in the serum levels of parathyroid hormone (PTH), but these are not in the hyperparathyroid range (5). This would suggest that secondary hyperparathyroidism is not a major determinant of the increased bone resorption. Glucocorticoids increase the expression of PTH and PTH-related peptide receptors, and enhanced sensitivity to PTH possibly plays a role in the observed bone resorption (6). Secondary hyperparathyroidism, however, is not likely to play a fundamental or lasting role in the metabolic disease observed (5). Histomorphometric analysis of bone biopsies from patients with hyperparathyroidism reveal increased remodeling, whereas analysis of biopsies from

## TABLE 12B.1
### PATHOPHYSIOLOGY OF GLUCOCORTICOID-INDUCED OSTEOPOROSIS

1. Glucocorticoids
   a. Direct skeletal effects
      Increased bone resorption
      Decreased bone formation
      Decreased IGF-I
   b. Indirect skeletal effects
      Possible transient hyperparathyroidism
      Hypogonadism
      Resistance to GH/IGF-I
   c. Effects on mineral and calcium metabolism
2. Underlying disease
   a. Inflammatory cytokines
      Increased resorption
      Decreased formation
   b. Disease state
   c. Other therapies

## TABLE 12B.2
### EFFECTS OF GLUCOCORTICOIDS ON CELLS OF THE OSTEOCLAST LINEAGE

1. Indirect effects
   Increased PTH levels or sensitivity
   Decreased estrogen and androgen levels
2. Direct effects
   Increased RANKL, CSF-1
   Decreased osteoprotegerin
   Osteoclast apoptosis

patients with GIOP eventually reveal decreased bone remodeling.

Glucocorticoids inhibit gonadotropin hormone secretion and can cause hypogonadism with a consequent bone loss caused by androgen or estrogen deficiency. Cytokines, such as interleukin-6 and tumor necrosis factor α, enhance bone resorption and play a role in the bone loss that follows estrogen deficiency (7–9). Glucocorticoids also have direct effects on skeletal cells leading to osteoclastogenesis and bone resorption. These are mediated by changes in the expression of the receptor activator of nuclear factor-κB ligand (RANKL) and of its decoy receptor osteoprotegerin (10,11). RANKL, secreted by osteoblasts, binds and activates its receptor, RANK, on the surface of osteoclast precursors and, in association with colony stimulating factor 1 (CSF 1), induces osteoclastogenesis (12). Osteoprotegerin binds RANKL, preventing RANKL from binding to its osteoclast receptor. Glucocorticoids increase the expression of RANKL and CSF-1 and decrease osteoprotegerin expression in osteoblasts and stromal cells (10,11). The consequence is an increase in the formation of osteoclasts capable of resorbing bone. Glucocorticoids have the potential to increase the number of osteoclasts by extending the life span of the cell, although this effect is primarily observed following bisphosphonate-induced osteoclastic apoptosis (13). Eventually, glucocorticoids deplete the osteoblastic population, and when this occurs, signals inducing osteoclastogenesis are lost with a consequent decrease in osteoclast number. Glucocorticoids also have been reported to induce osteoclast apoptosis, and this event may contribute to an eventual decrease in bone remodeling (14).

## EFFECTS OF GLUCOCORTICOIDS ON BONE MATRIX

The bone matrix is composed primarily by type-I collagen, which is synthesized by osteoblasts and degraded by proteases secreted by skeletal cells. Glucocorticoids inhibit type-I collagen synthesis by transcriptional and post-transcriptional mechanisms and regulate the synthesis of collagenases, which are matrix metalloproteinases (MMP) that cleave collagen fibrils and regulate matrix breakdown (15,16). Three collagenases have been described: collagenase 1 (MMP-1), collagenase 2 (MMP-8), and collagenase 3 (MMP-13) (16). Osteoblasts secrete collagenase 1 and 3, and these cleave type-I collagen fibrils with similar efficiency (17,18). Collagenases also play a central function in bone resorption, and mutations of the collagenase-3 cleavage site of the type-I collagen molecule and null mutations of the collagenase-3 gene result in impaired bone resorption and limited response to the resorptive actions of PTH (19). Glucocorticoids are known for their inhibitory effects on collagenase 1 transcription, leading to a decrease in matrix breakdown in articular joints (20). In contrast, glucocorticoids increase collagenase-3 mRNA and protease levels in osteoblasts by posttranscriptional mechanisms (15). Glucocorticoids prolong the half-life of collagenase-3 mRNA by three-fold and this effect may contribute to their effects on bone resorption. Recently, the mechanisms involved in collagenase-3 mRNA stabilization by glucocorticoids were explored. We demonstrated that ATTT (T,T)A sequences encoding AU-rich elements present in the 3′ untranslated region of the collagenase-3 RNA are responsible for transcript stabilization. Cortisol enhanced the binding of cytosolic proteins from osteoblasts to these sequences, and two proteins, vinculin and far upstream element (FUSE)-binding protein 2, bound to the 3′ untranslated region of collagenase 3 RNA. Vinculin, a cytoskeletal protein present in focal cell contacts, is considered to play a role in osteoclastic adhesion and function (21,22). The FUSE-binding proteins may act as transcription factors and regulate transcript stability (23,24). The decrease in type-I collagen synthesis and increase in collagenase-3 synthesis caused by glucocorticoids should result in a decrease in the collagen matrix available for mineralization and contribute to the bone loss of GIOP.

## EFFECTS OF GLUCOCORTICOIDS ON BONE FORMING CELLS

The number and function of cells present in the bone microenvironment determine skeletal homeostasis and changes in the number and function of cells of the osteoblastic lineage are critical to the effect of glucocorticoids in bone (Table 12B.3). Bone marrow stroma contain pluripotent cells with the potential to differentiate into various cells of the mesenchymal lineage, including osteoblasts and adipocytes (25,26). The ultimate cellular phenotype depends on extracellular and intracellular signals. Glucocorticoids have significant effects on cells of the osteoblastic lineage, depending on the stage of cell differentiation and specific test conditions. Although investigators have reported that glucocorticoids may induce osteoblast cell differentiation, this effect is inconsistent with the loss of cells of the osteoblastic lineage after glucocorticoid

**TABLE 12B.3**
### EFFECTS OF GLUCOCORTICOIDS ON CELLS OF THE OSTEOBLAST LINEAGE

1. Decreased cell number
    Impaired osteoblastogenesis
    Enhanced apoptosis
2. Decreased cell function
    Decreased type-I collagen synthesis
    Decreased IGF-I transcription

exposure (27,28). We have shown that glucocorticoids impair the differentiation of stromal cells toward cells of the osteoblastic lineage and prevent the terminal differentiation of quasimature osteoblastic cells, resulting in a decrease in the number of mature osteoblasts (29,30). Glucocorticoids induce apoptosis of mature osteoblasts and osteocytes, which, in association with the impairment in cell differentiation, causes a decrease in the number of bone forming cells (31).

Glucocorticoids shift the differentiation of stromal cells away from the osteoblastic and toward the adipocytic lineage. This shift involves the regulation of nuclear factors of the CCAAT/enhancer binding protein (C/EBP) family and of peroxisome proliferator activated receptor γ2 (PPARγ2) (29). C/EBPs are a family of transcription factors that regulate cell differentiation (32). To date, six C/EBPs have been characterized, α, β, δ, γ, ε, and ζ. The C/EBP proteins contain a highly conserved DNA-binding domain and a dimerization domain and can form homo- and heterodimers that bind to similar sequence motifs (32). C/EBPs are expressed by osteoblasts and adipocytes and are critical for adipocyte differentiation and maturation (33,34). Mice carrying null mutations of C/EBP α, β, and δ have reduced fat because of impaired adipocyte differentiation (35). Recently, we confirmed that glucocorticoids induce adipogenesis and enhance the expression of C/EBP α, β, and δ in cells of the osteoblastic lineage (29). Because these classic C/EBPs are essential for adipogenesis, the findings suggested that they play a role in the effect of glucocorticoids directing mesenchymal cells away from the osteoblastic and toward the adipocytic pathway. This was confirmed in *in vitro* studies where the overexpression of C/EBP homologous protein (CHOP) or growth arrest and DNA damage-inducible gene (GADD) 153, or DNA damage-inducible transcript 3 (DDIT 3), a transdominant negative inhibitor of classic C/EBPs, prevented adipogenesis and induced osteoblastic cell maturation (36,37). Glucocorticoids also regulate PPARγ2 directly and indirectly via C/EBPs, and PPARγ2 also plays a role in the adipogenic effect of glucocorticoids (29). The transcription factors playing a role in adipogenesis are also important in the downregulation of insulin-like growth factor (IGF)–I transcription by glucocorticoids (38).

The shift of osteoblast toward adipocyte differentiation caused by glucocorticoids appears to involve additional signals. These include the induction of Notch1, which enhances the effects of glucocorticoids favoring adipogenesis and opposing osteoblastogenesis (39,40). Notch are a family of four closely related genes, which are activated by proteolytic cleavage resulting in the release of their intracellular domain, following binding by their ligands, Delta 1 to 4 and Jagged/Serrate 1 and 2 (41–43). Overexpression of the constitutively active Notch1 intracellular domain impairs osteoblast differentiation, chondrocyte maturation, and myogenesis (40,44,45). Notch1 and 2 and their ligands, Delta 1 and Jagged 1, are expressed by osteoblasts, whereas Notch3 and 4 are not (39). Cortisol increases Notch1 and 2 transcription in osteoblasts but does not alter the expression of Notch ligands. Overexpression of Notch1 in stromal and osteoblastic cells mimics some effects of glucocorticoids, impairing osteoblastic maturation and favoring adipogenesis (40). Notch1 and Wnt have opposite effects on cell differentiation, because Wnt signaling inhibits adipogenesis and it has the potential to induce osteoblastic differentiation possibly by regulating bone morphogenic protein (BMP) signaling pathways (46). The signaling and inhibitory crosstalk between the Wnt and the Notch signaling pathways occurs at multiple levels and may be critical to their impact on the differentiation of cells of the osteoblastic lineage. Wnt binds to the Notch extracellular domain and the Wnt-dependent disheveled binds to the Notch intracellular domain (46,47). In addition, glycogen synthase kinase 3β, which inactivates the Wnt signaling β-catenin, modulates Notch stability (48). Furthermore, presenilins regulate β-catenin degradation and play a role in the activation of Notch (46). Recently, we demonstrated that Notch1 overexpression decreased Wnt-β-catenin signaling in cells of the osteoblastic lineage (40). The direct actions of glucocorticoids on the function of the osteoblast and the reduced population of bone forming cells, because of impaired maturation and enhanced apoptosis, are believed to play a fundamental role in the skeletal disease observed in patients treated with glucocorticoids.

## EFFECTS OF GLUCOCORTICOIDS ON SKELETAL GROWTH FACTORS

Although glucocorticoids have significant effects on the number and function of cells of the osteoblastic lineage, additional actions are less direct and involve the synthesis and activity of growth factors present in the bone microenvironment. Glucocorticoids modulate the binding of transforming growth factor β, shifting its binding from signaling to nonsignaling receptors (49). Their greatest impact, however, appears to be on IGF-I and its binding proteins (IGFBP). Glucocorticoids and IGF-I have opposite effects on bone formation, and IGF-I enhances the differentiated function of the osteoblast with a consequent increase in the formation of new bone (50). Consequently, it is not surprising that glucocorticoids downregulate the transcription of the IGF-I gene in osteoblasts and suppress IGF-I synthesis (38).

The levels of IGF-I in cultured osteoblasts and intact calvariae are decreased by glucocorticoids. The mechanisms involve the suppression of IGF-I gene transcription, and the effect is characterized by analysis of the rat IGF-I gene in cultured osteoblasts. The rat IGF-I gene consists of six exons with clusters of transcription initiation sites within alternative promoters in exons 1 and 2 (51). In osteoblasts, cortisol represses transcription of the IGF-I promoter, and mutation and electrophoretic mobility gel shift analyses demonstrated that a C/EBP binding site adjacent to the third start site of transcription was responsible for the effect of glucocorticoids (38). Electrophoretic mobility shift and supershift assays revealed that C/EBP α, β, and δ interacted with IGF-I promoter sequences, and cortisol increased C/EBP β and δ mRNA levels. The increased expression of C/EBP β and δ is in accordance with the effect of glucocorticoids directing pluripotent marrow stromal cells toward the adipocytic pathway, because C/EBP β and δ play a fundamental role in adipocytic cell differentiation (29).

Glucocorticoids have the potential to regulate IGF-I activity through their actions on the synthesis of IGFBPs. Glucocorticoids do not alter IGF-I receptor number or affinity in osteoblasts but decrease IGF-II receptor transcription (52). The function of this receptor is not clear, however, and it is not responsible for anabolic responses to IGF. The six known IGFBPs are expressed by osteoblasts, and glucocorticoids decrease the expression of IGFBP-3, -4, and -5 mRNAs and stimulate IGFBP-6 synthesis in osteoblasts (53). Until recently, the inhibitory effect on IGFBP-5 transcription was considered relevant to the mechanism of action of glucocorticoids in bone because IGFBP-5 has been reported to have anabolic effects on the skeleton (54). However, studies conducted in transgenic mice overexpressing IGFBP-5 under the control of the osteoblast-specific osteocalcin promoter failed to demonstrate an anabolic effect of IGFBP-5 on the skeleton (55). Overexpression of IGFBP-5 in the bone microenvironment resulted in osteopenia secondary to decreased bone formation. The inhibitory effect of glucocorticoids on IGFBP-5 expression, therefore, does not appear to have immediate relevance to their mechanism of action in bone. In addition to IGFBPs, there is an increasing family of IGFBP-related proteins (IGFBP-rP), which share biochemical and functional properties with the IGFBPs (56). IGFBP-rP1, the product of the mac25 gene, and IGFBP-rP2, or connective tissue growth factor (CTGF), are expressed by osteoblasts, and their synthesis is enhanced by glucocorticoids (57,58). At the present time, it is not known whether other IGFBP-rP genes are regulated by glucocorticoids in osteoblasts.

## ENZYMATIC ACTIVATION AND INACTIVATION OF GLUCOCORTICOIDS IN OSTEOBLASTS

Glucocorticoid activity is regulated at the level of its target tissues by the actions of two isoenzymes, 11β-hydroxysteroid dehydrogenase (11β-HSD) type 1 and type 2. These isoenzymes catalyze the interconversion of hormonally active cortisol and inactive cortisone and, as a result, modulate glucocorticoid activity (59,60). 11β-HSD type 1 (11β-HSD1), a low affinity nicotinamide adenine dinucleotide phosphate (NADP)-(H)-dependent enzyme, is bi-directional (dehydrogenase/reductase), although it displays primarily reductase activity converting cortisone to cortisol (59). 11β-HSD type 2 has exclusively dehydrogenase activity and inactivates glucocorticoids but does not play a functional role in the adult skeleton because it is expressed by fetal, not adult, bone (59). In contrast, 11β-HSD1 is widely expressed in glucocorticoid target tissues, including adult bone (61). Because 11β-HSD1 can activate inactive glucocorticoids, it can facilitate glucocorticoid action. Moreover, glucocorticoids enhance 11β-HSD1 activity, and as such it can act as a local amplifier of glucocorticoid action in target tissues. Differential expression of 11β-HSD1 may explain differential sensitivity of patients to the systemic effects of glucocorticoids.

## EFFECT OF GLUCOCORTICOIDS ON CARTILAGE CELLS

Children treated with glucocorticoids exhibit impaired growth, possibly because of the effects of glucocorticoids on the growth hormone (GH) IGF-I axis and their impact on the epiphyseal growth plate. Glucocorticoids decrease IGF-1 expression in liver cells, the main source of circulating IGF-I, but serum levels of IGF-I and GH often are normal in patients receiving glucocorticoids (62). Glucocorticoids impair IGF-I secretion at the tissue level in chondrocytes and osteoblasts, causing a generalized decrease in skeletal IGF-I levels, which may be responsible for some of their inhibitory actions on skeletal growth and bone mass (63). Glucocorticoids decrease chondrocyte cell replication, and this is in part because of tissue insensitivity to GH and IGF-I (63). The effects of glucocorticoids on GH and IGF-I receptors are variable, but these steroids can blunt the induction of GH and IGF-I receptors in chondrocytes. Decreased local IGF-I synthesis and cellular sensitivity to IGF-I in chondrocytes appear to be at the center of the actions of glucocorticoids on linear growth (64).

In conclusion, glucocorticoids have direct and indirect effect on skeletal cells, resulting in altered bone remodeling, osteoporosis, and impaired linear growth.

## ACKNOWLEDGMENTS

Work from the author's laboratory was supported by grant DK 45227 from the National Institute of Diabetes Digestive and Kidney Diseases. The author thanks Ms. Nancy Wallach for secretarial assistance.

## REFERENCES

1. Saag K. Glucocorticoid-induced osteoporosis. *Endocrinol Metab Clin North Am* 2003;32:135–157.
2. Canalis E, Giustina A. Glucocorticoid-induced osteoporosis: summary of a workshop. *J Clin Endocrinol Metab* 2001;86:5681–5685.
3. Carbonare LD, Arlot ME, Chavassieux PM, et al. Comparison of trabecular bone microarchitecture and remodeling in glucocorticoid-induced and postmenopausal osteoporosis. *J Bone Miner Res* 2001;16:97–103.
4. Hattersley AT, Meeran K, Burrin J, et al. The effect of long- and short-term corticosteroids on plasma calcitonin and parathyroid hormone levels. *Calcif Tissue Int* 1994;54:198–202.
5. Rubin MR, Bilezikian JP. Clinical review 151: The role of parathyroid hormone in the pathogenesis of glucocorticoid-induced osteoporosis: a re-examination of the evidence. *J Clin Endocrinol Metab* 2002;87:4033–4041.
6. Urena P, Iida-Klein A, Kong XF, et al. Regulation of parathyroid hormone (PTH)/PTH-related peptide receptor messenger ribonucleic acid by glucocorticoids and PTH in ROS17/2.8 and OK cells. *Endocrinology* 1994;134:451–456.
7. Jilka RL, Hangoc G, Girasole G, et al. Increased osteoclast development after estrogen loss: mediation by interleukin-6. *Science* 1992;257:88–91.
8. Srivastava S, Toraldo G, Weitzmann MN, et al. Estrogen decreases osteoclast formation by down-regulating receptor activator of NF-kappa B ligand (RANKL)-induced JNK activation. *J Biol Chem* 2001;276:8836–8840.
9. Cenci S, Toraldo G, Weitzmann MN, et al. Estrogen deficiency induces bone loss by increasing T cell proliferation and lifespan through IFN-{gamma}-induced class II transactivator. *Proc Natl Acad Sci U S A* 2003;100:10405–10410.
10. Hofbauer LC, Gori F, Riggs BL, et al. Stimulation of osteoprotegerin ligand and inhibition of osteoprotegerin production by glucocorticoids in human osteoblastic lineage cells: potential paracrine mechanisms of glucocorticoid-induced osteoporosis. *Endocrinology* 1999;140:4382–4389.
11. Rubin J, Biskobing DM, Jadhav L, et al. Dexamethasone promotes expression of membrane-bound macrophage colony-stimulating factor in murine osteoblast-like cells. *Endocrinology* 1998;139:1006–1012.
12. Suda T, Takahaski N, Udagawa N, et al. Modulation of osteoclast differentiation and function by the new members of the tumor necrosis factor receptor and ligand families. *Endocr Rev* 1999;20:345–357.
13. Weinstein RS, Chen JR, Powers CC, et al. Promotion of osteoclast survival and antagonism of bisphosphonate-induced osteoclast apoptosis by glucocorticoids. *J Clin Invest* 2002;109:1041–1048.
14. Dempster DW, Moonga BS, Stein LS, et al. Glucocorticoids inhibit bone resorption by isolated rat osteoclasts by enhancing apoptosis. *J Endocrinol* 1997;154:397–406.
15. Delany AM, Jeffrey JJ, Rydziel S, et al. Cortisol increases interstitial collagenase expression in osteoblasts by post-transcriptional mechanisms. *J Biol Chem* 1995;270:26607–26612.
16. Matrisian LM, Hogan BL. Growth factor-regulated proteases and extracellular matrix remodeling during mammalian development. *Curr Top Dev Biol* 1990;24:219–259.
17. Knauper V, Will H, Lopez-Otin C, et al. Cellular mechanisms for human procollagenase-3 (MMP-13) activation. *J Biol Chem* 1996;271:17124–17131.
18. Freije JMP, Diez-Itza I, Balbin M, et al. Molecular cloning and expression of collagenase 3, a novel human matrix metalloproteinase produced by breast carcinomas. *J Biol Chem* 1994;269:16766–16773.

19. Zhao W, Byrne MH, Boyce BF, et al. Bone resorption induced by parathyroid hormone is strikingly diminished in collagenase-resistant mutant mice. *J Clin Invest* 1999;103:517–524.

20. Jonat C, Rahmsdorf HJ, Park KK, et al. Antitumor promotion and anti-inflammation: down-modulation of AP-1 (Fos/Jun) activity by glucocorticoid hormone. *Cell* 1990;62:1189–1204.

21. Duong LT, Lakkakorpi I, Nakamura I, et al. Integrins and signaling in osteoclast function. *Matrix Biol* 2000;19:97–105.

22. Rodriguez-Fernandez JLR, Geiger B, Salomon D, et al. Suppression of vinculin expression by antisense transfection confers changes in cell morphology, motility, and anchorage-dependent growth of 3T3 cells. *J Cell Biol* 1993;122:1285–1294.

23. Davis-Smith T, Duncan RC, Zheng T, et al. The far upstream element—binding proteins compromise an ancient family of single-strand DNA-binding transactivators. *J Biol Chem* 1996;271: 31679–31687.

24. Siomi H, Choi M, Siomi MC, et al. Essential role for KH domains in RNA binding: impaired RNA binding by a mutation in the KH domain of FMR1 that causes fragile X syndrome. *Cell* 1994;77:33–39.

25. Bianco P, Robey PG. Marrow stromal stem cells. *J Clin Invest* 2000;105:1663–1668.

26. Canalis E, Economides AN, Gazzerro E. Bone morphogenetic proteins, their antagonists, and the skeleton. *Endocr Rev* 2003;24: 218–235.

27. Bellows CG, Aubin JE, Heersche JNM. Physiological concentrations of glucocorticoids stimulate formation of bone nodules from isolated rat calvaria cells in vitro. *Endocrinology* 1987;212: 1985–1992.

28. Shalhoub V, Conlon D, Tassinari M, et al. Glucocorticoids promote development of the osteoblast phenotype by selectively modulating expression of cell growth and differentiation associated genes. *J Cell Biochem* 1992;50:425–440.

29. Pereira RC, Delany AM, Canalis E. Effects of cortisol and bone morphogenetic protein-2 on stromal cell differentiation: correlation with CCAAT-enhancer binding protein expression. *Bone* 2002;30:685–691.

30. Pereira RMR, Delany AM, Canalis E. Cortisol inhibits the differentiation and apoptosis of osteoblasts in culture. *Bone* 2001;28:484–490.

31. Weinstein RS, Jilka RL, Parfitt AM, et al. Inhibition of osteoblastogenesis and promotion of apoptosis of osteoblasts and osteocytes by glucocorticoids. *J Clin Invest* 1998;102:274–282.

32. Ramji DP, Folka P. CCAAT/enhancer-binding proteins: structure, function and regulation. *Biochem J* 2002;365:561–575.

33. Wu Z, Bucher NLR, Farmer SR. Induction of peroxisome proliferator-activated receptor during the conversion of 3T3 fibroblasts into adipocytes is mediated by C/EBPβ, C/EBPδ and glucocorticoids. *Mol Cell Biol* 1996;16:4128–4136.

34. Darlington GJ, Ross SE, MacDougald OA. The role of C/EBP genes in adipocyte differentiation. *J Biol Chem* 1998;273:30057–30060.

35. Tanaka T, Yoshida N, Kishimoto T, et al. Defective adipocyte differentiation in mice lacking the C/EBPβ and/or C/EBPδ gene. *Eur Med Biol Org J* 1997;16:7432–7443.

36. Ron D, Habener JF. CHOP, a novel developmentally regulated nuclear protein that dimerizes with transcription factors C/EBP and LAP and functions as a dominant-negative inhibitor of gene transcription. *Genes Dev* 1992;6:439–453.

37. Batchvarova N, Wang XZ, Ron D. Inhibition of adipogenesis by the stress-induced protein CHOP (GADD153). *EMBO J* 1995;14: 4654–4661.

38. Delany AM, Durant D, Canalis E. Glucocorticoid suppression of IGF I transcription in osteoblasts. *Mol Endocrinol* 2001;15: 1781–1789.

39. Pereira RMR, Delany AM, Durant D, et al. Cortisol regulates the expression of Notch in osteoblasts. *J Cell Biochem* 2002;85: 252–258.

40. Sciaudone M, Gazzerro E, Priest L, et al. Notch 1 impairs osteoblastic cell differentiation. *Endocrinology* 2003;144:5631–5639.

41. Weinmaster G. Review: the ins and outs of notch signaling. *Mol Cell Neurosci* 1997;9:91–102.

42. Weinmaster G. Notch signal transduction: a real rip and more. *Curr Opin Genet Dev* 2000;10:363–369.

43. Mumm JS, Kopan R. Notch signaling: from the outside in. *Dev Biol* 2000;228:151–165.

44. Nofziger D, Miyamoto A, Lyons KM, et al. Notch signaling imposes two blocks in the differentiation of C2C12 myoblasts. *Development* 1999;126:1689–1702.

45. Crowe R, Zikherman J, Niswander L. Delta-1 negatively regulates the transition from prehypertrophic to hypertrophic chondrocytes during cartilage formation. *Development* 1999;126:987–998.

46. De Strooper B, Annaert W. Where Notch and Wnt signaling meet: the presenilin hub. *J Cell Biol* 2001;152:F17–20.

47. Axelrod JD, Matsuno K, Artavanis-Tsakonas S, et al. Interaction between Wingless and Notch signaling pathways mediated by Disheveled. *Science* 1996;271:1826–1832.

48. Foltz DR, Santiago MC, Berechid BE, et al. Glycogen synthase kinase-3β modulates Notch signaling and stability. *Curr Biol* 2002;12:1006–1011.

49. Centrella M, McCarthy TL, Canalis E. Glucocorticoid regulation of transforming growth factor-β1 (TGF-β1) activity and binding in osteoblast-enriched cultures from fetal rat bone. *Mol Cell Biol* 1991;11:4490–4496.

50. Hock JM, Centrella M, Canalis E. Insulin-like growth factor I (IGF-I) has independent effects on bone matrix formation and cell replication. *Endocrinology* 1988;122:22–27.

51. Adamo ML, Ben-Hur H, Roberts CT Jr, et al. Regulation of start site usage in the leader of exons of the rat insulin-like growth factor-I gene by development, fasting, and diabetes. *Mol Endocrinol* 1991;5:1677–1686.

52. Rydziel S, Canalis E. Cortisol represses insulin-like growth factor II receptor transcription in skeletal cell cultures. *Endocrinology* 1995;136:4254–4260.

53. Okazaki R, Rigg BL, Conover CA. Glucocorticoid regulation of insulin-like growth factor-binding protein expression in normal human osteoblast-like cells. *Endocrinology* 1994;134:126–132.

54. Andress DL, Birnbaum RS. Human osteoblast-derived insulin-like growth factor (IGF) binding protein-5 stimulates osteoblast mitogenesis and potentiates IGF action. *J Biol Chem* 1992;267: 22467–22472.

55. Devlin RD, Du Z, Buccilli V, et al. Transgenic mice overexpressing insulin-like growth factor binding protein-5 display transiently decreased osteoblastic function and osteopenia. *Endocrinology* 2002;143:3955–3962.

56. Baxter RC, Binoux MA, Clemmons DR, et al. Recommendations for nomenclature of the insulin-like growth factor binding protein superfamily. *Endocrinology* 1998;139:4036.

57. Pereira RC, Blanquaert F, Canalis E. Cortisol enhances the expression of mac25/insulin-like growth factor-binding protein-related protein-1 in cultured osteoblasts. *Endocrinology* 1999;140: 228–232.

58. Pereira RC, Durant D, Canalis E. Transcriptional regulation of connective tissue growth factor by cortisol in osteoblasts. *Am J Physiol Endocrinol Metab* 2000;279:E570–E576.

59. Diederich S, Quinkler M, Burkhardt P, et al. 11β hydroxysteroid dehydrogenase isoforms: tissue distribution and implications for clinical medicine. *Eur J Clin Invest* 2000;30:21–27.

60. Canalis E, Delany AM. 11b-Hydroxysteroid dehydrogenase, an amplifier of glucocorticoid action in osteoblasts. *J Bone Miner Res* 2002;17:987–990.

61. Cooper MS, Rabbitt EH, Goddard PE, et al. Autocrine activation of glucocorticoids in osteoblasts increase with age and glucocorticoid exposure. *J Bone Miner Res* 2002;17:979–986.

62. Reid IR, Gluckman PD, Ibbertson HK. Insulin-like growth factor I and bone turnover in glucocorticoid-treated and control subjects. *Clin Endocrinol (Oxf)* 1989;30:347–353.

63. Jux C, Leiber K, Hugel U, et al. Dexamethasone impairs growth hormone (GH)-stimulated growth by suppression of local insulin-like growth factor (IGF)-I production and expression of GH- and IGF-I receptor in cultured rat chondrocytes. *Endocrinology* 1998;139:3296–3305.

64. Canalis E. Inhibitory actions of glucocorticoids on skeletal growth. Is local insulin-like growth factor I to blame? *Endocrinology* 1998;139:3041–3042.

# Glucocorticoid-Induced Osteoporosis: Prevention and Treatment

*Jeffrey R. Curtis*    *Kenneth G. Saag*

Few medications have altered the management of rheumatic disease as dramatically as glucocorticoids. Despite more than 50 years of glucocorticoid use during which equally effective alternatives might have been developed, the unparalleled short-term benefit of glucocorticoids in reducing inflammation and controlling symptoms have perpetuated their widespread use. Indeed, recent evidence also supports a possible disease modifying role for low-dose glucocorticoid administration in rheumatoid arthritis (RA) (1–3). However, high rates of associated adverse events, particularly insufficiency fractures, all too commonly occur in patients on chronic glucocorticoid therapy (4,5). Physicians, therefore, need to carefully balance the desired benefits of glucocorticoid therapy against the potential toxicities including glucocorticoid-induced osteoporosis (GIOP).

Measures to reduce the risk of GIOP are appropriate for all patients on long-term glucocorticoids. While definitions of what constitutes chronic use remains controversial, continued use or anticipated use of 3 months or more constitutes a reasonable threshold for concern (6). Dose reduction or complete cessation of glucocorticoid therapy is always desirable (7), but this may not be achievable for many patients. Nonpharmacologic interventions such as smoking cessation, weight-bearing exercise, and fall-risk assessment should be provided to all patients at clinical risk for fracture. Therapeutic doses of calcium and vitamin D are necessary but may not be sufficient for patients receiving chronic glucocorticoids. Of the several prescrip-

tion medications that are used to prevent or treat GIOP, only the oral bisphosphonates alendronate (approved for treatment of GIOP) and risedronate (approved for both prevention and treatment of GIOP) are Food and Drug Administration (FDA) approved for use in the United States. However, biologic rationale and/or more limited scientific evidence exists for other agents including parenteral bisphosphonates, calcitonin, hormone replacement, selective estrogen-receptor modulators, thiazide diuretics, and human parathyroid hormone in the management of GIOP. This chapter reviews the evidence and guidelines for the prevention and treatment of GIOP with the use of both nonpharmacologic and pharmacologic medications. Significant practice pattern variations among healthcare providers in the use of these preventive therapies further highlights the importance of disseminating an increasingly large body of evidence into clinical practice.

## CALCIUM AND VITAMIN D

Calcium and vitamin D supplementation is advised in all GIOP management guidelines (8–11). Recommended daily calcium doses are at least 1,200 mg and in most guidelines, 1,500 mg. Because the calcium content of foodstuffs in the average adult diet is insufficient to meet this target for most glucocorticoid users, the majority of calcium needs to come from oral supplements. Calcium alone, however, has only modest beneficial effect on bone turnover in glucocorticoid-treated patients (12), and calcium monotherapy is insufficient to prevent or treat GIOP. In conjunction with calcium, a variety of vitamin-D preparations including ergocalciferol and activated forms of vitamin D such as calcitriol are available. Studies supporting recommendations for calcium and vitamin-D supplementation in GIOP include a 2-year trial of 65 RA patients treated chronically with low-dose prednisone (approximately 5 mg/day) randomized to 1,000 mg of calcium carbonate and 500 IU of ergocalciferol versus placebo (13). Those given daily supplements gained 0.7% and 0.9% annually in lumbar spine and greater trochanter bone mineral density (BMD) compared to losses of −2.0% and −0.9% at these sites in the placebo group. Data from the placebo arm of bisphosphonate clinical trials also demonstrated relative BMD preservation, more so in the spine than the hip, in patients receiving daily calcium and inactive vitamin D (14–17). These patients in clinical trials included many at lower risk of fractures such as premenopausal women and those with normal BMD at study entry. Most but not all studies of active vitamin-D metabolites such as calcitriol and alfacalcidiol have showed similar preservation or only modest BMD losses in glucocorticoid treated patients (18–22).

Results from several calcium and vitamin-D studies in GIOP are summarized in meta-analyses (23,24). One meta-analysis (Fig. 12C.1) found a pooled effect size of 0.6 [95% confidence interval (CI):0.3-0.9] in lumbar spine BMD improvement with the use of vitamin D compared to calcium alone or no treatment. Consideration of only active vitamin-D metabolites did not alter these conclusions. Most subsequent work has demonstrated at best only modest differences between active and inactive forms of vitamin D. In a 2-year trial, patients receiving average daily doses of prednisone of 12 to 16 mg were randomized to calcitriol (0.5 to 0.75 mg/day), erogocalciferol (10,000 IU three times weekly), and calcium (600 mg/day) or daily alendronate with calcium (600 mg) (25). Significant improvements in lumbar spine BMD were observed in the alendronate plus calcium group (+5.9%) compared to

modest losses in both the calcitriol group (−0.7%) and ergocalciferol group (−0.5%). Nonsignificant changes in femoral neck BMD of +0.5%, −2.2%, and −3.2% were observed, respectively, in the alendronate, calcitriol, and ergocalciferol groups. Prevalent glucocorticoid users receiving calcitriol trended towards less BMD loss than those receiving ergocalciferol at the lumbar spine (+0.3 versus −0.03%) and the femoral neck (−1.7 versus −3.1%). The authors also found more bone loss across all three groups in patients receiving ≤6 months of glucocorticoid therapy at baseline than in users receiving ≥6 months of glucocorticoid therapy. In these incident glucocorticoid users experiencing high rates of bone turnover, the difference between the two forms of vitamin D was negligible. In contrast, other investigators have shown improved lumbar spine BMD and reduced fracture risk with alfacalcidiol plus calcium compared to ergocalciferol plus calcium (26,27). Regardless of the preparation of vitamin D used, which also may be influenced by product availability, high fracture rates were observed in most of these studies, especially in patients older than age 50 or with previous fragility fractures. For the majority of individuals, calcium and vitamin-D supplementation is necessary but not sufficient to reduce GIOP-related fracture morbidity.

## GUIDELINES FOR PHARMACOLOGIC INTERVENTION

Abnormalities in bone quality associated with initiation and, in particular, with use of higher-dose glucocorticoids can occur even before deleterious effects on BMD are observed (6,28–31). For this reason, GIOP guidelines differ modestly in their BMD criteria recommending treatment for new versus existing glucocorticoid users. The American College of Rheumatology (ACR) Ad Hoc Guidelines Committee, for example, recommends pharmacologic therapy for prevalent glucocorticoid users receiving prednisone doses of ≥5 mg/day who have a T score below −1.0 (10,32). The ACR also recommends bisphosphonates for all new glucocorticoid users who expect to continue therapy for more than 3 months, although caution is advised in premenopausal women. For patients already taking a dosage of glucocorticoids over 15 mg/day of prednisone or for patients receiving lower doses (≥7.5 mg/day) but at high risk of future fracture, U.K. and Dutch expert panels support bisphosphonate use even in the absence of a bone mass measurement (11,33). High-risk groups include postmenopausal women, men ≥70, and individuals with a history of previous fragility fracture. An algorithm for the evaluation and prevention of GIOP was recently published by the Dutch Society for Rheumatology and is presented in Figure 12C.2. In situations where bone mass measurement is impractical or unavailable, the Department of Veterans Affairs recommends empiric therapy with bisphosphonates when doses of prednisone

### Meta-Analysis of Vitamin D for GIOP Comparisons to No Rx/Calcium

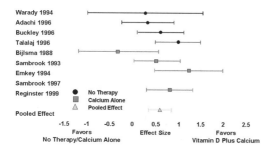

**Figure 12C.1** Meta-analysis of the effects on BMD of calcium and vitamin D compared to calcium alone or no treatment in glucocorticoid-induced osteoporosis.

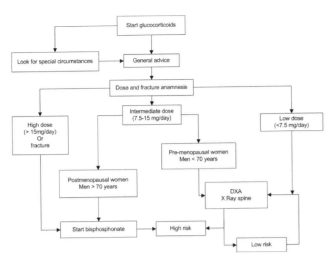

**Figure 12C.2** Guidelines from the Dutch Society for Rheumatology for the Prevention of Glucocorticoid-Induced Osteoporosis.

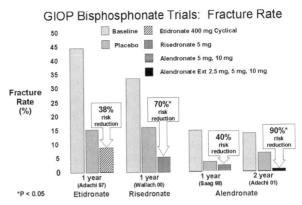

**Figure 12C.3** Efficacy of oral bisphosphonates in reducing fracture risk in glucocorticoid-induced osteoporosis.

≥7.5mg/day are prescribed for more than 3 months (34). Because bone turnover for new glucocorticoid users exceeds age-related bone loss, repeat BMD testing at approximately 1 year is justifiable either to monitor the response to pharmacologic therapy or to reevaluate the decision to defer such therapy (8,10,11). Although markers of bone formation and resorption predict fracture in high-risk patients including chronic glucocorticoid users (35,36), the clinical utility of bone biomarkers in patients receiving antiresorptive therapies is uncertain and remains largely investigational.

## Bisphosphonates

The advent of bisphosphonates has changed GIOP management dramatically. Cyclic etidronate, alendronate, and risedronate in GIOP significantly increase BMD (14–17,37–53). For example, in a second year extension to a multinational GIOP study, changes in BMD at the lumbar spine (3.85% to 0.68%) and femoral neck (0.61% to 0.66%) in the 10 mg daily alendronate-treatment group were greater compared to the placebo-treated group (−0.77 to 0.64% and −2.93 to 0.86%, respectively). Data from this trial and from a combined report of two risedronate trials demonstrated a significant reduction in a small number of overall fractures (14,15,17,39). Fracture risk reduction for these two studies and trends seen in other oral bisphosphonate studies range from 38% to 90% (Fig. 12C.3). The magnitude of decreased fracture risk is in contrast to the 1% to 4% gains in lumbar spine BMD seen at 1 to 2 years in most bisphosphonate trials. This discordance may support a role of bisphosphonates in not only reducing fracture risk by increasing BMD but also by improving bone quality, perhaps through reduced turnover (54). Based on the absolute fracture rates from clinical trials, the number of postmenopausal women needed to treat

to prevent one fragility fracture per year ranges from 8 to 26 (55). Toxicity with oral bisphosphonate therapy is low, even among high-risk GIOP commonly coprescribed non-steroidal antiinflammatory agents. The alendronate GIOP study (15,16) has been the only alendronate clinical trial to demonstrate a significant increased risk of nonserious upper gastrointestinal (Gl) events in patients randomized to 10 mg but not to 5 mg of alendronate. Weekly administration of bisphosphonates may somewhat attenuate nuisance GI side effects (56–60), and serious esophageal sequelae remain rare (61,62).

Off-label use of parenteral bisphosphonates, including pamidronate and zolendronate, may be considered for patients on glucocorticoids who cannot tolerate oral bisphosphonates. In small GIOP studies, quarterly infusions of intravenous pamidronate effected greater increases in lumbar spine and femoral neck BMD compared to patients receiving only calcium (63–67). Similar to past claims for calcitonin in postmenopausal osteoporosis (68–70), pamidronate may also reduce back pain associated with osteoporotic fractures (71). Zolendronate has not been studied for GIOP, but postmenopausal osteoporosis data showing efficacy with annual dosing compared to more frequent administration (72) suggest promise in glucocorticoid treated patients as well. A once yearly administration, if proved effective at fracture risk reduction, could fill a niche for selected GIOP patients. The newest internationally marketed bisphosphonate, ibandronate, has been studied as both oral and intravenous preparations. Preclinical data from animal models document ibandronate's ability to significantly reduce bone turnover and increase BMD in GIOP (73). Ibandronate is now approved for daily oral use in the United States but is not marketed, and intermittent parenteral dosing is being studied. An ibandronate trial of 115 patients with established GIOP (T score ≤ 2.5) randomized patients to receive either 500 mg of calcium and 1 microgram of alfacalcidiol daily or calcium and quarterly infusions of 2 mg intravenous ibandronate (74,75). At 3 years, lumbar spine BMD changes in the ibandronate group were significantly greater (13.3% to 7.2%) than in the alfacalcidiol group (2.6% to 2.3%). Respective changes in the femoral neck were 5.2% to 2.8% versus 1.9% to 1.6%. A total of 18 incident vertebral and 29 nonvertebral fractures occurred over the 3-year period. Although not specifically powered to detect a reduction in fracture risk, the incidence of new vertebral fractures in the alfacalcidiol group (22.8%) was statistically greater than in the ibandronate group (8.6%) ($p = 0.04$), a 62% relative risk reduction. There was no significant difference in the rate of nonvertebral fractures with the use of ibandronate.

Given the prolonged skeletal retention of bisphosphonates, the optimal duration of bisphosphonates therapy is controversial. One observational study of patients receiving mean prednisone doses of 9 mg/day for more than 1 year and who discontinued alendronate showed a −5.1% change in lumbar spine BMD and a −9.2% change at the femoral neck at 1 year (76). In contrast, patients who continued receiving both glucocorticoids and alendronate experienced minimal BMD change at the lumbar spine (+0.1%) and the femoral neck (−0.9%). Having now passed the 10-year mark in accumulating efficacy and safety data for oral bisphosphonates (61), the recommendation found in expert guidelines to continue therapy to prevent or treat GIOP for as long as glucocorticoids are prescribed (10) seems justified for many patients.

## Calcitonin

In contrast to the bisphosphonate data, evidence supporting the use of calcitonin for GIOP is more limited. In a GIOP prevention study, Adachi and colleagues (77) found a nonsignificant reduction (−1.3%) in BMD at 1 year in 31 patients treated with nasal calcitonin compared to a more substantial loss of BMD (−5.0%) in placebo-treated patients. While results of another prevention study of 64 sarcoid patients treated for 2 years were similar (78), no benefit was observed in a randomized, controlled trial of polymyalgia rheumatica patients treated with calcitonin (79). Results from three treatment studies of calcitonin in GIOP were similarly mixed (80–82). At best, calcitonin is a weak antiresorptive agent with mixed evidence regarding its ability to preserve bone mass in glucocorticoid treated patients. Perhaps more importantly, no reduction in fracture risk in GIOP has been documented to date. Calcitonin is generally very well tolerated with rhinitis as the only common adverse event. Calcitonin is currently a second or third line agent for use in GIOP patients that are not candidates for other approaches.

## Hormone Therapy: Estrogen, Selective Estrogen Receptor Modulators, and Testosterone

Recent data from the Women's Health Initiative (83) showing an increased risk of breast cancer and cardiovascular disease has dramatically dampened enthusiasm for the long-term use of estrogen. Nevertheless, estrogens are still considered for symptomatic postmenopausal women who may experience significant short-term improvements in climacteric symptoms and quality of life with hormone therapy (HT). In GIOP, a small head-to-head trial of transdermal estradiol (50 μg/day) or calcium supplementation (400 mg/day) in postmenopausal women with RA showed greater increases in lumbar spine BMD (3.75%, 95% CI:+0.72, +6.78) than in women receiving only calcium, although changes in femoral neck BMD (1.62%, 95% CI:−1.27, +4.51) were not different between the two groups (84). Biomarkers reflecting increased bone resorption were most elevated in glucocorticoid-treated women and fell significantly in both glucocorticoid and nonglucocorticoid users following HT use (85). Two small observational studies also document the benefit of hormonal replacement theory for GIOP (86,87). Estrogens should not be used in rheumatic disease patients who are hypercoagulable (such as those with antiphospholipid antibody syndrome), and its use in systemic lupus erythematosis (SLE) is also not recommended.

Similar to the HT data for women, improvements in lumbar spine BMD at 1 year (5.0% ± 1.4%) in hypogonadal asthmatic men treated with testosterone have been described (88). In this study, the control group not receiving testosterone experienced no significant change in BMD. Increases in lean body mass in the testosterone-treated patients were documented as well. Head-to-head comparisons of testosterone versus alendronate in small animal studies of GIOP suggest that both have efficacy in mitigating glucocorticoid-associated bone loss, but the efficacy of alendronate was greater than testosterone (89). Despite potential concerns related to the long-term administration of testosterone in men (90), including prostate cancer and the absence of long-term cardiovascular data, screening for hypogonadism and testosterone replacement should be considered in men receiving chronic glucocorticoid therapy (10).

The conclusions from these small studies of hormonal agents suggest modest efficacy in reducing glucocorticoid-associated BMD loss with the use of HT or testosterone in hypogonadal patients. The patients in these studies were treated with only low-to-moderate doses of glucocorticoids, and the efficacy of hormonal therapy in preventing BMD loss when patients are treated with higher glucocorticoid doses is unknown. Moreover, in studies of postmenopausal osteoporosis, the improvements in BMD associated with HRT are rapidly reversible upon discontinuation of therapy (90,91). Loss of BMD may even be more rapid in glucocorticoid treated patients discontinuing HT.

In contrast to the evidence supporting the use of HT and testosterone in GIOP, no data on selective estrogen receptor modulators (SERMs) is currently available. SERMs may be a reasonable choice for younger women or those for whom bisphosphonates are contraindicated, but lack of both BMD and fracture data in glucocorticoid-treated patients should make prescribers cautious. Because current data in postmenopausal osteoporosis studies suggest that raloxifene is likely a somewhat weaker antiresorptive agent than a bisphosphonate, proven therapies for prevention and treatment of GIOP should be preferred until new evidence becomes available. Similar to estrogens, SERMS slightly increase the risk of thromboembolic disease. Although in contrast to estrogen, they are not associated with breast tenderness, they lead to hot flushes in some patients. With an ever increasing number of alternate bone agents available for consideration, and unknown long-term safety, it is likely that SERMs and other hormonal therapy will play a diminishing role for GIOP prevention in the future.

## Thiazides

Systemic glucocorticoid use impairs gastrointestinal absorption and increases renal excretion of calcium (92,93). For this reason, a 24-hour urine collection to measure calcium, sodium, and creatinine may be useful to determine whether restricting sodium intake, increasing calcium intake, or administering a thiazide to decrease hypercalciuria may be appropriate. The ratio of urinary calcium to creatinine may be used as a rough estimate of daily calcium excretion, if collection of a 24-hour urine sample is not feasible. Only one study of 16 patients has specifically examined the role of thiazides diuretics in GIOP (93). In conjunction with restriction of dietary sodium to 1,150 mg per day, hydochlorothiazide at a dose of 50 mg twice daily improved calcium absorption and reduced urinary calcium excretion to the levels of nonglucocorticoid-treated patients. Whether a smaller dose of hydrochlorothiazide might be as effective in improving calcium balance as the doses used in this study is uncertain, but repeating urine electrolytes to compare with pretreatment values may be helpful in determining response. A relative paucity of data combined with symptomatic adverse effects of thiazides, at least at higher doses, limit enthusiasm for their routine use in GIOP prevention.

## Parathyroid Hormone

While several antiresorptive therapies have proved benefit in GIOP, most fail to address the defect in osteoblastic bone formation seen with glucocorticoid use. An agent that could stimulate osteoblast function and/or extend lifespan would clearly have a major role in GIOP. Teriparatide, a recombinant peptide containing the first 34 amino acids of human parathyroid hormone, is a subcutaneously administered anabolic agent effective in fracture risk reduction among both high-risk postmenopausal and male osteoporosis (94,95), and it may play a future role in GIOP. Because of concerns regarding the risk of osteosarcoma from rat models, teriparatide should not be used in patients at potential increased risk for bone tumors such as those with Paget's disease, prior skeletal radiation, and

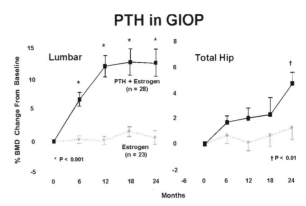

**Figure 12C.4** Improvements in BMD with teriparatide and estrogen compared to estrogen alone in glucocorticoid-treated women.

children with open epiphyses. Side effects associated with teriparatide include leg cramps, nausea, headache, and dizziness. The cost for teriparatide is approximately $500 to $600 per month in the United States.

No human parathyroid hormone (hPTH) formulation is yet indicated for prevention or treatment of GIOP. A 12-month trial of women with low bone mass (T score $\leq -2.5$) who had been receiving glucocorticoids for an average of 12 to 15 years at doses of 8 to 9 mg of prednisone daily, compared hPTH to placebo, with both groups receiving calcium, vitamin D, and estrogen (96,97). BMD at the lumbar spine assessed by dual energy x-ray absorptiometry (DXA) rapidly increased in the combination hPTH and estrogen group compared to the estrogen alone group (Fig. 12C.4). Increases in total hip BMD were delayed in the combination group but were significantly different at 24 months. Only one vertebral and four nonvertebral fractures occurred during 2 years of follow-up, so conclusions could not be drawn on fracture efficacy. Aside from its ability to increase BMD, subsequent work suggests that hPTH may reduce fracture risk by increasing bone cross-sectional area, thus increasing compressive strength (98). Improvements both in BMD and cross-sectional area may act in concert to reduce fractures. Additional trials of hPTH are currently underway to assess their relative efficacy in improving BMD in GIOP and for other indications.

## PRACTICE PATTERN VARIATIONS IN PHARMACOLOGIC THERAPIES USED FOR GIOP

Despite advances both in screening technologies and medical therapies to prevent and treat GIOP, population-based studies both in the United States and internationally suggest that fewer than one-third of chronic glucocorticoid users receive prescription therapies to prevent or treat GIOP (99–108). Despite being at greatest risk for fracture, patients older than 70 years of age and those with more comorbidities are generally less likely to receive effective interventions to prevent fractures than patients age 50 to 70 and those with fewer concomitant medical conditions (105,108). While substantial practice pattern variation between physician specialties in GIOP management has been observed, with rheumatologists often outperforming other specialty and general medicine colleagues, absolute rates of screening and treatment among all physicians are generally low (<50%) even for simple interventions such as calcium and vitamin D supplementation. Although a variety of reasons might account for low rates of GIOP screening and treatment, physicians may under appreciate the magnitude of GIOP-related fracture risk (109).

### Improving Quality of Care for GIOP

A variety of efforts have been made to improve the quality of care in GIOP. An intervention in Southern Tasmania, Australia, provided educational materials, GIOP guidelines, and academic detailing to both physicians and pharmacies within the region and assessed pre- and postintervention changes in calcium and vitamin-D supplementation and prescription therapy (110). An adjacent region (Northern Tasmania) was used as the control. Substantial improvements in the use of calcium supplementation (5% to 19%) and pharmacologic therapies (31% to 57%) were observed in hospitalized patients between the pre- and post-intervention time periods. Additionally, regional use of GIOP preventive therapies increased more in the intervention region compared to the control region, although patient level data was not available. The study was limited by assessment of only hospitalized patients and lack of patient or provider-level randomization. Nevertheless, the results suggest that evidence-based guidelines and locally endorsed educational materials in conjunction with academic detailing to both physicians and pharmacists may be effective in improving GIOP management.

Another trial randomized 21 rheumatologists caring for 373 chronic glucocorticoid users to an intervention consisting of a lecture, discussion, and confidential physician audit of practice patterns (111). In this one academic medical center, no differences in the rates of BMD testing or prescription therapies were observed in the intervention compared to the control group for BMD testing or prescription therapies for GIOP. These negative results were disappointing, although changing practicing physician behavior has been long recognized as a difficult problem (112,113). Nevertheless, the substantial morbidity and mortality related to fractures along with good clinical evidence that treatments do work should make GIOP prevention and treatment a high priority for providers caring for patients receiving glucocorticoids chronically. Novel strategies to improve suboptimal GIOP management are badly needed to reduce the disparities between evidence-based GIOP guidelines and actual practice.

## COST EFFECTIVENESS OF TREATMENT

Drug costs and potential adverse events have been described as barriers to adherence to osteoporosis guidelines (114). Despite the availability of effective therapies for GIOP, it is possible that cost concerns, in part, cause physicians to struggle with the need for prescriptions therapies in patients perceived to be at low risk for fracture. One analysis concluded that the cost effectiveness of both empiric bisphosphonates [$224,300/quality adjusted life years (QALY)] and bisphosphonates for patients with T scores $\leq -1.0$ ($92,600/QALY) was unacceptable compared to watchful waiting until a fracture occurred (115). However, the assumptions used were quite conservative, assuming a fracture rate of only 6.4% in untreated patients and a relative risk reduction of fracture with alendronate of only 12.5%. Assuming a 10-year fracture risk reduction of 50% with the use of alendronate, the cost per QALY decreased to of $18,700; more within the range of other accepted medical interventions. Sensitivity analysis using the higher baseline fracture rates observed in bisphosphonate clinical trials of GIOP (10% to 20%) made bisphosphonate treatment even more cost effective.

A more recent cost-effective analysis of calcium, vitamin D, and alendronate in women treated with chronic glucocorticoids demonstrated cost effectiveness of calcium and vitamin D supplementation in women of all age groups except women 30 years old with normal bone density (116). Based on the assumptions of this model, the cost per vertebral fracture avoided with bisphosphonate therapy over a 10-year period was in line with other medical therapies only for older women (70 years of age) with low bone mass at baseline (T score = −2.0). Bisphosphonate treatment was more reasonable (<$8,000 per vertebral fracture avoided) for younger women with higher BMD when the lifetime risk of fracture was considered.

## CONCLUSIONS

Effective therapies to prevent and treat GIOP such as the use of sufficient calcium, vitamin D, and early prescription for bisphosphonates can result in a lower risk of insufficiency fractures. Newer medications with convenient dosing schedules such as parenteral bisphosphonates and anabolic agents that rapidly improve BMD and bone quality such as parathyroid hormone offer hope for a broader range of treatment options in the near future. Despite accumulating evidence, GIOP therapies are underutilized for many patients, and physicians do not consistently recognize or appreciate early, accelerated bone loss and increased fracture risk associated with glucocorticoid use. Despite substantial strides already, further work is needed to improve the efficacy, effectiveness, and ultimately the cost effectiveness of prevention and treatment of GIOP.

# REFERENCES

1. Kirwan JR, Arthritis and Rheumatism Council Low Dose Glucocorticoid Study Group. The effect of glucocorticoids on joint destruction in rheumatoid arthritis. *N Engl J Med* 1995;333:142–146.
2. Kirwan JR, Russell AS. Systemic glucocorticoid treatment in rheumatoid arthritis—a debate. *Scand J Rheumatol* 1998;27: 247–251.
3. van Everdingen AA, Jacobs JWG, van Reesema DR, Bijlsma JWJ. Low dose prednisone therapy for patients with early active rheumatoid arthritis: clinical efficacy, disease modifying properties and side effects. A double-blind placebo-controlled clinical trial. *Ann Intern Med* 2002;136:1–12.
4. Saag KG, Koehnke R, Caldwell JR, et al. Low dose long-term corticosteroid therapy in rheumatoid arthritis: an analysis of serious adverse events. *Am J Med* 1994;96:115–123.
5. Michel BA, Bloch DA, Wolfe F, Fries J. Fractures in rheumatoid arthritis: an evaluation of associated risk factors. *J Rheum* 1993;20:1666–1669.
6. van Staa T, Leufkens H, Abenhaim L, et al. Use of oral corticosteroids and risk of fractures. *J Bone Miner Res* 2000;15(6): 993–1000.
7. Pocock NA, Eisman JA, Dunstan CR, et al. Recovery from steroid-induced osteoporosis. *Ann Intern Med* 1987;107:319.
8. Adachi JD, Olszynski WP, Hanley DA, et al. Management of corticosteroid-induced osteoporosis. *Sem Arth Rheum* 2000;29(4): 228–251.
9. Adler R, Hochberg MC. Suggested guidelines for evaluation and treatment of glucocorticoid-induced osteoporosis for the Department of Veterans Affairs. *Arch Int Med* 2003;163(21): 2619–2624.
10. American College of Rheumatology Ad Hoc Committee on Glucocorticoid-Induced Osteoporosis. Recommendations for the prevention and treatment of glucocorticoid-induced osteoporosis. *Arthritis Rheum* 2001;44:1496–1503.
11. Bone & Tooth Society of Great Britain. *Glucocorticoid-Induced Osteoporosis: Guidelines for Prevention & Treatment.* 2002.
12. Lane N, Goldring S, Stewart J, Morris S. Biochemical markers of bone turnover in glucocorticoid treated patients are altered by calcium supplementation: preliminary results from the ACTIVATE trial. *Arthritis Rheum* 2003;48(9):S498.
13. Buckley LM, Leib ES, Cartularo KS, et al. Calcium and vitamin D3 supplementation prevents bone loss in the spine secondary to low-dose corticosteroids in patients with rheumatoid arthritis. *Ann Intern Med* 1996;125:961–968.
14. Wallach S, Cohen S, Reid DM, et al. Effects of risedronate treatment on bone density and vertebral fracture in patients on corticosteroid therapy. *Calcif Tissue Int* 2000;67:277–285.
15. Adachi R, Saag K, Emkey R, et al. Effects of alendronate for two years on BMD and fractures in patients receiving glucocorticoids. *Arthritis Rheum* 2001;44:202–211.
16. Saag KG, Emkey R, Schnitzer T, et al. Alendronate for the treatment and prevention of glucocorticoid-induced osteoporosis. *N Engl J Med* 1998;339:292–299.
17. Reid DM, Hughes R, Laan RF. Efficacy and safety of daily risedronate in the treatment of corticosteroid-induced osteoporosis in men and women: a randomized trial. *J Bone Min Res* 2000;15: 1006–1013.
18. Sambrook P, Birmingham J, Kelly P, et al. Prevention of corticosteroid osteoporosis. A comparison of calcium, calcitriol, and calcitonin. *N Engl J Med* 1993;328:1747–1752.
19. Dykman T, Haralson K, Gluck O, et al. Effect of oral 1,25-dihydroxyvitamin D and calcium on glucocorticoid-induced osteopenia in patients with rheumatic diseases. *Arthritis Rheum* 1984;27(12):1336–1343.
20. Braun JJ, Birkenhager-Frenkel DH, Rietvoeld AH, et al. Influence of 1 alpha-(OH)D3 administration on bone and bone mineral metabolism in patients on chronic glucocorticoid treatment; A double blind controlled study. *Clin Endocrinol* 1983;18:265–273.
21. Reginster JY, Kuntz D, Verdickt W, et al. Prophylactic use of alfacalcidol in corticosteroid-induced osteoporosis. *Osteoporos Int* 1999;9:75–81.
22. Bijlsma JWJ, Raymakers JA, Mosch C, et al. Effect of oral calcium and vitamin D on glucocorticoid-induced osteopenia. *Clin Exper Rheumatol* 1988;6:113–119.
23. Homik J, Suarez-Almazor M, Shea B, et al. Calcium and vitamin D for corticosteroid-induced osteoporosis (Cochrane Review). *The Cochrane Library.* 1999;Vol.Issue 1. Oxford: Update Software.
24. Amin S, LaValley MP, Simms RW, Felson DT. The role of vitamin D in corticosteroid-induced osteoporosis. *Arthritis Rheum* 1999;42(8):1740–1751.
25. Sambrook PN, Kotowicz M, Nash P, et al. Prevention and treatment of glucocorticoid-induced osteoporosis: a comparison of calcitriol, vitamin D plus calcium, and alendronate plus calcium. *J Bone Miner Res* 2003;18(5):919–924.
26. Ringe J, Dorst A, Faber H, et al. Superiority of alfacalcidol over plain vitamin D in the treatment of glucocorticoid-induced osteoporosis. *Rheumatology Int* 2004;24(2):63–70.
27. Ringe J, Coster A, Meng T, et al. Treatment of glucocorticoid-induced osteoporosis with alfacalcidol/calcium versus vitamin D/calcium. *Calcif Tissue Int* 1999;65(4):337–340.
28. van Everdingen AA, Siewertsz van Reesema DR, Jacobs JW, Bijlsma JW. Low-dose glucocorticoids in early rheumatoid arthritis: discordant effects on bone mineral density and fractures? *Clin Exp Rheumatol* 2003;21(2):155–160.
29. van Staa T, Leufkens H, Cooper C. The epidemiology of corticosteroid induced osteoporosis: a meta-analysis. *Osteoporos Int* 2002;13:777–787.
30. van Staa TP, Laan RF, Barton IP, et al. Bone density threshold and other predictors of vertebral fracture in patients receiving oral glucocorticoid therapy. *Arthritis Rheum* 2003;48(11):3224–3229.
31. van Staa TP, Leukens HGM, Abenhaim L, et al. Oral corticosteroids and fracture risk: relationship to daily and cumulative doses. *Rheumatology (Oxf)* 2000;39:1383–1389.
32. American College of Rheumatology Task Force on Osteoporosis Guidelines. Recommendations for the prevention and treatment of glucocorticoid-induced osteoporosis. *Arthritis Rheum* 1996;39: 1791–1801.
33. Geusens P, de Nijs RNJ, Lems WF, et al. Prevention of glucocorticoid osteoporosis: a consensus document of the Dutch Society for Rheumatology. *Ann Rheum Dis* 2004;63:324–325.
34. Adler RA, Hochberg MC. Suggested guidelines for evaluation and treatment of glucocorticoid-induced osteoporosis for the Department of Veterans Affairs. *Arch Intern Med* 2003;163(21): 2619–2624.
35. Van Staa T, Eastell R, Barton IP, et al. The value of bone turnover markers in the prediction of vertebral fracture in patients using oral glucocorticoids. *J Bone Min Res* 2003;18(S2):S66.
36. Eastell R, Barton I, Hannon R, et al. Relationship of Early Changes in Bone Resorption to the reduction in fracture risk with risedronate. *J Bone Min Res* 2003;18(6):1051–1056.
37. Adachi JD, Roux C, Pitt PI, et al. A pooled data analysis on the use of intermittent cyclical etidronate therapy for the prevention and treatment of corticosteroid induced bone loss. *J Rheumatol* 2000;27(10):2424–2431.
38. Reid D, Cohen C, Pack S, et al. Risedronate reduces the incidence of vertebral fractures in patients on chronic corticosteroid therapy. *Arthritis Rheum* 1998;41:S136.
39. Cohen S, Levy RM, Keller M, et al. Risedronate therapy prevents corticosteroid-induced bone loss: a twelve-month, multicenter, randomized, double-blind, placebo-controlled, parallel-group study. *Arthritis Rheum* 1999;42(11):2309–2318.
40. Roux C, Oriente P, Laan R, et al. Randomized trial of effect of cyclical etidronate in the prevention of corticosteroid-induced bone loss. *J Clin Endocrinol Metab* 1998;83:1128–1133.
41. Loddenkemper K, Grauer A, Burmester GR, Buttgereit F. Calcium, vitamin D and etidronate for the prevention and treatment of corticosteroid-induced osteoporosis in patients with rheumatic diseases. *Clin Exp Rheumatol* 2003;21(1):19–26.
42. Sebaldt RJ, Ioannidis G, Adachi JD, et al. 36 month intermittent cyclical etidronate treatment in patients with established corticosteroid induced osteoporosis. *J Rheumatol* 1999;26:1545–1549.
43. Pitt P, Todd P, Webber D, et al. A double blind placebo controlled study to determine the effects of intermittent cyclical etidronate on bone mineral density in patients on long term oral corticosteroid treatment. *Thorax* 1998;53:351–356.

44. Geusens P, Dequeker J, Vanhoof J, et al. Cyclical etidronate increases bone density in the spine and hip of postmenopausal women receiving long term corticosteroid treatment. A double blind, randomised placebo controlled study. *Ann Rheum Dis* 1998;57:724–727.

45. Wolfhagen FH, vanBuuren HR, denOuden JW, et al. Cyclic etidronate in the prevention of bone loss in corticosteroid-treated primary biliary cirrhosis. *J Hepatol* 1997;26:325–330.

46. Adachi JD, Bensen WG, Brown J, et al. Intermittent etidronate therapy to prevent corticosteroid-induced osteoporosis. *N Engl J Med* 1997;337:382–387.

47. Struys A, Snelder AA, Mulder H. Cyclical etidronate reverses bone loss of the spine and proximal femur in patients with established corticosteroid-induced osteoporosis. *Am J Med* 1995;99:235–242.

48. Diamond T, McGuigan L, Barbagallo S, Bryant C. Cyclical etidronate plus ergocalciferol prevents glucocorticoid-induced bone loss in postmenopausal women. *Am J Med* 1995;98:459–463.

49. Skingle SJ, Crisp AJ. Increased bone density in patients on steroids with etidronate. *Lancet* 1994;344:543.

50. Mulder H, Struys A. Intermittent cyclical etidronate in the prevention of corticosteroid-induced bone loss. *Br J Rheumatol* 1994;33:348–350.

51. Adachi JD, Cranney A, Goldsmith CH, et al. Intermittent cyclic therapy with etidronate in the prevention of corticosteroid induced bone loss. *J Rheumatol* 1994;21:1922–1926.

52. Gonnelli S, Rottoli P, Cepollaro C, et al. Prevention of corticosteroid-induced osteoporosis with alendronate in sarcoid patients. *Calcif Tissue Int* 1997;6:382–385.

53. Jenkins EA, Walker-Bone KE, Wood A, et al. The prevention of corticosteroid-induced bone loss with intermittent cyclical etidronate. *Scand J Rheumatol* 1999;28:152–156.

54. Riggs L, Melton L. Bone turnover matters: The raloxifene treatment paradox of dramatic decreases in vertebral fractures without commensurate increases in bone density. *J Bone Min Res* 2002;17(1):11–14.

55. Sambrook PN. Corticosteroid osteoporosis: practical implications of recent trials. *J Bone Min Res* 2000;15(9):1645–1649.

56. Sambrook P. Once weekly alendronate. *Drugs Today (Barc)* 2003;39(5):339–346.

57. Blumel J, Castelo-Branco C, de la Cuadra G, et al. Alendronate daily, weekly in conventional tablets and weekly in enteric tablets: preliminary study on the effects in bone turnover markers and incidence of side effects. *J Obstet Gynaecol* 2003;23(3):278–281.

58. Lanza F, Sahba B, Schwarts H, et al. The upper GI safety and tolerability of oral alendronate at a dose of 70 milligrams once weekly: a placebo-controlled endoscopy study. *Am J Gastroenterol* 2002;97(1):58–64.

59. Greenspan S, Field-Munves E, Tonino RP, et al. Tolerability of once-weekly alendronate in patients with osteoporosis: a randomized, double-blind, placebo-controlled study. *Mayo Clin Proc* 2002;77(10):1044–1052.

60. Schnitzer T, Bone H, Crepaldi G, et al. Therapeutic equivalence of alendronate 70 mg once-weekly and alendronate 10 mg daily in the treatment of osteoporosis. Alendronate Once-Weekly Study Group. *Aging* 2000;12(1):1–12.

61. Bone HG, Hosking D, Devogelaer J-P, et al. Ten years' experience with alendronate for osteoporosis in postmenopausal women. *N Engl J Med* 2004;350(12):1189–1199.

62. Donahue JG, Chan KA, Andrade SE, et al. Gastric and duodenal safety of daily alendronate. *Arch Intern Med* 2002;162(8):936–942.

63. Boutsen Y, Jamart J, Esselinckx W, et al. Primary prevention of glucocorticoid-induced osteoporosis with intermittent intravenous pamidronate: a randomized trial. *Calcif Tissue Int* 1997;61:266–271.

64. Boutsen Y, Jamart J, Esselnickx W, Devogelaer JP. Primary prevention of glucocorticoid-induced osteoporosis with intravenous pamidronate and calcium: a prospective controlled 1-year study comparing a single infusion, an infusion given once every 3 months, and calcium alone. *J Bone Miner Res* 2001;16(1):104–112.

65. Gallacher SJ, Fenner JAK, Anderson K, et al. Intravenous pamidronate in the treatment of osteoporosis associated with corticosteroid dependent lung disease: an open pilot study. *Thorax* 1992;47:932–936.

66. Valkema R, Vismans F-JE, Papapoulos SE, et al. Maintained improvement in calcium balance and bone mineral content in patients with osteoporosis treated with the bisphosphonate APD. *Bone Miner* 1989;5:183–192.

67. Reid IR, King AR, Alexander CJ, Ibbertson HK. Prevention of steroid-induced osteoporosis with (3-amino-1-hydroxypropylidene)-1, 1-bisphosphonate (APD). *Lancet* 1988;1:143–146.

68. Lyritis GP, Tsakalabos S, Magiasis B, et al. Analgesic effect of salmon calcitonin on osteoporotic vertebral fractures. Double-blind, placebo-controlled study. *Calcif Tissue Int* 1991;49:369–372.

69. Lyritis GP, Paspati I, Karachalios T, et al. Pain relief from nasal salmon calcitonin in osteoporotic vertebral crush fractures. A double blind, placebo controlled clinical study. *Acta Orthop Scand Suppl* 1997;275:112–114.

70. Pun KK, Chan LWL. Analgesic effect of intranasal salmon calcitonin in the treatment of osteoporotic vertebral fractures. *Clin Therapeutics* 1989;11(2).

71. Gangji V, Appelboom T. Analgesic effect of intravenous pamidronate on chronic back pain due to osteoporotic vertebral fractures. *Clin Rheumatol* 1999;18:266–267.

72. Reid IR, Brown JP, Burckhardt P, et al. Intravenous zoledronic acid in postmenopausal women with low bone mineral density. *N Engl J Med* 2002;346:653–661.

73. Bauss F, Russell R. Ibandronate in osteoporosis: preclinical data and rationale for intermittent dosing. *Osteoporos Int* 2004; (in press).

74. Ringe JD, Dorst A, Faber H, et al. Intermittent intravenous ibandronate injections reduce vertebral fracture risk in corticosteroid-induced osteoporosis: results from a long-term comparative study. *Osteoporos Int* 2003;14(10):801–807.

75. Ringe JD, Dorst A, Faber H, et al. Three-monthly ibandronate bolus injection offers favourable tolerability and sustained efficacy advantage over two years in established corticosteroid-induced osteoporosis. *Rheumatology (Oxf)* 2003;42(6):743–749.

76. Emkey R, Delmas PD, Goemaere S, et al. Changes in bone mineral density following discontinuation or continuation of alendronate therapy in glucocorticoid-treated patients: a retrospective, observational study. *Arthritis Rheum* 2003;48(4):1102–1108.

77. Adachi JD, Bensen WG, Bell MJ, et al. Salmon calcitonin nasal spray in the prevention of corticosteroid-induced osteoporosis. *Br J Rheumatol* 1997;36(2):255–257.

78. Montemurro L, Schiraldi G, Fraioli P, et al. Prevention of corticosteroid-induced osteoporosis with salmon calcitonin in sarcoid patients. *Calcif Tissue Int* 1991;49:71–76.

79. Healey JH, Paget SA, Williams-Russo P, et al. A randomized controlled trial of salmon calcitonin to prevent bone loss in corticosteroid-treated temporal arteritis and polymyalgia rheumatica. *Calcif Tissue Int* 1996;58:73–80.

80. Kotaniemi A, Piirainen H, Paimela L, et al. Is continuous intranasal salmon calcitonin effective in treating axial bone loss in patients with active rheumatoid arthritis receiving low dose glucocorticoid therapy? *J Rheumatol* 1996;23:1875–1879.

81. Luengo M, Pons F, Martinez de Osaba MJ, Picado C. Prevention of further bone mass loss by nasal calcitonin in patients on long term glucocorticoid therapy for asthma: a two year follow up study. *Thorax* 1994;49:1099.

82. Ringe J-D, Welzel D. Salmon calcitonin in the therapy of corticosteroid-induced osteoporosis. *Eur J Clin Pharmacol* 1987;33:35–39.

83. Writing Group for the Women's Health Initiative Investigators. Risks and benefits of estrogen plus progestin in healthy postmenopausal women: Principal results from the Women's Health Initiative Randomized Controlled Trial. *JAMA* 2002;288:321–333.

84. Hall GM, Daniels M, Doyle DV, Spector TD. Effect of hormone replacement therapy on bone mass in rheumatoid arthritis patients treated with and without steroids. *Arthritis Rheum* 1994;37:1499–505.

85. Hall G, Spector T, Delmas P. Markers of bone metabolism in postmenopausal women with rheumatoid arthritis. Effects of corticosteroids and hormone replacement therapy. *Arthritis Rheum* 1995;38(7):902–906.

86. Lukert BP, Johnson BE, Robinson RG. Estrogen and progesterone replacement therapy reduces glucocorticoid-induced bone loss. *J Bone Miner Res* 1992;7:1063–1069.

87. Sambrook P, Birmingham J, Champion D, et al. Postmenopausal bone loss in rheumatoid arthritis: effect of estrogens and androgens. *J Rheumatol* 1992;19:357–361.

88. Reid IR, Wattie DJ, Evans MC, Stapleton JP. Testosterone therapy in glucocorticoid-treated men. *Arch Intern Med* 1996;156: 1173–1177.

89. Wimalawansa S, Simmons D. Prevention of corticosteroid-induced bone loss with alendronate. *Proc Soc Exp Biol Med* 1998;217(2):162–167.

90. Rhoden E, Morgentaler A. Medical Progress: Risks of testosterone-replacement therapy and recommendations for monitoring. *N Engl J Med* 2004;350:482–492.

91. Greenspan S, Emkey R, Bone H, et al. Significant differential effects of alendronate, estrogen, or combination therapy on the rate of bone loss after discontinuation of treatment of postmenopausal osteoporosis: a randomized, double-blind, placebo-controlled trial. *Ann Intern Med* 2002;137:875–883.

92. Adams JS, Song CF, Kantorovich V. Rapid recovery of bone mass in hypercalciuric, osteoporotic men treated with hydrochlorothiazide. *Ann Intern Med* 1999;130:658–660.

93. Adams JS, Wahl TO, Lukert BP. Effects of hydrochlorothiazide and dietary sodium restriction on calcium metabolism in corticosteroid treated patients. *Metabolism* 1981;30:217–221.

94. Orwoll ES, Scheele WH, Paul S, et al. The effect of teriparatide [human parathyroid hormone (1–34)] therapy on bone density in men with osteoporosis. *J Bone Min Res* 2003;18(1):9–17.

95. Neer R, Arnaud C, Zanchetta J, et al. Effect of parathyroid hormone (1–34) on fractures and bone mineral density in postmenopausal women with osteoporosis. *N Engl J Med* 2001; 344(19):1434–1441.

96. Lane N, Sanchez S, Modin G, et al. Bone mass continues to increase at the hip after parathyroid hormone treatment is discontinued in glucocorticoid induced osteoporosis: results of a randomized controlled clinical trial. *J Bone Min Res* 2000; 15(5):944–951.

97. Lane NE, Sanchez S, Modin GW, et al. Parathyroid hormone treatment can reverse corticosteroid-induced osteoporosis. Results of a randomized controlled clinical trial. *J Clin Invest* 1998;102(8):1627–1633.

98. Rehman Q, Lang T, Arnaud C, et al. Daily treatment with parathyroid hormone is associated with an increase in vertebral cross-sectional area in postmenopausal women with glucocorticoid-induced osteoporosis. *Osteoporos Int* 2003;14(1):77–81.

99. Hart S, Green B. Osteoporosis prophylaxis during corticosteroid treatment: failure to prescribe. *Postgrad Med J* 2002;78(918): 242–243.

100. Gudbjornsson B, Juliusson UI, Gudjonsson FV. Prevalence of long term steroid treatment and the frequency of decision making to prevent steroid induced osteoporosis in daily clinical practice. *Ann Rheum Dis* 2002;61(1):32–36.

101. Walsh LJ, Wong CA, Pringle M, Tattersfield AE. Use of oral corticosteroids in the community and the prevention of secondary osteoporosis: a cross sectional study. *BMJ* 1996;313:344–346.

102. Mudano A, Allison J, Hill J, et al. Variations in glucocorticoid induced osteoporosis prevention in a managed care cohort. *J Rheumatol* 2001;28(6):1298–1305.

103. Yood RA, Harrold LR, Fish L, et al. Prevention of glucocorticoid-induced osteoporosis: experience in a managed care setting. *Arch Intern Med* 2001;161:1322–1327.

104. Osiri M, Saag KG, Ford AM, Moreland LW. Practice pattern variation among internal medicine specialists in the prevention of glucocorticoid-induced osteoporosis. *J Clin Rheumatol* 2000;6: 117–122.

105. Chantler IW, Davie MW, Evans SF, Rees JS. Oral corticosteroid prescribing in women over 50, use of fracture prevention therapy, and bone densitometry service. *Ann Rheum Dis* 2003;62(4): 350–352.

106. Peat ID, Healy S, Reid DM, et al. Steroid induced osteoporosis: an opportunity for prevention? *Ann Rheum Dis* 1995;54:66–68.

107. Buckley LM, Marquez M, Feezor R, et al. Prevention of corticosteroid-induced osteoporosis: results of a patient survey. *Arthritis Rheum* 1999;42(8):1736–1739.

108. Solomon DH, Katz J, Jacobs JW, et al. Management of glucocorticoid induced osteoporosis in patients with rheumatoid arthritis. *Arthritis Rheum* 2002;46(12):3136–3142.

109. Buckley LM, Marquez M, Hudson JO, et al. Variations in physician perceptions of the risk of osteoporosis in corticosteroid users by physician specialty. *J Rheumatol* 1998;25:2195–2202.

110. Naunton M, Peterson GM, Jones G, et al. Multifaceted educational program increases prescribing of preventive medication for corticosteroid induced osteoporosis. *J Rheumatol* 2004;31(3): 550–556.

111. Solomon D, Katz J, La Tourette A, Coblyn J. A multifaceted intervention to improve rheumatologists' management of glucocorticoid induced osteoporosis: a randomized controlled trial. *Arth Care Res* 2004;(in press).

112. Davis D, Thomson M, Oxman A, Haynes R. Changing physician performance. A systematic review of the effect of continuing medical education strategies. *JAMA* 1995;274:700–705.

113. O'Brien T, Oxman A, Davis D, et al. Educational outreach visits: effects on professional practice and health care outcomes [Cochrane Review]. *Cochrane Database Syst Rev* 2000;2(CD000409).

114. Simonelli C, Killeen K, Mehle S, Swanson L. Barriers to osteoporosis identification and treatment among primary care physicians and orthopedic surgeons. *Mayo Clin Proc* 2002;77: 334–338.

115. Solomon DH, Kuntz KK. Should postmenopausal women with rheumatoid arthritis who are starting corticosteroid treatment be screened for osteoporosis? *Arthritis Rheum* 2000;43:1967–1975.

116. Buckley LM, Hillner BE. A cost effectiveness analysis of calcium and vitamin D supplementation, etidronate, and alendronate in the prevention of vertebral fractures in women treated with glucocorticoids. *J Rheumatol* 2003;30(1):132–138.

# Drug-Induced Bone Loss

**13**

*Jonathan Adachi*

Glucocorticoids are a well-known cause of secondary osteoporosis. Many other medications are potential threats to skeletal health in patients with rheumatic diseases and are reviewed in this chapter.

## HEPARIN, LOW-MOLECULAR-WEIGHT HEPARINS AND WARFARIN

Rheumatic patients with thromboembolic phenomena and coagulopathies such as the antiphospholipid antibody syndrome may be treated with heparin, low-molecular-weight heparins (LMWHs), or warfarin. In addition to decreasing osteoblastic protein and collagen synthesis, heparin enhances Interleukin 11–induced expression of receptor activator of nuclear factor-κB ligand (RANKL) leading to osteoclast formation. An increased risk of symptomatic vertebral fractures has been described during pregnancy and postpartum in 2.2% of women undergoing prophylaxis with heparin (1). In general, fractures are unlikely in patients receiving less than 15,000 units per day for less than 3 months (2). LMWHs have been reported as less deleterious to bone then unfractionated heparin; however, long-term exposure to LMWHs can cause a modest decrease in bone mineral density (BMD) and a lumbar fragility fracture has been reported in a young patient exposed to this type of anticoagulation. Most investigators believe that LMWHs have similar effects on the skeleton as heparin and that the potential differences are related to dosage and duration of exposure.

Warfarin inhibits vitamin K–dependent gamma-carboxylation of clotting factors and osteocalcin, a noncollagenous skeletal protein. Warfarin has not been shown consistently to lower BMD or increase fracture risk.

## ANTICONVULSANTS

Chronic anticonvulsant therapy has been associated with reduced BMD and an increased risk of fractures (3). Individuals with epilepsy, especially those taking phenytoin, have an increase in fracture risk, although the increased fracture frequency may be related to seizures (4). Phenytoin, phenobarbital, and carbamazepine may induce hepatic cytochrome $P_{450}$ activity and accelerate catabolism of 25-hydroxyvitamin D. As a result, patients may present with hypocalcemia, an elevated serum alkaline phosphatase, and elevated serum parathyroid hormone levels. Bone loss can occur in the absence of reduced serum 25-hydroxyvitamin D. Phenytoin has been demonstrated to reduce intestinal calcium absorption and increase bone resorption (3). Valproic acid may lead to bone loss by inducing a renal leak of calcium and phosphorus. Gabapentin, lamotrigine, and felbamate have not yet reported to have adverse effect on bone.

High-dose, multiple anticonvulsant drug regimens (such as combination phenytoin and phenobarbital), long duration of anticonvulsant therapy, low calcium intake, and/or poor vitamin-D intake or exposure (in elderly or institutionalized patients) may worsen the effect of these drugs on the skeleton. Hypovitaminosis D may also lead to a clinically significant proximal myopathy, increasing the risk for falls.

## THYROID HORMONE THERAPY

Excessive thyroid hormone causes high bone turnover through an increase in activation frequency of bone remodeling units. There is more bone loss in cortical than in trabecular bone (5).

Thyroid stimulating hormone (TSH) oversuppression with thyroxine therapy has been associated with reduced BMD in some studies (6) but not in others (7). A systematic review concluded that thyroid hormone therapy without oversuppression of TSH does not negatively effect BMD (8). TSH suppression in premenopausal women does not significantly reduce BMD, but oversuppression in postmenopausal women is associated with significant bone loss (9).

The risk for hip fracture has been found to be higher in women with a history of hyperthyroidism, and men taking thyroid hormone may be at increased risk of fracture (10). To prevent bone loss during thyroid hormone therapy, serum free thyroxine and TSH should be monitored using the most sensitive techniques, and the thyroid replacement dosage should be adjusted to avoid hyperthyroidism.

## METHOTREXATE

Histomorphometric studies in rats treated with methotrexate (MTX) have shown decreased bone formation and increased bone resorption (11). Clinical reports that MTX might cause low bone density and/or fractures came from children treated with high-dose MTX for leukemia (12). Whether bone loss and fractures were caused by MTX, concurrent prednisone therapy, immobility, or the disease state is not clear.

There is very little evidence for a role of MTX causing osteoporosis in rheumatic patients. In one study, low-dose MTX was not associated with bone loss at the femoral neck or lumbar spine in patients not treated with concurrent glucocorticoids (13). A prospective case-control study of patients with either psoriatic or rheumatoid arthritis showed that lower doses of MTX do not have an adverse effect on BMD in patients either at cortical or trabecular sites (14). In a study of 116 nonglucocorticoid-treated RA patients, no adverse effect of low-dose MTX (mean 10 mg/week) was found (15).

## CALMODULIN-CALCINEURIN PHOSPHATASE INHIBITORS

Calmodulin-calcineurin phosphatase inhibitors (cyclosporine A and tacrolimus) have also been used in the treatment of rheumatoid arthritis and other autoimmune diseases. Whether cyclosporine or tacrolimus cause bone loss in human beings is difficult to ascertain, as they are generally given in addition to glucocorticoids (16). In rats, cyclosporine and tacrolimus induce increased bone turnover, elevated osteocalcin, and trabecular bone loss (17).

## DEPOT MEDROXYPROGESTERONE ACETATE

Depot medroxyprogesterone acetate (DMPA) is an injectable contraceptive that works by inhibiting pituitary gonadotropin secretion, resulting in suppression of ovulation and ovarian estrogen secretion. DMPA use has been associated with significant bone loss (18). The greatest loss appears to occur in the first year of use, although bone loss can continue to occur for 3 to 4 years after initiation of DMPA. The extent of loss is comparable to that seen in early menopause.

## AROMATASE INHIBITORS

Aromatase inhibitors such as anastrozole and letrozole block the conversion of androgen to estrogen in peripheral tissues and are being increasingly used for the treatment of advanced breast cancer in postmenopausal women (18,19). A trial comparing tamoxifen and anastrozole demonstrated increased bone loss and fractures in those treated with the aromatase inhibitor (20). Trials of concurrent administration of bisphosphonates with aromatase inhibitors are currently underway.

## LUTEINIZING HORMONE-RELEASING HORMONE AGONISTS

Luteinizing hormone-releasing hormone agonists (LHRH-a), used as treatment for prostate carcinoma, advanced breast cancer, and several gynecologic conditions act to stimulate gonadotropins and down-regulate anterior pituitary LHRH receptors, resulting in the suppression of sex steroids and alterations in bone metabolism.

Loss of both bone and lean body mass has been reported in men treated with LHRH-a (21), and there may be an increased incidence of fractures in these patients. Both intravenous pamidronate (60 mg every 3 months) (22) and intravenous zoledronate (4 mg every 3 months) (23) have prevented bone loss induced by androgen ablation. Similar studies have not yet been performed with oral bisphosphonates.

## CONCLUDING REMARKS

An increased awareness of the potential causes of secondary osteoporosis can aid in the prevention and treatment of bone loss. Regular monitoring of the skeletal status of patients being treated with medications known to cause bone loss would be advisable to identify individuals who are at risk of osteoporosis and to initiate appropriate therapeutic or preventative measures.

## REFERENCES

1. Dahlman TC. Osteoporotic fractures and the recurrence of thromboembolism during pregnancy and the puerperium in 184 women undergoing thromboprophylaxis with heparin. *Am J Obstet Gynecol* 1993;168:1265–1270.

2. Tannirandorn P, Epstein S. Drug-induced bone loss. *Osteoporos Int* 2000;11:637–659.

3. Weinstein RS, Bryce GF, Sappington LJ, et al. Decreased serum ionized calcium and normal vitamin D metabolite levels with anticonvulsant drug treatment. *J Clin Endocrinol Metab* 1984;58(6):1003–1009.

4. Morrell MJ. Reproductive and metabolic disorders in women with epilepsy. *Epilepsia* 2003;44(4S):11–20.

5. Sheppard MC, Holder R, Franklyn JA. Levothyroxine treatment and occurrence of fracture of the hip. *Arch Intern Med* 2002;162(3):338–343.

6. Kung AW, Yeung SS. Prevention of bone loss induced by thyroxine suppressive therapy in postmenopausal women: the effect of calcium and calcitonin. *J Clin Endocrinol Metab* 1996;81(3):1232–1236.

7. Marcocci C, Golia F, Bruno-Bossio G, et al. Carefully monitored levothyroxine suppressive therapy is not associated with bone loss in premenopausal women. *J Clin Endocrinol Metab* 1994;78(4):818–823.

8. Greenspan SL, Greenspan FS. The effect of thyroid hormone on skeletal integrity. *Ann Intern Med* 1999;130(9):750–758.

9. Faber J, Galloe AM. Changes in bone mass during prolonged subclinical hyperthyroidism due to L-thyroxine treatment: a meta-analysis. *Eur J Endocrinol* 1994;130(4):350–356.

10. Sheppard MC, Holder R, Franklyn JA. Levothyroxine treatment and occurrence of fracture of the hip. *Arch Intern Med* 2002;162(3):338–343.

11. May KP, West SG, McDermott MT, Huffer WE. The effect of low-dose methotrexate on bone metabolism and histomorphometry in rats. *Arthritis Rheum* 1994;37:201–206.

12. Ragab AH, Frech RS, Vietti T. Osteoporostic fractures secondary to methotrexate therapy of acute leukemia in remission. *Cancer* 1970;25:580–585.

13. Buckley LM, Leib ES, Cartularo KS, et al. Effects of low dose methotrexate on the bone mineral density of patients with rheumatoid arthritis. *J Rheumatol* 1997;24;8:1489–1494.

14. Minaur NJ, Kounali D, Vedi S, et al. Methotrexate in the treatment of rheumatoid arthritis. II. In vivo effects on bone mineral density. *Rheumatology* 2002;41;7:741–749.

15. Cranney AB, McKendry RJ, Wells GA, et al. The effect of low dose methotrexate on bone density. *J Rheumatol* 2001;28(11):2395–2399.

16. Mikuls TR, Julian BA, Bartolucci A, Saag KG. Bone mineral density changes within six months of renal transplantation. *Transplantation* 2003;75(1):49–54.

17. Epstein S. Post-transplantation bone disease: the role of immunosuppressive agents and the skeleton. *J Bone Miner Res* 1996;11:1–7.

18. Cromer BA. Bone mineral density in adolescent and young adult women on injectable or oral contraception. *Curr Opin Obstet Gynecol* 2003;15:353–357.

19. The ATAC Trialist's Group. Anastrozole alone or in combination with tamoxifen versus tamoxifen alone for adjuvant treatment of postmenopausal women with early breast cancer: first results of the ATAC randomised trial. *Lancet* 2002;359:2131–2139.

20. Goss PR, Ingle JN, Martino S, et al. A randomized trial of letrozole in postmenopausal women after five years of tamoxifen therapy for early-stage breast cancer. *N Engl J Med* 2003;349:1793–1802.

21. Berruti A, Dogliotti L, Terrone C, et al. Changes in bone mineral density, lean body mass and fat content as measured by dual energy x-ray absorptiometry in patients with prostate cancer without apparent bone metastases given androgen deprivation therapy. *J Urol* 2002;167(6):2361–2367.

22. Smith MR, McGovern FJ, Zietman AL, et al. Pamidronate to prevent bone loss during androgen deprivation therapy for prostate cancer. *N Engl J Med* 2001;345:948–955.

23. Smith RF, Eastman J, Gleason DM, et al. Randomized controlled trial of zoledronic acid to prevent bone loss in men receiving androgen deprivation therapy for nonmetastatic prostate cancer. *J Urol* 2003;169:2008–2012.

# Management of Bone Loss in Patients with Rheumatic Diseases

# Disease-Modifying Antirheumatic Drugs and Biological Therapy in Prevention of Bone Erosions

*Vibeke Strand*

Recently approved disease-modifying antirheumatic drugs (DMARDs), biologic and synthetic, and methotrexate (MTX) and sulfasalazine have all been demonstrated to retard radiographic progression in patients with active rheumatoid arthritis (RA). These data are summarized in two recent reviews, as well as assessment of radiographic damage over 3 years in the Combinatietherapie Bij Reumatoide Artritis (COBRA) study, comparing step-down therapy with sulfasalazine alone (1–3). Leflunomide, etanercept, infliximab, and adalimumab (both infliximab and adalimumab in combination with MTX) are approved for inhibiting radiographic progression; anakinra is labeled for slowing structural damage in patients with active RA (4–10).

## RADIOGRAPHIC PROGRESSION: EROSIONS AND JOINT SPACE NARROWING

All trials have demonstrated that radiographic progression occurs both by erosions and joint space narrowing (JSN). Although several studies have demonstrated that erosions tend to progress more rapidly than JSN in patients with early disease (<3 years duration), others have shown more progression by JSN as disease duration increases. Some have postulated that erosions and JSN reflect different underlying pathophysiological processes (11). Others have suggested that it may require more time to demonstrate radiographic improvement or worsening with erosions than JSN. Regardless, both erosions and JSN clearly should be assessed when measuring radiographic progression, as recommended by a National Institutes of Health (NIH) consensus conference (12).

Most recent randomized controlled trials have used the (modified) Sharp scoring method, which summarizes both erosions and JSN and includes assessment of both hands and feet (1,2). In comparison, the Larsen/Scott method predominantly scores erosions (13). In most studies, two or more observers independently scored radiographs in blinded fashion. A report by the international Outcome Measures in Rheumatology Clinical Trials (OMERACT) consensus effort indicated that statistical assessment of the smallest detectable difference (SDD) beyond chance using the Sharp method, 5.0 points, closely matched the amount of progression that a panel of experts determined should indicate addition or change in therapy, for example, the minimum clinically important difference (MCID) (14). In comparison, SDDs using the Larsen method are too large to correspond to MCID; they are not sufficiently sensitive to reflect clinically meaningful changes.

In these study populations, the extent of damage at baseline was not normally distributed at baseline, and radiographic progression was highly skewed. Even patients with long disease duration and extensive damage, as in the Anti-Tumor Necrosis Factor Trial in RA with Concomitant Therapy (ATTRACT) trial, rarely had radiographic scores exceeding 60% to 75% of maximum possible values at baseline (6). This apparent limitation in progression remains unexplained. Certain joints may account for the majority of radiographic progression, thereby limiting the total amount of damage observed.

## HEALING OR REVERSAL OF DAMAGE

As accepted scoring methods randomize both treatment and order in which radiographs are assessed, negative scores do not necessarily indicate reversal of damage (15). If scored at baseline and 12 months, and again at 24 months, x-rays are read first in pairs and then rerandomized in groups of three. Although paired readings blinded to sequence have been shown to offer greater power to detect a treatment effect, it is not possible for this method to definitively demonstrate improvement or "healing" (16,17). A recent report showed that assessment of radiographs in chronological order was the most sensitive way to detect change, and sensitivity increased over time (3). Another OMERACT consensus effort established that healing, reversal of erosions, could be demonstrated by chronological assessment of radiographs, even with MTX therapy (19,20).

## QUANTIFICATION OF RADIOLOGICAL SCORES

Either means and standard deviations or medians and interquartile ranges of changes from baseline in radiographic scores may be utilized for primary analyses, but both should be reported, preferably with box-whisker plots to indicate the skewed distribution of data (12). Presentation of both mean and median changes allows better comprehension of the heterogeneity of the data, as well as magnitude of treatment effects.

Additional analyses recommended at the NIH consensus conference included several definitions of no radiographic progression: the number (%) of patients with ≤0 change in total Sharp scores compared with baseline; the number (%) of patients with no newly eroded joints, and the number (%) of patients with ≤0 change in erosion scores. As discussed by Landewe, et al. (19), a low cutoff level of "0" does not accommodate the SDD, or measurement error, especially when more than one assessor scores radiographic change, as was true in most recent trials (20).

The NIH consensus conference agreed that missing data should not be imputed, and statistical analyses should be

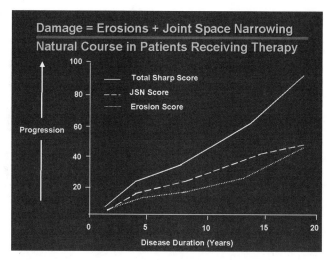

**Figure 14.1** Wolfe and Sharp (22) followed radiographic progression in a cohort of 256 rheumatoid arthritis patients longitudinally for up to 19 years. Progression was evident both by erosions and joint space narrowing. As this was a large cohort, mean changes in total Sharp scores were linear over time.

applied to support validity of the data (12). Sensitivity analyses were performed in most of these trials to account for early protocol discontinuations. Worst values from the placebo group were substituted for missing values in the active treatment arms, and best values from active treatment for missing values in placebo confirmed robustness of the data in trials where as many as 30% of patients did not have 12-month radiographs because of early withdrawals (1,4–7).

To demonstrate linear changes over time, treatment groups must be sufficient size to account for variability in progression rates (Fig. 14.1) (21,22). The effect of active treatment on progression of erosions appears to be more pronounced during the second 6 to 12 months of therapy compared with the first 6-month period, whereas the slope of the line reflecting changes in JSN remains similar. This is illustrated by graphic displays of changes in total Sharp scores over time in the etanercept group in Early Rheumatoid Arthritis (ERA), adalimumab DE019, active-controlled trial of patients receiving infliximab for the treatment of RA of early onset (ASPIRE), and Trial of Etanercept and Methotrexate with Radiographic Patient Outcomes (TEMPO) trials (Figs. 14.3–14.6) (5,7,23,24). These observations may reflect a lag time before radiographs are able to demonstrate change, the underlying disease pathophysiology, or differing treatment effects.

## PREVENTION OF DAMAGE

*Prevention* is a regulatory term that is difficult to define when considering a progressive disease of 20 to 30 years duration (25). Is prevention of further damage as meaningful

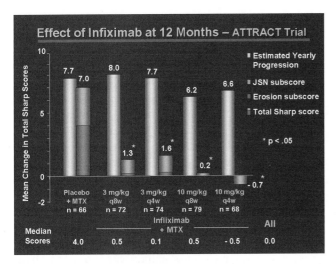

**Figure 14.2** Anti–Tumor Necrosis Factor Trial in RA with Concomitant Therapy (ATTRACT) examining the effects of infliximab on radiographic progression at 12 months in patients failing treatment with methotrexate (MTX) (6). Comparisons of observed versus predicted changes in erosion and joint space narrowing (JSN) subscores and total Sharp scores between baseline and the end point are shown. Estimated yearly progression for each treatment group was calculated by dividing the mean baseline scores by the mean duration of disease. Note the good agreement between estimated yearly progression and mean change in total Sharp score in the placebo + MTX treatment group. PL = placebo; q8w = every 8 weeks; q4w = every 4 weeks.

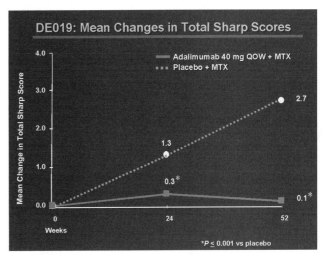

**Figure 14.4** Mean changes in total Sharp scores over 6 and 12 months in protocol DE019, examining the effects of adalimumab on radiographic progression in patients failing treatment with methotrexate (MTX) (7). Rescue therapy was allowed on or after 8 weeks for defined lack of response. Radiographic progression in the placebo + MTX group, therefore, did not approach the estimated yearly progression rate of 6.1, yet was statistically significantly more than in the combined treatment groups of patients receiving 40 mg every other week or 20 mg weekly of adalimumab + MTX. In the active treatment group, mean change in total Sharp score was less at 12 than at 6 months.

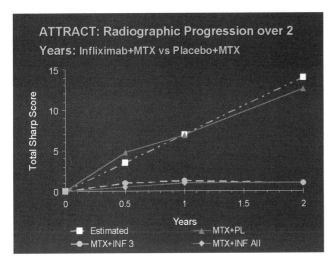

**Figure 14.3** Anti–Tumor Necrosis Factor Trial in RA with Concomitant Therapy (ATTRACT) examining the effects of infliximab on radiographic progression over 2 years in patients failing treatment with methotrexate (MTX) (1). Comparisons of observed versus predicted changes in erosion and joint space narrowing (JSN) subscores and total Sharp scores between baseline and end point are shown. Estimated yearly progression for each treatment group was calculated by dividing the mean baseline scores by the mean duration of disease. Again note the good agreement between estimated yearly progression and mean changes in total Sharp score in the placebo + MTX treatment group over 2 years.

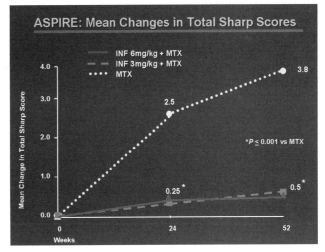

**Figure 14.5** Mean changes in total Sharp scores over 6 and 12 months in the Active controlled trial of patients receiving infliximab for the treatment of RA of early onset [ASPIRE] trial, examining the effects of methotrexate compared with Infliximab 3 mg or 6 mg plus methotrexate on radiographic progression in patients with early RA (23). Mean changes in total Sharp scores were statistically greater in patients receiving MTX monotherapy, suggesting an additive effect of combination therapy with a TNF inhibitor. Note that in the Infliximab 6 mg+MTX combination group, the mean change in total Sharp score over 6 to 12 was less than from 0 to 6 months.

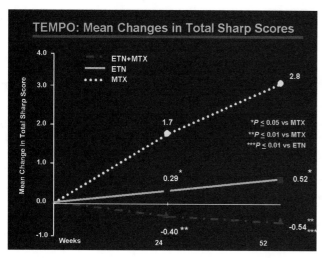

**Figure 14.6** Mean changes in total Sharp scores over 6 and 12 months in the Trial of Etanercept and Methotrexate with Radiographic Patient Outcomes (TEMPO) trial, examining the effects of methotrexate compared with etanercept or the combination of methotrexate + etanercept on radiographic progression in patients with rheumatoid arthritis (RA) of mean 6.6 years duration (24). Mean changes in total Sharp scores were statistically greater in patients receiving methotrexate (MTX) monotherapy than in either etanercept monotherapy or combination treatment groups at 6 and 12 months. Note that in the etanercept + MTX combination group, the mean change in total Sharp score was statistically less than in the etanercept monotherapy group at 12 months, indicating an additive, if not synergistic, effect.

as preventing the initial occurrence of erosions and JSN? Inhibition or slowing best describe observed radiographic effects in recent trials, especially when patients with early disease were selected on the basis of seropositivity or presence of erosions at baseline. Although prevention implies maintaining a state of no damage, ongoing studies with magnetic resonance imaging and ultrasound in early arthritis cohorts without evidence of joint damage will be required before trials can be designed to establish such a claim (26–28).

## CHALLENGES IN INTERPRETING RADIOGRAPHIC DATA

Interpreting radiographic data in terms of clinical practice poses certain difficulties. Without head-to-head comparisons, it is difficult to compare data across different protocol populations: patients with early versus established disease, aggressive versus nonprogressive disease, and those receiving monotherapy versus combination with failed DMARD treatment. These studies represent a "snapshot in time" of disease effects of many years duration. Baseline radiographic damage appears to be the best predictor of future progression and, in individual patients and patient populations, may significantly influence response to an effective therapy (29–31). In contrast, patients who do not

develop radiographic damage in the first several years of active disease are less likely to do so later.

Another challenge when interpreting x-ray data is to understand radiographic progression in the control populations in the various protocols. Few treatment groups have received pure placebo therapy (only three recent trials)(4,8,9) even for a limited period of time; most comparisons are "against" placebo plus failed-background DMARD therapy or active controls. Given the differences in protocol populations, it is not appropriate to directly compare changes in total Sharp scores across trials. However, it is possible to use as a benchmark the "estimated yearly progression rate" of radiographic damage, based on previous x-ray damage, assuming that patients had remained on their previous treatment regimen or continued untreated. This value is obtained by dividing baseline mean Sharp scores in a treatment group by mean disease duration, thereby allowing rough numerical comparisons with observed change scores (1). Estimated progression rates are only estimates and should not be used for statistical comparisons. Despite common baseline demographics and disease characteristics across treatment groups in certain protocols, it is clear each represent unique populations, as estimated yearly progression rates differ. Of interest, mean changes in total Sharp scores in the pure placebo treatment groups in three of four recent trials approximated or exceeded estimated yearly progression rates for each protocol, serving as reasonable benchmarks for comparison of treatment effects across trials (Figs. 14.2, 14.3) (4,6,9). In the one exception, alternate therapy was offered, and approximately 60% of patients initially assigned to the placebo group had received active therapy for a mean of 6 to 7 months when follow-up radiographs were obtained at 12 months (1,4).

Recent placebo-controlled trials have allowed rescue with active therapy as early as 8 or 12 weeks (Fig. 14.4) (7,10). To demonstrate benefit in this setting, studying drug administration over a full 12 months must result in better radiographic outcomes than active treatment over only 7 to 10 months. With better and more effective treatments, and trials limited to active comparators, one may expect that radiographic changes will be even lower in future trials. Then estimated yearly progression rates may only identify differences between protocol populations, overestimating radiographic changes even in the control group (7,10,23).

## META-ANALYSES ON RADIOGRAPHIC PROGRESSION

In an attempt to compare treatment effects on radiographic progression, Jones, et al. (32), performed a meta-analysis of randomized, placebo-controlled trials in RA. In an accompanying editorial, Landewe, et al. discussed several limitations of this analysis (19). Comparing or pooling trial data is appropriate only if clinical and statistical homogeneity are present. Not only were protocol populations clinically different, baseline and radiographic progression data were heterogeneous. Changes from baseline in all studies were skewed, making it inappropriate to utilize untransformed radiographic data. The authors defined patients as progressors and nonprogressors, based exclusively on erosion scores, despite consensus that both erosions and JSN should be assessed. Landewe, et al. elegantly argue that the arbitrary definition of >0 change in erosion scores chosen to identify progressors failed to account for interobserver variability or measurement error, e.g. SDD. Further, this meta-analysis did not account for selective dropouts in these trials, as discussed above.

Other errors in the interpretation of trial data also confound this meta-analysis. Although data with most active DMARDs, including cyclosporine, infliximab, sulfasalazine, leflunomide, MTX, intramuscular gold, and corticosteroids indicated equivalent therapeutic effect, Jones, et al. (32), stated that infliximab was statistically superior to MTX. This conclusion must be viewed with caution, as the ATTRACT trial compared infliximab with placebo, in patients already failing MTX, demonstrating that infliximab was superior to placebo as an add-on therapy (Figs. 14.2 and 14.3) (1,2,6). They also failed to note that 60% of patients randomized to placebo in the trial comparing MTX with leflunomide in MTX naïve patients had received active treatment for a mean of 7 to 8 months, thereby accounting for the low rate of radiographic progression in this "placebo" group (1,4).

## RELATIONSHIP OF CLINICAL AND RADIOGRAPHIC RESPONSE

Finally, poor correlations between clinical and radiographic responses further confound clinical interpretation of these data. As Scott, et al. (33), elegantly demonstrated in a meta-analysis of several longitudinal studies, radiographic damage and impairment in physical function are not closely correlated until patients have had the disease 8 to 15 years. Only weak correlations between American College of Rheumatology response rates and decreases in C-reactive protein (CRP) levels were shown in several trials; others emphasized beneficial treatment effects on radiographic progression even in patients without apparent clinical responses (4,5,34,35). Clinically, a patient can be responding to therapy, yet still show progression of radiographic damage (36). One must, therefore, clinically evaluate both signs and symptoms and radiographs on a regular basis.

## REFERENCES

1. Strand V, Sharp JT. Radiographic data from recent randomized controlled trials in rheumatoid arthritis. *Arthritis Rheum* 2003;48:21–34.
2. Ory PA. Interpreting radiographic data in rheumatoid arthritis. *Ann Rheum Dis* 2003;62:597–604.
3. Landewe RB, Boers M, van der Heijde D, et al. COBRA combination therapy in patients with early rheumatoid arthritis: long term structural benefits of a brief intervention. *Arthritis Rheum* 2002;46:347–356.
4. Sharp JT, Strand V, Leung H, et al. Treatment with leflunomide slows radiographic progression of rheumatoid arthritis: results from three randomized controlled trials of leflunomide in patients with active rheumatoid arthritis. *Arthritis Rheum* 2000;43:495–505.
5. Bathon JM, Martin RW, Fleischmann RM, et al. A comparison of etanercept and methotrexate in patients with early rheumatoid arthritis. *N Engl J Med* 2000;343:1586–1593.
6. Lipsky PE, van der Heijde DMFM, St. Clair EW, et al. Infliximab and methotrexate in the treatment of rheumatoid arthritis. *N Engl J Med* 2000;343:1594–1602.
7. Keystone EC, Kavanaugh AF, Sharp JT, et al. Radiographic, clinical and functional outcomes with adalimumab (a human anti-TNF monoclonal antibody) in the treatment of patients with active rheumatoid arthritis on concomitant methotrexate therapy: a randomized, placebo-controlled, 52-week trial. *Arthritis Rheum* 2004;50(5):1400–1411.
8. Bresnihan B, Alvaro-Gracia JM, Cobby M, et al. Treatment of rheumatoid arthritis with recombinant human interleukin-1 receptor antagonist. *Arthritis Rheum* 1998;41:2196–2204.
9. Jiang Y, Genant HK, Watt I, et al. A multicenter, double-blind, dose-ranging, randomized, placebo-controlled study of recombinant human interleukin-1 receptor antagonist in patients with rheumatoid arthritis: radiologic progression and correlation of Genant and Larsen scores. *Arthritis Rheum* 2000;43:1001–1009.
10. Shergy W, Cohen S, Greenwald M, et al. Anakinra inhibits the progression of radiographically measured joint destruction in rheumatoid arthritis. *Arthritis Rheum* 2002;46:S "late breaking."
11. Kirwan J. Links between radiological change and other outcomes in rheumatoid arthritis. *J Rheumatol* 2001;28:881–886.
12. van der Heijde DM, van Leeuwen MA, van Riel PL, van de Putte LB. Radiographic progression on radiographs of the hands and feet during the first 3 years of rheumatoid arthritis measured according to Sharp's method (van der Heijde modification). *J Rheumatol* 1995;22:1792–1796.
13. Scott DL, Houssien D, Laasonen L. Proposed modification to Larsen's scoring method for hand and wrist radiographs. *Br J Rheumatol* 1995;34:56.
14. Bruynesteyn K, van der Heijde D, Boers M, et al. Determination of the minimal clinically important difference in rheumatoid arthritis joint damage of the Sharp/van der Heijde and Larsen/Scott scoring methods by clinical experts and comparison with the smallest detectable difference. *Arthritis Rheum* 2002;46:913–920.
15. Salaffi F, Carotti M. Interobserver variation in quantitative analysis of hand radiographs in rheumatoid arthritis: a comparison of 3 different reading procedures. *J Rheumatology* 1997;24:2055–2056.
16. Ferrara R, Priolo F, Cammisa M, et al. Clinical trials in rheumatoid arthritis: methodological suggestions for assessing radiographs arising from the GRISAR Study. Gruppo Reumatologi Italiani Studio Artrite Reumatoide. *Ann Rheum Dis* 1997;56:608–612.
17. van der Heijde D, Boonen A, Boers M, et al. Reading radiographs in chronological order, in pairs or as single films has important implications for the discriminative power of rheumatoid arthritis clinical trials. *Rheumatology* 1999;38:1213–1220.
18. Sharp JT, van Der Heijde D, Boers M, et al. Subcommittee on Healing of Erosions of the OMERACT Imaging Committee. Repair of erosions in rheumatoid arthritis does occur. Results from 2 studies by the OMERACT Subcommittee on Healing of Erosions. *J Rheumatol* 2003;30:1102–1107.
19. Landewe RBM, Boers M, van der Heijde. How to interpret radiological progression in randomized clinical trials? *Rheumatol* 2003;42:2–5.
20. Lassere M, van der Heijde D, Johnson KR. Robustness and generalizability of smallest detectable difference in radiological progression. *J Rheumatol* 2001;28:911–913.
21. Sharp JT, Wolfe F, Corbett M, et al. Radiological progression in rheumatoid arthritis: how many patients are required in a

treatment trial to test disease modification? *Ann Rheum Dis* 1993;52:332–337.

22. Wolfe F, Sharp JT. Radiographic outcome of recent-onset rheumatoid arthritis: a 19-year study of radiographic progression. *Arthritis Rheum* 1998;41:1571–1582.

23. Smolen JS, Emery P, Bathon J, et al. Treatment of early rheumatoid arthritis with infliximab plus methotrexate or methotrexate alone: preliminary results of the ASPIRE trial. *Ann Rheum Dis* 2003;62:S64.

24. Klareskog L, van der Heijde D, de Jager J, et al. Therapeutic effect of the combination of etanercept and methotrexate compared with each treatment alone in patients with rheumatoid arthritis: double-blind randomised controlled trial. *Lancet* 2004;363:675–681.

25. Department of Health and Human Services (US), Food and Drug Administration, Guidance for Industry. *Clinical development programs for drugs, devices, and biological products for the treatment of rheumatoid arthritis (RA)*. Washington (DC): Department of Health and Human Services, 1999.

26. McQueen FM, Benton N, Crabbe J, et al. What is the fate of erosions in early rheumatoid arthritis? Tracking individual lesions using x-rays and magnetic resonance imaging over the first two years of disease. *Ann Rheum Dis* 2001;60:859–868.

27. McGonagle D, Conaghan PG, O'Connor P, et al. The relationship between synovitis and bone changes in early untreated rheumatoid arthritis: a controlled magnetic resonance imaging study. *Arthritis Rheum* 1999;42:1706–1711.

28. Karlund M, Ostergaard M, Jensen KE, et al. Magnetic resonance imaging, radiography, and scintigraphy of the finger joints: one year follow up of patients with early arthritis. *Ann Rheum Dis* 2000;59:521–528.

29. van der Heijde DM, Landewe RB, Lipsky PE, Maini RN. Radiological progression rate at baseline predicts treatment differences: results from the ATTRACT trial. *Arthritis Rheum* 2001;44:S80 (abst).

30. Landewe RB, van der Heijde DM, Verhoeven A, et al. Radiological progression rate at baseline predicts treatment differences: results from the COBRA trial. *Arthritis Rheum* 2001;44:S371 (abst).

31. Strand V, Landewe R, van der Heijde D. Using estimated yearly progression rates to compare radiographic data across recent randomized controlled trials in rheumatoid arthritis. *Ann Rheum Dis* 2002;61:ii64–ii66.

32. Jones G, Halbert H, Crotty M, et al. The effect of treatment on radiological progression in rheumatoid arthritis: a systemic review of randomized placebo-controlled trials. *Rheumatology* 2003;42:6–13.

33. Scott DL, Pugner K, Kaarela K, et al. Review: The links between joint damage and disability in rheumatoid arthritis. *Rheumatology* 2000;39:122–132.

34. Boers M, for the COBRA Study Group. Demonstration of response in rheumatoid arthritis patients who are nonresponders according to the American College of Rheumatology 20% criteria: the paradox of beneficial treatment effects in nonresponders in the ATTRACT trial. *Arthritis Rheum* 2001;44:2703–2704.

35. Keystone E, Han C, Keenan GF, et al. Infliximab plus methotrexate prevents structural damage progres-sion in rheumatoid arthritis patients which was independent of clinical response. *Arthritis Rheum* 2001;44:S81.

36. Molenaar ETH, Voskuyl AE, Dinant HJ, et al. Progression of radiographic damage in patients with rheumatoid arthritis in clinical remission. *Arthritis Rheum* 2004;50:36–42.

# Exercise and Rehabilitation in Patients with Osteoporosis and Arthritis

**15**

*Robert L. Swezey*

## OSTEOPOROSIS, ARTHRITIS, AND FRACTURES

In osteoporosis, the main therapeutic goal is the prevention of fractures and their attendant mortality and morbidity (pain, disability, depression, dependency), especially in rheumatic disorders (1).

Three major components of osteoporosis fracture prevention include proper nutrition, pharmacological agents to maintain or increase bone mass, and exercise and safety measures. Nutritional measures such as calcium and vitamin D have been shown to play a role in fracture prevention. Vitamin D not only enhances bone mineralization but also plays a significant role in muscular function and balance regulation (2). This is of particular importance to our fall/fracture-susceptible aging population, who are often vitamin D deficient (3). Medications include bisphosphonates, hormone therapy (HT), selective estrogen receptor modulators (SERMS), calcitonin, and teriparatide (parathyroid hormone). These are covered separately in other chapters of this book. Exercise and safety measures for patients with osteoporosis are reviewed in this chapter.

Although atraumatic spinal fractures may occur, most fractures are a consequence of falling. Osteoporosis in patients with arthritis is compounded by muscle weakness, joint contractures, deformity, and balance problems, all of which can lead to falls and fractures (4).

Other systemic illnesses frequently accompany arthritic disorders and osteoporosis. Cardiovascular, pulmonary, gastrointestinal, urological disorders, central nervous system conditions, visual impairments, auditory and labyrinthine dysfunction, and medication side effects all potentially contribute to imbalance and the risk of falls and fractures (5–7).

## SAFETY MEASURES IN FRACTURE PREVENTION

Most accidents and falls occur in the home; therefore, one must first review safety and ergonomic issues critical to fall prevention (8). Home safety hazards are well known and include loose rugs and wires, slippery floors, poor lighting, unstable seating, lack of bathroom and stairway rails, and absence of handles and assistive devices for reaching and grasping. Occupational therapy and home nurse visits may be crucial to achieving a successful ergonomic and safe fracture-prevention environment.

To prevent joint pain or instability from predisposing one to otherwise avoidable falls, there are a number of useful and often essential orthotics and assistive devices. Slip proof shoes, braces, crutches, canes, walkers, and wheel chairs may be necessary to help prevent falls and fractures. In patients who have already sustained either hip or vertebral fractures, instruction in the proper use of walkers, canes, or crutches should be taught. Following vertebral compression fractures, standard walkers without wheels should be avoided because of the increased load on the spine when the walker is lifted. These patients should be offered walkers with wheels and brakes that allow patients to transfer body loads off of their fractured vertebra and onto the walker, keeping their spine erect (9).

Although falls are complex events secondary to a number of both extrinsic and intrinsic factors, a number of trials have suggested that therapeutic exercise can reduce the risk of falling (10,11). The use of hip protector pads can, if worn, offer additional protection against hip fractures in the event of a fall (12).

## EXERCISE TO IMPROVE BACK PAIN AND POSTURAL DEFORMITY

Initial treatment for the acute pain caused by vertebral fracture includes analgesics, avoidance of constipation, especially in patients using narcotics, rest, and often bracing. Physical therapy for the patient with acute back pain includes instruction on proper posture and principles to avoid excessive back strain during transfers and other normal activities. Resistive or strengthening exercises should be avoided for the first few months following fracture. Canes or walkers with wheels may be helpful to avoid loading the vertebral column.

Treatment for chronic back pain resulting from vertebral fractures includes analgesics and a therapeutic exercise program to strengthen the extensor muscles of the spine (13,14). Flexion and forceful rotation of the spine should be avoided as these motions produce high vertebral body compressive loads (15), but gentle flexion and rotation range of motion exercises can be performed safely with the spine unloaded (lying down). Proper posture and positioning should be continually reinforced.

A kyphotic deformity often results from vertebral compression fractures, many of which are painless or "silent." Bracing, exercise, and postural training can to some extent minimize this postural deformity (16). Postural training and conditioning with back extensor strengthening exercise may help minimize pain in patients with kyphosis. In addition, good mattress support and ergonomic posture seating for home, office, and automobile may be beneficial.

## OTHER TYPES OF EXERCISE

Many patients with arthritis can readily employ and enjoy walking (17) and pool therapy (18). Despite all of the range of motion, general conditioning, and cardiovascular and psychological benefits that can be derived, water exercises benefit neither bone strengthening nor osteoporosis.

Brief isometric resistive exercises utilizing an inflated vinyl ball easily adapted to arthritis patients can provide protective muscle and osseous strengthening in a home program (14,17,25).

Tai chi can provide balance and range of motion exercises within the capabilities of many patients with arthritis (19–21). Yoga can provide postural and range of motion stretching, as well as meditation, for those who can participate but does not directly address issues related to strengthening. The Alexander technique (22) is a well-established postural training method. This requires close supervision and patience. Balance and postural enhancements are the major benefits, but it does not offer any significant strengthening component to muscle or bone.

Rolfing is a fairly widely used exercise system that emphasizes slowly working with gravity to enhance stretching and musculoskeletal alignment and function (23). It is not designed to enhance bone strength but may be of some benefit to balance.

Pilates exercises consist of a variety of stretching and resistance movements and postures (24). They emphasize body awareness and are designed to stretch and strengthen virtually all muscle groups. They can be performed at home and require supervised instruction and monitoring. Specialized Pilates exercise equipment may or may not be used. The various positions and postures may preclude participation by patients with arthritic diseases and their specific efficacy on strengthening, bone mineralization, or fracture prevention has not been studied.

## OTHER THERAPEUTIC MODALITIES

An integral part of rehabilitative therapy, particularly for rheumatologic diseases, is pain control and the use of various modalities to supplement or offset pharmacological analgesic treatments for pain. Time honored heat or cold applications can still play a role in easing arthritic and posttraumatic pain syndromes. More sophisticated, and sometimes more effective, are the use of ultrasound, diathermy, laser or transcutaneous electrical stimulation devices. These modalities, often in conjunction with corsets, splints, braces, pharmacological therapy, and acupuncture can play a useful role in easing pain, promoting activity, facilitating exercise, and improving morale and quality of life.

## REFERENCES

1. Swezey RL. Rehabilitation medicine and arthritis. In: McCarty DJ, Koopman WJ, eds. *Arthritis and allied conditions: a textbook of rheumatology.* Philadelphia: Lea & Febiger, 1993.
2. Bischoff HE, et al. Effects of vitamin D and calcium supplementation on falls: a randomized controlled trial. *J Bone Miner Res* 2003;18:343–351.

3. LeBoff MS, Kohlmeier L, Hurwitz S, et al. Occult vitamin D deficiency in postmenopausal US women with acute hip fracture. *JAMA* 1999;281:1505–1511.

4. Akesson K. Principles of bone and joint disease control programs—osteoporosis. *J Rheumatol* 2003;30(suppl 67):S21–S25.

5. Cummings SR, Nevitt MC, Browner WS, et al. Risk factors for hip fracture in white women. Study of Osteoporotic Fractures Research Group. *N Engl J Med* 1995;332:363–372.

6. Brown JS, Vittinghoff E, Wyman JF, et al. Urinary incontinence: does it increase risk for falls and fractures? Study of Osteoporotic Fractures Research Group. *J Am Geriat Soc* 2000;48:721–725.

7. Cumming RG. Epidemiology of medication-related falls and fractures in the elderly. *Drugs Aging* 1998;12:43–53.

8. Norton R, Campbell AJ, Lee-Joe T, et al. Circumstances of falls resulting in hip fractures among older people. *J Am Geriatr Soc* 1997;45:1108–1112.

9. Bonner FJ, Sinaki M, Grabois M, et al. Health professional's guide to rehabilitation of the patient with osteoporosis. *Osteoporos Int* 2003;14(suppl 2);S1–S22.

10. Gregg EW, Pereira MA, Caspersen CJ. Physical activity, falls, and fractures among adults: a review of the epidemiological evidence. *J Am Geriatr Soc* 2000;48:883–893.

11. Henderson NK, White CP, Eisman JA. The role of exercise and fall risk reduction in the prevention of osteoporosis. *Endocrinol Metab Clin North Am* 1998;27:369–381.

12. Kannus P, Parkkari J, Niemi S, et al. Prevention of hip fracture in elderly people with use of a hip protector. *N Engl J Med* 2000;343:1506–1513.

13. Malmos B, Mortenson L, Jensen MB, Charles P. Positive effects of physiotherapy on chronic pain and performance in osteoporosis. *Osteoporosis Int* 1998;8:215–221.

14. Swezey RL, Swezey A, Adams J. Isometric progressive resistive exercise for osteoporosis. *J Rheumatol* 2000;27(5):1260–1264.

15. Sinaki M, Mikkelsen BA. Postmenopausal spinal osteoporosis: flexion vs extension exercises. *Arch Phys Med Rehabil* 1984; 65593–65596.

16. Kaplan RS, Sinaki M, Hameister M. Effect of back supports on back strength in patients with osteoporosis: a pilot study. *Mayo Clin Proc* 1996;17:235–241.

17. Swezey RL. Exercise for osteoporosis—is walking enough? *Spine* 1996;21:2809–2813.

18. Semble EL, Loeser RF, Wise CM. Therapeutic exercise for rheumatoid arthritis and osteoarthritis. *Semin Arthritis Rheum* 1990;20:32–40.

19. Qin L, Au S, Choy W, et al. Regular Tai Chi Chuan exercise may retard bone loss in postmenopausal women: a case-control study. *Arch Phys Med Rehabil* 2002;83:1355–1359.

20. Kirsteins AE, Dietz F, Hwang SM. Evaluating the safety and potential use of a weight-bearing exercise, Tai-Chi Chuan, for rheumatoid arthritis patients. *Am J Phys Med Rehabil* 1990;70;136–141.

21. Lan C, Lai J, Chen S, Wong M. Tai Chi to improve muscular strength and endurance in elderly individuals: a pilot study. *Arch Phys Med Rehabil* 2000;81:604–607.

22. MacDonald G. *Illustrated elements of alexander technique.* Hammersmith, London: Harper Collins, 2002.

23. Rolf I. Rolfing and physical reality. Rochester, Vermont: Healing Arts Press, 1990.

24. Trentman CPT. Pilates: core stability. *Advance for Physical Therapists & PT Assistants* 2002;Dec 9:35–37.

25. Ronenn R. Exercise and inflammatory disease. *Arthritis Rheum* 2003;49(2):263–266.

# Estrogens and Rheumatic Diseases

*Jeffrey R. Lisse*

The use of estrogen compounds in rheumatic patients remains controversial. This chapter summarizes the information available on the effects of estrogen (ET) on bone loss and fractures and estrogen therapy's effects on the major rheumatic diseases.

## ESTROGENS AND FRACTURES

Until a few years ago, ET was considered the method of choice for the prevention and treatment of osteoporosis. This was based on both the wealth of retrospective data suggesting fracture reduction in women who took estrogen and presumed extraskeletal benefits of ET (also based on retrospective data).

Estrogen use has declined sharply because of results of and early termination of the estrogen-progesterone hormonal therapy (HT) arm of the Women's Health Initiative (WHI), which demonstrated that the global adverse events of HT exceeded the benefits (1). The WHI was a double-blind, controlled, randomized trial of 16,608 women between the ages of 50 and 79. The estrogen plus progestin (E+P) arm was designed to determine the effects of oral estrogen (conjugated equine estrogen, CEE, 0.625 mg/day) and progesterone (medroxyprogesterone, MPA, 2.5 mg/day) compared with placebo on a number of chronic diseases of postmenopausal women. After 5.2 years, the Data and Safety Monitoring Board decided to halt this arm of this trial because the global index of harm exceeded the benefit to participants. However, this was the first prospective demonstration that estrogen significantly decreases fractures (2). Hip and clinical vertebral fractures were reduced by 34% (Fig. 16.1), and total osteoporotic fractures were reduced by 24%. Seven hundred thirty-three women (8.6%) in the E+P group and 896 (11.1%) women in the placebo group experienced a fracture [hazard ratio (HR) = 0.76; 95% confidence interval (CI): 0.69–0.83]. Stratification by age, baseline bone mineral density (BMD), personal and family history of fracture, body mass index, smoking status, history of falls, or past use of hormone therapy did not reveal any significant differences. There were 52 hip fractures in the treatment group and 73 in the placebo group. One hundred eighty-nine women had lower arm and wrist fractures and 245 did in the placebo group. There were 41 clinical vertebral fractures in the treatment group and 60 in the placebo group.

One thousand twenty-four women of a total 16,608 had BMD measurements. Total hip BMD in the E+P group improved by 3.7% by year 3 compared to a 0.14% improvement in the placebo (calcium and vitamin D) group ($p = 0.01$) In the lumbar spine, after 6 years BMD increased 7.5% in the women on E+P compared to 2.6% in the control group.

The estrogen-only arm of the WHI (10,739 hysterectomized women) demonstrated a decrease in the risk of hip fracture by 39% (HR = 0.61; 95% CI:0.41–0.91) compared to placebo (3). Clinical vertebral fractures were also reduced ($p = 0.02$). Total osteoporotic fractures were 139 in the ET group and 195 in the placebo arm ($p < 0.001$). As in the estrogen-progesterone arm of the WHI, there was a significant increase in the risk of stroke (HR = 1.39, 95% CI:1.10–1.77). The risk of deep venous thrombosis was also increased for women taking estrogen therapy. In this study, the risk of invasive breast cancer and coronary heart disease was not increased with estrogen.

A large, population-based prospective study designed to investigate the health effects of estrogen therapy (The Million Women's Study) confirmed the beneficial effects of hormone therapy on fracture protection (4). Current users of hormone therapy had a significant reduction of fractures

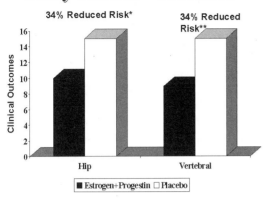

# WHI Estrogen+Progestin Trial Study Results - Fractures

34% Reduced Risk*          34% Reduced Risk**

*Hip Fractures: HR 0.66; Nominal 95% CI (0.45-0.98), Adjusted 95% CI (0.33-1.33)
**Vertebral Fractures: HR 0.66; Nominal 95% CI (0.44-0.98), Adjusted 95% CI (0.32-1.34)
Writing Group for the Women's Health Initiative. *JAMA.* 2002;288:321-333.

**Figure 16.1** The estrogen plus progestin cohort experienced fewer hip fractures and clinical vertebral fractures by one-third compared with placebo. Both of these results were statistically significant ($p < 0.05$). The reductions in other osteoporotic fractures (23%) and total fractures (24%) were also statistically significant.

[relative risk (RR) = 0.62; 95% CI, 0.58–0.66; $p < 0.001$]. This protective effect was evident shortly after hormone therapy was begun. Increased duration of use of HT resulted in greater reduction in fracture risk.

To determine the effects of lower doses of estrogen and estrogen plus progesterone, the HOPE (Women's Health, Osteoporosis, Progestin, Estrogen) trial was performed (5). Eight hundred twenty-two healthy postmenopausal women aged 40 to 65 years who were within 4 years of their last menstrual period were randomly assigned to receive CEEs, 0.625; CEEs, 0.625 and MPA, 2.5; CEEs, 0.45; CEEs, 0.45 and MPA, 2.5; CEEs, 0.45 and MPA, 1.5; CEEs, 0.3; CEEs; 0.3 and MPA, 1.5 (all doses in mg/d), or placebo for 2 years.

At 24 months, women assigned to all of the active treatment groups had significant gains from baseline ($p < .001$) in spine and hip bone mineral density (BMD). These changes were significantly different from those in the placebo group ($p < .001$). Osteocalcin and N-telopeptides of type-I collagen were significantly reduced from baseline ($p < .001$) for all active treatment groups at all time points; no changes were found for the placebo group. Therefore, dosages of CEEs or CEEs and MPA lower than 0.625 mg/d effectively increase BMD and bone mineral content (BMC) in early postmenopausal women.

The ultra-low estradiol (ULTRA) trial examined 417 women over 60 years of age with hip BMD Z scores above −2.0 and intact uteri who were randomized to 0.0125 mg of transdermal estradiol or placebo for 2 years (6). At 2 years, BMD in the lumbar spine increased 2.4% and hip BMD 1.5% compared to placebo ($p < 0.1$). This effect was greater in women with undetectable baseline estrogen levels. Ultra-low transdermal estrogen improved BMD without causing endometrial proliferation.

Because of the results of the estrogen/progesterone arm of the WHI, a large percent of women taking these compounds have discontinued their use. This discontinuation puts these women at high risk for accelerated bone loss. In a 5-year, randomized, prospective study, the treatment effect of estrogen replacement therapy/hormone replacement therapy (ERT/HRT) and the effect of discontinuation of therapy for 2 more years on BMD and markers of bone remodeling in 489 elderly women was studied (7). After discontinuing therapy for 2 years, there was rapid bone loss, and most of the decrease in BMD occurred in the first year. In the ERT/HRT group, spine BMD increased 5.5% in year 3, decreased 3.2% in year 4, and decreased 0.7% in year 5; femoral neck BMD increased 3.7% in year 3, decreased 2.5% in year 4, and decreased 0.4% in year 5. These results suggest that discontinuation of ERT/HRT in elderly women leads to a decrease in much of the BMD gained in treatment. Such patients should have bone density measurements at the time of discontinuation and alternative therapies should be considered.

## ESTROGENS AND AUTOIMMUNITY

Certain autoimmune diseases, most notably systemic lupus erythematosus (SLE) and rheumatoid arthritis, occur more frequently in women. In humans, the effect of estrogens in autoimmune diseases is associated with an increase in disease incidence rather than severity. An increase in incidence is more likely to involve a threshold response, while an increase in severity would be more likely with upregulation of the immune process (8). Estrogens are felt to inhibit cellular immunity (Th1-associated responses), and stimulate humoral immunity (Th2-associated responses). This may explain some of the variation in estrogen effects with different autoimmune diseases.

## ESTROGEN TREATMENT IN SYSTEMIC LUPUS ERYTHEMATOSUS

Evidence for estrogens enhancing autoimmunity in SLE comes from several sources. SLE occurs most frequently in women of childbearing age (9,10). One animal model of SLE, the New Zealand Black (NZB)/New Zealand White (NZW) cross hybrid, has a higher occurrence of disease in females, and manipulation of sex hormones affects disease severity (11). In this model, estrogens worsen the disease, while androgens ameliorate it. Other animal models of SLE are not affected by hormonal manipulation, however, and there is no consistent increase in disease prevalence in females.

As mentioned, the prevalence of SLE in postpubertal patients is much higher in women, with ratios between

7 to 1 and 20 to 1 in women compared to men (9). SLE patients have normal serum levels of estrogens, although there is some evidence that their metabolism of estrogens may be altered (12). Elevated hydroxylation of estradiol has been noted not only in SLE patients but also in unaffected, first-degree relatives (13).

Clinically, the use of estrogens in SLE patients has been discouraged, although data supporting this is not conclusive. The Safety of Estrogen in Lupus Erythematosus: National Assessment (SELENA) Trial was designed to examine whether estrogen plus medroxyprogesterone would cause an exacerbation of lupus disease symptoms. Patients with a history of thrombosis or significant levels of antiphospholipid antibodies were excluded. The results demonstrated no difference in severe flares between estrogen/progesterone therapy, but mild to moderate flares were increased 34% ($p = 0.01$) in the hormone therapy arm (14).

Birth control pills have been implicated in exacerbations of disease, but prospective clinical trials are lacking (15). One study found an increased risk of developing SLE in past users of oral contraceptives (16). The strongest recommendation against the use of estrogens is in the subgroup of SLE patients with antiphospholipid antibody syndrome and in those with antiphospholipid markers without thrombosis (17).

## ESTROGEN TREATMENT IN RHEUMATOID ARTHRITIS

In postmenopausal women, two prospective studies examining the effect of estrogen on rheumatoid arthritis (RA) disease activity have been reported. A double-blind, placebo-controlled trial was performed on 40 women with RA, using 2 mg/day of estradiol valerate (18). Outcome measurements included visual analog scales for pain, erythrocyte sedimentation rates, health assessment questionnaires, and articular indices. No statistically significant differences were noted in any of the above between the two groups. A second study involved 200 postmenopausal RA patients using transdermal estrogen (19). The study duration was 6 months. No significant differences were noted in any of the above indices of disease activity. Compliance with the study protocol was low, but patients with increased serum estradiol (indicating compliance) had improvement in their self-reported feelings of well being.

Studies have reported an increase of BMD in the lumbar spine and maintenance of BMD in the femoral neck with transdermal estrogen in patients with RA (20). Estrogen therapy also has been demonstrated to decrease markers on bone resorption in patients with RA whether or not they received glucocorticoid therapy (21). Estrogen replacement, therefore, increases BMD in RA, decreases bone resorptive markers, and does not appear to affect disease activity (22).

## ESTROGEN TREATMENT IN OSTEOARTHRITIS

An epidemiologic study performed on 1003 women in the United Kingdom found a significant 31% decrease in knee osteoarthritis (OA) as measured by Kellgren and Lawrence classification in current users of HT (23). The cohort of 4,366 patients over age 65 years in the Study of Osteoporotic Fractures had pelvic radiographs to evaluate OA of the hip (24). Current users of estrogen had a significant reduced risk of any OA of the hip with an adjusted odds ratio of 0.62 (95% CI:0.49–0.86) and moderate to severe manifestations of OA with an odds ratio (OR) of 0.54 (95% CI: 0.33–0.88). Estrogen use for more than 10 years displayed the greatest benefit.

In contrast, a cross-sectional study of the Framingham population showed no protective effect for radiographic OA of the knee in estrogen users (odds ratio of 0.66) (25). A longitudinal study was performed on the same population, examining 551 women aged 63 to 91 years (26). The subjects were classified as never, past, and current users. Radiographs were performed 8 years apart. Adjusted relative risks for the development of OA were 0.8 for past and 0.4 for current versus never users (not statistically significant).

The only controlled trial in humans has not been supportive of a protective effect. The 4-year Heart and Estrogen/progestin Replacement Study (HERS) reported no difference between HT users and nonusers in the prevalence of knee pain, severity of pain, or disability scores in postmenopausal women (27).

Risk factors for OA appear to differ for different joints. Most of the epidemiologic data favors a protective effect of estrogen therapy on the development of OA in the hip.

## REFERENCES

1. Writing Group for the Women's Health Initiative. Risks and benefits of estrogen plus progestin in healthy postmenopausal women: principal results from the Women's Health Initiative Randomized Trial. *JAMA* 2002;288:321–333.
2. Cauley JA, Robbins J, Chen Z, Cummings SR. Effects of estrogen plus progestin on risks of fracture and bone mineral density. The Women's Health Initiative Randomized Trial. *JAMA* 2003:290; 1729–1738.
3. The Women's Health initiative Steering Committee. Effects of conjugated equine estrogen in postmenopausal women with hysterectomy: the Women's Health Initiative randomized controlled trial. *JAMA* 2004;291(14):1769–1771.
4. Banks E, Beral V, Reeves G, et al. Fracture incidence in relation to the pattern of use of hormone therapy in postmenopausal women. *JAMA* 2004;291(18):2212–2220.
5. Lindsay R, Gallagher JC, Kleerekoper M, Pickar JH. Effect of lower doses of conjugated equine estrogens with and without medroxyprogesterone acetate on bone in early postmenopausal women. *JAMA* 2002;287(20):2668–2676.
6. Ettinger B, Ensrud KE, Wallace R, et al. Effects of ultralow-dose transermal estradiol on bone mineral density: a randomized clinical trial. *Obstet Gynecol* 2004;104(3):443–451.
7. Gallagher JC, Rapuri PB, Haynatzki G, Detter JR. Effect of discontinuation of estrogen, calcitriol, and the combination of both on

bone density and bone markers. *J Clin Endocrinol Metab* 2002;87(11):4914–4923.

8. Lockshin MD. Sex ratio and rheumatic disease: excerpts from an Institute of Medicine report. *Lupus* 2002;11:662–666.

9. Lahita RG. Sex hormones and systemic lupus erythematosus. *Rheum Dis Clin North Am* 2000;26:951–968.

10. Beeson PB. Age and sex associations of 40 autoimmune diseases. *Am J Med* 1994;96:457–462.

11. Siiteri PK, Jones LA, Roubinian J, et al. Sex steroids and the immune system. I. Sex difference in autoimmune disease in NZB/NZW hybrid mice. *J Steroid Biochem Mol Biol* 1980;12:425–432.

12. Lahita RG. Sex steroids and SLE: metabolism of androgens to estrogens. *Lupus* 1992;1:125–127.

13. Lahita RG, Bradlow HL, Fishman J, et al. Estrogen metabolism in systemic lupus erythematosus: patients and family members. *Arthitis Rheum* 1982;25:843–846.

14. Buyon J, Petri M, Kim M, et al. Estrogen/cyclic progesterone replacement is associated with an increased rate of mild/moderate flares in the SLE patients in the SELENA trial. *Arthritis Rheum* 2003;48(12):3659–3660.

15. Petri M, Robinson C. Oral contraceptives and systemic lupus erythematosus. *Arthritis Rheum* 1997;40:797–803.

16. Sanchez-Guerrero J, Karlson EW, Liang MH, et al. Past use of oral contraceptives and the risk of developing systemic lupus erythematosus. *Arthitis Rheum* 1997;40:804–808.

17. Ostensen M. Use of estrogen in women with systemic lupus erythematosus—should, or should not? *Tidsskr Nor Laegeforen* 1999;116:3237–3239.

18. Van der Brink HR, van Everdingen AA, van Wijk MJG, et al. Adjuvant estrogen therapy does not influence disease activity in postmenopausal female patients with RA. *Ann Rheum Dis* 1993;52:862–865.

19. Hall GM, Daniels M, Huskisson EC, Spector TD. A randomized controlled trial of the effect of hormone replacement therapy on disease activity in postmenopausal RA. *Ann Rheum Dis* 1994;53:112–116.

20. Hall GM, Daniels M, Doyle DV, Spector TD. Effect of hormone replacement therapy on bone mass in rheumatoid arthritis patients treated with and without steroids. *Arthritis Rheum* 1994;37(10):1499–1505.

21. Hall GM, Spector TD, Delmas PD. Markers of bone metabolism in postmenopausal women with rheumatoid arthritis. Effects of corticosteroids and hormone replacement therapy. *Arthritis Rheum* 1995;38(7):902–906.

22. Bijlsma JWJ, Jacobs JWG. Hormonal preservation of bone in rheumatoid arthritis. *Rheum Clin North Am* 2000;26:897–910.

23. Spector TD, Nandra, Hart DJ, Doyle DV. Is hormone replacement therapy protective for hand and knee osteoarthritis in women? The Chingford study. *Ann Rheum Dis* 1997;56:432–434.

24. Nevitt MC, Felson DT, Williams EN, et al. The effects of estrogen plus progestin on knee symptoms and related disability in postmenopausal women. *Arthritis Rheum* 2001;44:811–818.

25. Hannan MT, Felson DT, Anderson JJ. Estrogen use and radiographic osteoarthritis of the knee in women. *Arthritis Rheum* 1990;33:525–532.

26. Zhang Y, McAlindon TE, Hannan MT, et al. Estrogen replacement therapy and worsening of radiographic knee osteoarthritis. *Arthritis Rheum* 1998;41:1867–1873.

27. Oliveria SA, Felson DT, Klein RA, et al. Estrogen replacement therapy and the development of osteoarthritis. *Epidemiology* 1996;7:415–419.

# Calcitonin in the Treatment of Rheumatic Diseases

## 17

*Stuart L. Silverman*

Calcitonin inhibits activity of osteoclasts by binding to osteoclast receptors. Nasal spray calcitonin (NS-CT) has been available for the treatment of postmenopausal osteoporosis since 1995 in the United States.

## THE PREVENT RECURRENCE OF OSTEOPOROTIC FRACTURE STUDY

The Prevent Recurrence of Osteoporotic Fracture (PROOF) study (1) was a 5-year, multicenter, double-blind randomized study begun in 1991 to examine the efficacy of nasal spray salmon calcitonin (NS-CT) in patients with one to five prior vertebral fractures and low vertebral bone mass (T score < −2.0). Of the original 1,255 postmenopausal women, mean age 68, 817 had one to five prevalent vertebral fractures with follow-up x-rays. Patients were randomized to placebo or one of three doses of NS-CT daily, 100, 200, or 400 IU. All patients received supplements of 1,000 mg elemental calcium and 400 IU vitamin D daily plus the usual dietary calcium for a mean total calcium intake of 1,800 mg. Baseline variables were similar across each of the four arms. Of the patients, 62% completed the 3 years of the trial.

Lumbar vertebral bone density increased 1.2% in the 200-IU group in the first year and was a significant change compared to control only at 1 year. There was no further increase in lumbar bone mineral density (BMD) after 1 year. There was a mean reduction in serum C telopeptide (CTX) from baseline of 25% at 12 months, which was sustained at 20% throughout the 5 years in both the 200-IU group and 400-IU group.

Using an intent-to-treat analysis of all randomized patients with one to five prevalent vertebral fractures at baseline who had follow-up x-rays, there was significant 36% vertebral fracture reduction seen in the 200-IU group with a 36% reduction in relative risk compared to placebo of 0.64 ($p$ = .03) and a 45% reduction in the number of patients with multiple new vertebral fractures. These reductions were seen only in the 200-IU group and surprisingly not in the 400-IU group. Significant vertebral fracture reduction was seen with the 200-IU dose by year 3 and was sustained through year 5. Reduction in vertebral fracture risk was independent of age, years since menopause, number of prevalent fractures, baseline bone markers, and baseline spinal BMD (2). The PROOF study was not powered to detect nonvertebral fracture reduction.

There are two major limitations of the PROOF study. There was a high discontinuation rate of 59% for the 5 years of the study, and a dose-response curve of nasal calcitonin for fracture reduction was not seen. Although there was significant reduction in serum CTX and a significant increase in lumbar spine BMD compared to the control group in years 1 and 2 in the 400-IU group, there was no significant fracture reduction in this group.

## EFFECT OF NS-CT ON BONE MARKERS

Nasal spray calcitonin modestly reduces both urine and serum markers of bone turnover within 4 to 8 weeks (3,4). The response is dependent on continued treatment with nasal calcitonin. After cessation of treatment, all markers return to baseline over a subsequent 12-week period. In

PROOF, patients with the highest levels of baseline bone turnover had the greatest reduction in bone markers (1).

## USE OF NS-CT IN MEN WITH IDIOPATHIC OSTEOPOROSIS

Trovas, et al. (5) studied the efficacy of 200-IU NS-CT in a 1-year, randomized, double-blind, placebo controlled study of 28 men with idiopathic osteoporosis. The subjects ranged in age from 27 to 74 years (mean 52.4). All the men received a daily supplement of 500 mg of calcium. There was a significant increase from baseline in lumbar spine BMD of $7.1 \pm 1.7\%$ in the group receiving calcitonin compared to an increase of $2.4 \pm 1.5\%$ in the placebo group ($p < 0.05$). NS-CT may be an alternative therapy in men unable to tolerate other therapies for osteoporosis.

## USE OF CALCITONIN IN GLUCOCORTICOID-INDUCED OSTEOPOROSIS

A few small studies demonstrate that nasal calcitonin may maintain lumbar spine BMD in patients who have been treated with glucocorticoids (6). No data on hip BMD or fracture reduction with calcitonin in glucocorticoid-induced osteoporosis (GIOP) is available. At this time, NS-CT is not considered a first-line agent for treatment of GIOP.

## ANALGESIC EFFECTS OF CALCITONIN

Intramuscular or nasal salmon calcitonin has been reported to be analgesic for both the acute and chronic pain of vertebral fracture (7–9). The American Food and Drug Administration (FDA) has not approved calcitonin for analgesia. The mechanism of bone pain relief due to calcitonin is not known but appears to be a central effect, operating through both opioid and nonopioid mechanisms (7).

## SIDE EFFECTS AND ADMINISTRATION OF NS-CT

In the PROOF study, the only adverse effect that was significantly increased compared to placebo was rhinitis. Patients may develop antibodies to calcitonin under treatment. Binding antibodies with titers of greater than 1:1000 were observed in approximately 20% of patients in the PROOF study. The presence of these antibodies did not appear to affect fracture efficacy.

The recommended dose of NS-CT is 200 IU daily administered intranasally in alternating nostrils. The medication should be refrigerated until opened and then kept at room temperature and covered to avoid evaporation and condensation on the glass surface of the bottle.

Recent research has focused on an oral delivery system for calcitonin. An oral calcitonin is feasible and has been found to be well absorbed and to reduce markers of bone turnover (10).

## USE OF CALCITONIN IN COMBINATION THERAPY IN OSTEOPOROSIS

Meschia, et al. (11) combined eel calcitonin and hormone therapy with a significant 10% gain in lumbar spine bone mass at 1 year. Hodsman, et al. (12) found that the increase in BMD with sequential calcitonin and parathyroid hormone (PTH) was no better than with PTH alone.

## SUMMARY OF CALCITONIN IN THE TREATMENT OF POSTMENOPAUSAL OSTEOPOROSIS

Calcitonin is FDA approved for the treatment of postmenopausal osteoporosis but not for prevention. The preferred delivery system is nasal. Nasal calcitonin is safe and well tolerated. Calcitonin produces small increments in bone mass of the spine and modestly reduces bone turnover in women with osteoporosis. Calcitonin reduces vertebral fracture risk similar to other antiresorptive agents but has not been demonstrated to reduce nonvertebral (including hip) fracture risk.

## CALCITONIN IN THE TREATMENT OF PAGET'S DISEASE

Historically, calcitonin was one of the first therapies for Paget's disease (13). The newer bisphosphonates offer both greater effectiveness and ease of use (14). Only parenteral (not nasal spray) calcitonin is approved for treatment of Paget's disease. The usual starting dose is 100 IU daily. Biochemical benefit may occur after 3 to 6 months of treatment. At that point, the dosing frequency may be reduced to every other day or three times weekly at doses of 50 to 100 IU. Escape from calcitonin may result from down regulation of receptors or development of neutralizing antibodies. Side effects include flushing and local injection site reactions.

## CALCITONIN IN THE TREATMENT OF COMPLEX REGIONAL PAIN SYNDROME TYPE I

Complex regional pain syndrome type I (CRPS1), formerly known as reflex sympathetic dystrophy or RSD, is a painful neuropathic disorder that develops after trauma affecting the limbs without overt nerve injury. Although a neuropathic disorder, CRPS1 is also associated with changes in bone.

CPRS1 has a wide spectrum of clinical manifestations (15). These include pain, hyperthermia, and cutaneous changes of the affected limb. This syndrome is associated with soft tissue injury, fractures, myocardial infarctions, and cerebrovascular accidents. No precipitating event is identified in up to one-third of patients.

The pathogenesis of CRPS1 may involve alterations in the sympathetic nervous system, regional inflammation, and bone. There is increased sympathetic innervation and decreased perfusion of the affected limb (16). There is evidence for local inflammation as judged by increased levels of bradykinin and calcitonin gene-related peptide (17). CRPS1 is also characterized by bone involvement. Arriagada and Arinoviche (18) studied bone involvement in 12 patients and 18 controls using dual energy x-ray absorptiometry (DXA). BMD and bone mineral content (BMC) were significantly lower in the involved side compared to the contralateral normal limb (28.4% and 45.1%, respectively). Controls only showed a minimal variation of 2.17% in BMD and 4.38% in BMC between right and left measures. The difference between patients and controls was highly significant ($p < 0.001$). A second measurement of BMD and BMC was made in 8 patients following treatment (prednisone or calcitonin) and showed increments in both variables, which was significant in the affected limbs (20.1%). This suggests that DXA is an appropriate technique to evaluate regional bone mass in patients with CPRS1 and to aid in monitoring.

Physical therapy, analgesics, nonsteroidal antiinflammatory drugs, vasodilators, regional nerve blocks, sympathectomy, glucocorticoids, bisphosphonates, and calcitonin have been utilized for the treatment of CPRS1. In a meta-analysis of various treatments for CPRS1 (19), calcitonin was found to have a significant effect. However, the proper therapy for this condition remains controversial, and no single agent has been shown to be universally efficacious.

# REFERENCES

1. Chesnut CH, Silverman SL, Andriano K, et al, for the PROOF Study Group. Prospective, randomized trial of nasal spray calcitonin in postmenopausal women with established osteoporosis: the PROOF Study. *Am J Med* 2000;109:267–276.

2. Chesnut C, Silverman SL, Andriano K, et al, for the Proof Study Group. Salmon calcitonin nasal spray reduces the rate of new vertebral fractures independently of known major pretreatment risk factors. *Bone* 1998;23(5):S290.

3. Kraenzlin ME, Seibel MJ, Trechsel U, et al. The effect of intranasal salmon calcitonin on postmenopausal bone turnover as assessed by biochemical markers: evidence of maximal effect after 8 weeks of continuous treatment. *Calcif Tissue Int* 1996;58:216–220.

4. Ongpghiphadhanakul B, Piaseu N, Chailurkit L, Rajatanavin R. Suppression of bone resorption in early postmenopausal women by intranasal salmon calcitonin in relation to dosage and basal bone turnover. Calcif Tissue Int 1998;62:379–382.

5. Trovas GP, Lyritis GP, Gallants A, et al. A randomized trial of nasal spray salmon calcitonin in men with idiopathic osteoporosis: effects on bone mineral density and bone markers. *J Bone Miner Res* 2002;17:521–527.

6. Sambrook P, Birmingham J, Kelly P, et al. Prevention of corticosteroid osteoporosis: a comparison of calcium, calcitriol and calcitonin. *N Engl J Med* 1993;328:1747–1752.

7. Silverman SL, Azria M. The analgesic role of calcitonin following osteoporotic fracture. *Osteoporos Int* 2002;13:858–867.

8. Combe B, Cohen C, Aubin F. Equivalence of nasal spray and subcutaneous formulations of salmon calcitonin. *Calcif Tissue Int* 1997;61:10–15.

9. Pun KK., Chan LW. Analgesic effect of intranasal salmon calcitonin in the treatment of osteoporotic vertebral fractures. *Clin Therapeutics* 1989;11:205–209.

10. Safety and efficacy of a novel salmon calcitonin (s CT) Technology-based oral formulation in healthy postmenopausal women: acute and 3-month effects on biomarkers of bone turnover. *J Bone Miner Res* 2004;Sept 19(9):1531–1538.

11. Meschia M, Brincat M, Barabcini P, et al. A clinical trial on the effects of a combination of elcatonin (carbocalcitonin) and conjugated estrogens on vertebral bone mass in early postmenopausal women. *Calcif Tissue Int* 1993;53:17–20.

12. Hodsman AB, Steer BM, Fraher LJ, Drost DJ. Bone densitometric and histomorphometric responses to sequential human parathyroid hormone (1–38) and salmon calcitonin in osteoporotic patients. *J Bone Miner Res* 1991;14:67–83.

13. DeRose J, Singer FR, Avramides A, et al. Response of Paget's disease to porcine and salmon calcitonins: effects of long term treatment. *Am J Med* 1974;56:858–866.

14. Lyles KW, Siris ES, Singer FR, Meunier PJ. A clinical approach to the diagnosis and management of Paget's disease of bone. *J Bone Miner Res* 2001;16:1379–1387.

15. Schwartzman RJ. Reflex sympathetic dystrophy. *Curr Opin Neurol Neurosurg* 1993;6:531–536.

16. Goldstein DS, Tack C, Li ST. Sympathetic innervation and function in reflex sympathetic dystrophy. *Ann Neurol* 2000;48:49–59.

17. Blair SJ, Chintagada M, Hoppenstehdt D, et al. Role of neuropeptides in pathogenesis of reflex sympathetic dystrophy. *Acta Orthop Belg* 1998;64:448–451.

18. Arriagada, M, Arinoviche, R. X-ray bone densitometry in the diagnosis and follow-up of reflex sympathetic dystrophy syndrome. *J Rheumatol* 1994:498–500.

19. Perez, RS, Kwakkel, G, Zuurmond, WW, de Lange, JJ. Treatment of reflex sympathetic dystrophy (CRPS type 1): a research synthesis of 21 randomized clinical trials. *J Pain Symptom Manage* 2001;Jun 21:511–526.

# The Use of Bisphosphonates in Rheumatic Disease and Osteoporosis

18

*Chad Deal*

The first report of the biologic characteristics of bisphosphonates (called diphosphonates at that time) appeared in 1968. Bisphosphonates, analogs of pyrophosphates, were developed to produce an oral agent that would resist hydrolysis and have physiochemical activities of pyrophosphates, including avid binding to bone and physiologic regulation of calcification. Bisphosphonates were found to inhibit bone resorption effectively in animals by suppressing the recruitment and activity of osteoclasts and shortening their lifespan. This was first reported in human beings in 1971 (1). The nonnitrogen containing bisphosphonate, etidronate, was the first used to treat Paget's disease and was followed by other bisphosphonates. The first studies in osteoporosis were performed in the 1970s with etidronate. Subsequent studies lead to the approval of alendronate for postmenopausal osteoporosis in 1995, risedronate in 2000, and ibandronate in 2003. In addition to postmenopausal osteoporosis, various bisphosphonates are approved for male osteoporosis, glucocorticoid-induced osteoporosis, Paget's disease, hypercalcemia of malignancy, tumoral osteolysis, bony metastasis, and multiple myeloma. They have been used in a variety of other conditions including fibrous dysplasia, osteogenesis imperfecta, hyperparathyroidism, paraplegia, myositis ossificans progressiva, heterotopic ossification, otosclerosis, and hypercalcemia from prolonged bed rest and for destructive arthropathies (2).

## MECHANISM OF ACTION

Bisphosphonates are stable synthetic analogs of pyrophosphate. Their primary effect is to suppress osteoclast-mediated bone resorption. They bind avidly to bone; this property is primarily related to the R1 side chain (Fig. 18.1) (an OH group for amino bisphosphonates), which functions as a "bone hook." The R2 side chain determines the compound's potency as an antiresorptive agent and contains the nitrogen group common to all potent bisphosphonate compounds (Table 18.1). Nonnitrogen containing bisphosphonates (etidronate, tiludronate, and clodronate) are metabolized to cytotoxic ATP-bisphosphonate analogs that inhibit cell function and lead to apoptosis and cell death of osteoclasts. The nitrogen-containing bisphosphonates (alendronate, risedronate, ibandronate, and zolendronate) interfere with the mevalonate pathway by inhibiting farnesyl pyrophoshate. This prevents protein prenylation, the attachment of a lipid anchor in membranes, which inhibits osteoclast recruitment, differentiation, formation of the ruffled border, and acid production and induces apoptosis. While didronel is deposited diffusely on bone surfaces, nitrogen-containing bisphosphonates are preferentially deposited in areas under osteoclasts. Drug that is not taken up by an osteoclast is encased in bone, inactive until it is unroofed during a remodeling event.

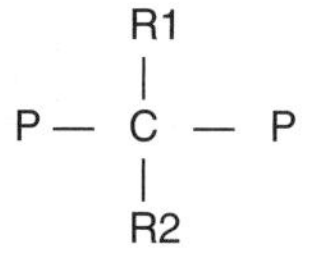

$$P — \overset{\overset{\displaystyle R1}{|}}{\underset{\underset{\displaystyle R2}{|}}{C}} — P$$

**Figure 18.1** The structure of bisphosphonates substitutes the oxygen of P-O-P with a carbon to form P-C-P. The R1 side chain is the bone hook, and the R2 side chain determines potency.

The suppression of osteoclasts decreases bone turnover, decreasing the number and activity of the bone remodeling units (BMUs), the functional unit that is responsible for the continuous process of bone resorption followed by formation. Remodeling is important for removing microdamage that accumulates in the skeleton. These remodeling sites are a source of trabecular perforations as well as microcracks and stress risers, weak areas that can propagate in bone and result in increased fragility and fractures. The decrease in resorption with bisphosphonate therapy occurs quickly, by 1 to 3 months. Because of the coupling of formation and resorption, the inhibition of resorption results in a decrease in bone formation, which is maximal at 6 to 12 months. Inhibition of resorption before formation allows the "remodeling space," the cavities created by the BMUs, to fill, which results in a brisk rise in bone mass in the first 1 to 2 years of therapy. Subsequent increase in bone mass occurs at a slower rate, approximately 0.6% to 0.8% per year through 10 years for alendronate and is, in part, related to an increase in matrix mineralization (a result of the decrease in turnover, which allows more complete secondary mineralization of bone) and to a decrease in cortical porosity. The continued rise in bone density out to 10 years, although small, may suggest a modest effect on osteoblasts.

The mechanism of fracture reduction is multifactorial. It is estimated that approximately 25% of the observed fracture risk reduction is related to bone mass increases. Other factors that may be important include decreased turnover, changes in mineralization and collagen, and cellular effects. Current evidence suggests that there may be a threshold effect both for decrease in turnover and increase in bone mass beyond which no further fracture reduction occurs (3). The search for more potent bisphosphonates, therefore, is not likely to produce additional fracture reduction and could impair repair of microdamage.

Bisphosphonates are poorly absorbed with less than 0.7% of the administered dose absorbed into the bloodstream. Food and liquids (except water) inhibit the absorption within the first 120 minutes after dosing. Alendronate absorption is 40% to 50% less when food is consumed 30 to 60 minutes after a dose compared to 120 minutes after dosing. A meal 2 hours before dosing also results in poor absorption, thus, the recommendation that they be taken after an overnight fast with no food or liquid other than water for a minimum of 30 minutes.

Because over 50% of administered bisphosphonates are excreted unmetabolized in the urine, patients with impaired renal function, that is, creatinine clearances less than 30 to 35 ml/minute, would be expected to retain a greater amount of the bisphosphonates in the skeleton. Greater retention of drug in these patients could reduce turnover to a degree that would impair the ability to remove and repair microdamage. A subset of patients with renal impairment have renal osteodystrophy and adynamic bone, characterized by a marked decrease in bone turnover. The use of bisphosphonates for them could further decrease turnover and cause accumulation of microcracks and increase skeletal fragility. There have been reports of adynamic bone and microdamage accumulation with high doses of pamidronate (4 to 5 times the dose given in osteogenesis imperfecta) in a child (4) and in dogs given doses of alendronate 5 to 10 times the clinically recommended doses for human beings (5).

Bone remodeling is required to repair skeletal microdamage. In osteopetrosis, osteoclast function is impaired and resorption is low, and although bone mass is high, microdamage accumulates and bone is fragile. Oversuppression of bone with bisphosphonates could

## TABLE 18.1
### STRUCTURE OF BISPHOSPHONATES

| Nonnitrogen bisphosphonates | R1 | R2 |
|---|---|---|
| Etidronate | OH | CH |
| Clodronate | Cl | Cl |
| Tiludronate | H | $SC_6H_3Cl$ |
| **Nitrogen bisphosphonates** | | |
| Pamidronate | OH | $CH_2CH_2NH_2$ |
| Alendronate | OH | $CH_2CH_2CH_2NH_2$ |
| Risedronate | OH | $CH_2$-3-pyridinyl |
| Zolendronate | OH | $CH_2C3N_2H_3$ |
| Ibandronate | OH | $(CH_2)2N(CH_3)(CH_2)5$ |

theoretically impair this normal remodeling process. With bisphosphonate therapy, turnover is reduced by 3 months to the middle-to-lower range of normal premenopausal turnover. With continued bisphosphonate treatment and continued incorporation into the skeleton, no further reduction in turnover occurs, suggesting the drug is buried in bone and becomes inactive. There is no evidence that bisphosphonates when used in currently recommended doses reduce bone turnover to a dangerous level, and there is no evidence for accumulation of microdamage at doses used in clinical practice. Histomorphometric data does sometimes show more striking inhibition of skeletal turnover with these drugs, but biopsy data in a small number of patients treated for 5 or more years is available and do not show significant microdamage accumulation. Combination therapy with a bisphosphonate and estrogen or raloxifene further reduces turnover and may be more of a long-term concern. With the intravenous bisphosphonate zolendronate, less is known about the long-term effect on turnover and the appropriate dose or interval of dosing; thus, caution is required.

Bone biopsies from alendronate-treated patients compared to placebo-treated patients demonstrate decreased cortical porosity (7.5% in placebo and 4% in alendronate) and increased uniformity of mineralization with a slight increase in mineral per unit volume (6). Because the cortical shell provides most of the bending strength of bone,

this observed reduction in porosity could account for a portion of the antifracture efficacy of alendronate.

Bone biopsies in risedronate-treated patients show preservation of skeletal microarchitecture with an increase in trabecular bone volume, trabecular thickness, trabecular number, and connectivity. (7)

## INDICATIONS—CLINICAL TRIALS

Bisphosphonates are indicated for the prevention and treatment of osteoporosis, steroid-induced osteoporosis, Paget's disease, hypercalcemia of malignancy, multiple myeloma, and metastases to bone. Bisphosphonates decrease fracture risk in patients at high risk for fracture including those with low bone mass, prevalent fractures, and other risk factors for fracture. The increased bone mass seen with these agents accounts for only 17% to 28% of the observed fracture reduction (8). Stable bone mass appears to result in fracture reduction, and larger increases in bone mass do not necessarily result in increasing fracture reduction. Factors other than bone density that may account for fracture reduction include a decrease in bone turnover, decreasing the number of "stress raisers" where microcracks may propagate resulting in fragility fractures. Other properties such as degree of mineralization, crystal size, and collagen crosslinking have important effects on fracture risk (9).

## TABLE 18.2
### BISPHOSPHONATE PIVOTAL TRIALS

**1. Vertebral fractures**

| | | # of Patients in Trial | Prev Fx | Duration | Fx Reduction | Ref |
|---|---|---|---|---|---|---|
| Alendronate | | | | | | |
| | FIT1 | 2,027 | Y | 3 yr | 47% | 23 |
| | FIT2 | 4,432 | N | 4 yr | 44% | 20 |
| Risedronate | | | | | | |
| | VERT-NA | 1,628 | Y | 3 yr | 41% | 37 |
| | VERT-MN | 814 | Y | 3 yr | 49% | 38 |
| Etidronate | | 423 | Y | 2 yr | 56% | 11 |
| Ibandronate | MN,NA | 2,946 | Y | 3 yr | 62%,50% | 49(a) |

**2. Hip fractures**

| | | # of Patients in Trial | Prev Fx | Duration | Fx Reduction | Ref |
|---|---|---|---|---|---|---|
| Alendronate | | | | | | |
| | FIT1 | 2,027 | Y | 3 yr | 51% | 23 |
| | FIT2 | 4,432 | N | 4 yr | 56% | |
| 20(b) | | | | | | |
| Risedronate | | | | | | |
| | HIP | 9,331 | | 3 yr | 30% | 41(c) |
| | | 5,455 | | 3 yr | 40% | (d) |
| | | 1,128 | | 3 yr | 60% | (e) |
| | | 3,886 | | 3 yr | 20% | (f) |

a) Combined multinational, North American, daily and intermittent dosing
b) post hoc analysis hip T-score <–2.5
c) intention-to-treat analysis
d) age 70-79 y/o , hip T-score <–2.5
e) post hoc analysis, with vert fracture
f) >80 y/o with risk factors

## TABLE 18.3
### GLUCOCORTICOID TRIALS

| | # of Patients in Trial | Prev Fx | Duration | Fx Reduction | Ref |
|---|---|---|---|---|---|
| 1. Alendronate | 447 | 15-17% | 48wks | 38% | 32(a) |
| | | | | 66% | (b) |
| 2. Risedronate | 290 | 33% | 1yr | 70% | 42(c) |
| | 224 | 31% | 1yr | 71% | 43(d) |
| | 518 | | 1yr | 70% | 44(e) |
| 3. Etidronate | 141 | 45% | 1yr | 40% | 14 (f) |
| 4. Ibandronate | 115 | 91% | 3yr | 62% | 55(g) |

a) p = 0.18
b) p = 0.05 post hoc analysis in postmenopausal women
c) GC > 6m p = .042 in combined 2.5-mg and 5-mg groups
d) GC < 3m p = .072
e) Pooled analysis, 70% in 5mg (p = 0.01), 58% in 2.5mg (p = 0.08)
f) P = 0.08
g) 2mg iv q3m vs po alfacalcidol 1mcg, p = 0.043

## Etidronate

Etidronate is the oldest bisphosphonate in use and is approved for treatment of postmenopausal osteoporosis in 27 countries although it is not FDA approved in the United States. A 2-year study demonstrated that etidronate prevented early postmenopausal bone loss (10). Trials have demonstrated vertebral fracture reduction in high-risk populations (11,12). The weight of the evidence supports its efficacy in reducing vertebral fractures in patients with osteoporosis. A meta-analysis reported a 37% reduction in vertebral fracture (13). Unlike alendronate and risedronate, etidronate can inhibit mineralization and cause osteomalacia. The patient takes etidronate for 14 days every 3 months instead of continuously to avoid a mineralization defect. Etidronate has not been shown to reduce nonvertebral fractures. Etidronate has also been shown to prevent bone loss in steroid-treated men and women (14). Its use for Paget's disease, at 400 mg per day for 6 months, has largely been supplanted by more potent bisphosphonates.

## Alendronate

Alendronate was approved for prevention and treatment of osteoporosis in 1995. Alendronate was shown to increase bone density in a dose-dependent fashion for 2 years in postmenopausal women without osteoporosis (15,16). In women under 60 years with normal bone mass, the effect of estrogen was slightly greater than 5 mg alendronate (17). Approval of 5 mg for prevention and 10 mg for treatment has been supplanted by weekly doses of 35 mg or 70 mg, which were shown to result in increases in bone mass equal to 5 mg or 10 mg per day (the study was not powered to evaluate fracture reduction) (18). In postmenopausal women with low bone mass and prevalent vertebral fracture (N = 2027) (FIT 1) treated for 3 years, alendronate was shown to reduce vertebral, hip, and wrist fractures by 50% and multiple vertebral fractures by 89%; all nonvertebral fractures were reduced from 14.7% to 11.9% (a 19% reduction) (19). In women without fractures but low bone mass treated for 4 years, a 44% reduction in vertebral fractures was noted ($p = .001$) (FIT 2). A *post hoc* analysis of this trial using patients with a T score of less than −2.5 (20) showed a 36% reduction in clinical osteoporotic fractures but no reduction in nonvertebral fractures in patients with a T score above −2.5. (21). Hip fractures were reduced by 50% in FIT 1, a population with prevalent fractures and a mean hip T score of −1.6. A lower bone mass with a T score below −2.5 is required to prevent hip fractures in women without vertebral fractures.

A rapid onset of fracture reduction was demonstrated in the Fosamax International Trial (FOSIT). Patients with a T score below −2.0 had a significant 47% reduction in clinical nonvertebral fractures by 12 months with alendronate (22). A *post hoc* analysis of FIT cohorts reported significant reduction in clinical vertebral fractures at 12 months in women with at least one vertebral fracture or femoral neck T score less than or equal to −2.5 (23). In a meta-analysis of several alendronate trials, clinical vertebral fractures were reduced at 1 year and hip fractures by 18 months (24).

Treatment with alendronate for 7 years resulted in a continuous increase in bone mass during the 7 years; however, the effect on fractures beyond 3 years could not be assessed because of the lack of a placebo control group beyond that interval (25). (Continued placebo treatment was felt not to be ethical.) However, analysis of fracture rates in the latter years of the trial appear to be similar to those in the first 3 years.

Ten years of treatment with 10 mg alendronate increased spine bone density by 13.7% with the greatest rate of rise early. After the initial 18 months the average increase was 0.73% per year (26). In patients treated for 5 years (20 mg daily for 2 years and 5 mg daily for 3 years) and discontinued for 2 years, bone mass in the spine was stable for 2 years, while hip density began to decline. Discontinuation of alendronate at 5 years resulted in an increase in urine N-telopeptide type 2 collagen (NTX) from −73% of baseline to −57.9% after 2 years off the drug. Bone-specific alkaline phosphatase increased from −55% of baseline to −36.7%. Another long-term study followed women under age 60 treated daily with 2.5 to 20 mg alendronate for 2, 4, or 6 years followed by no treatment for 7, 5, or 3 years. Even those treated for 2 years had higher bone mass 7 years after withdrawal than those receiving placebo (3.8% higher) although below the baseline bone density 9 years earlier. In patients treated daily with 20 mg alendronate for 2 years and nothing for 7 years, bone density was about 5% higher than baseline (27). The FIT long-term extension trial (FLEX) enrolled 1,099 women treated with alendronate for an average of 5 years in a 3-year extension. After 8.6 years the average increase in bone mass was 12.9%. After 3 years off alendronate, spine density declined −0.42%, hip density declined −2.39%, and NTX increased 25% (75% below pretreatment levels) (28). If patients discontinue alendronate after 10 years of treatment, the equivalent of an estimated 2.5 mg of drug would be released from the skeleton daily.

In early postmenopausal women with normal bone mass, bone-density increases were equal in women given 20 mg alendronate daily for 2 years followed by 3 years of placebo and women given 5 mg daily for 5 years. However, in patients who discontinued alendronate after 2 years of 20 mg per day, bone loss resumed at a normal postmenopausal rate, suggesting that longer term treatment is necessary in early postmenopausal women and that the residual effect of alendronate on bone mass and turnover seen with longer-term treatment is not present in early postmenopausal women treated for only 2 years (29). Alendronate has been shown to prevent bone loss associated with discontinuation of hormone replacement therapy (30).

In men with a T score of less than −2.0 treated for 2 years with daily 10 mg of alendronate, bone mass increased in both the spine and hip and vertebral fracture reduction was demonstrated (31). In 477 patients treated with alendronate for 48 weeks who recently started steroids bone loss was prevented and vertebral fracture was reduced (32). In fracture patients alendronate has been shown to decrease the number of days at bed rest and in the hospital (33).

## Risedronate

Risedronate was approved for prevention and treatment of osteoporosis in 2000. In a trial of women age 40 to 60 with normal bone density and in women with low bone mass, 5 mg daily of risedronate for 2 years was shown to increase bone mass in the spine and hip (34,35). Weekly dosing with 35 mg was shown to have equivalent bone density increases to 5 mg per day (36). The major fracture prevention trails for risedronate were the Vertebral Efficacy with Risedronate Trials (VERT). (North American, NA, and multinational, MN, cohorts were enrolled.) In postmenopausal women with previous fractures treated with 5 mg daily for 3 years, vertebral fractures were reduced by 41% and 49% and nonvertebral fractures were reduced by 33% and 39%. Multiple vertebral fractures were reduced by 77% and 96% (37,38). Spine x-rays at 1 year on the entire cohort demonstrated vertebral fracture reduction of 61% and 65%. *Post hoc* analysis reported a significant reduction in clinical vertebral fracture with risedronate at 6 months (39). An extension of the MN trial followed patients (with a placebo control) an additional 2 years (5 years total) and demonstrated a 50% reduction in vertebral fractures in years 3 to 5. This is the only bisphosphonate trial with a placebo group beyond 3 years (40). In this trial, 814 women were randomized, 472 completed 3 years, and 265 were enrolled in a 2-year extension (130 placebo and 135 risedronate). During years 3 to 5, there was a 59% reduction in vertebral fractures (*p* = .01) and a 41% reduction in nonvertebral fracture (*p* = not significant, NS). Over 5 years, lumbar spine bone density increased 9.3%. A further 2-year extension without a placebo group showed an increase BMD of 11.5% over 7 years, and vertebral fracture rate in years 5 to 7 was 3.8%, similar to the rate with risedronate in years 0 to 3 and 3 to 5 (28).

The only randomized, controlled trial with hip fracture as a primary end point was conducted with risedronate (41). In this trial, 9,331 patients were enrolled based on age, 70 to 79, with low bone mass (group 1) or over age 80 without measuring bone density (group 2). An intention-to-treat analysis of the entire cohort showed a reduction in hip fracture of 30% (*p* = .02). In group 1, a 40% reduction was seen, and in a *post hoc* analysis of group-1 patients with vertebral fracture, a 60% reduction was seen. In group 2 a 20% reduction in hip fractures were seen (*p* = NS) (42). Based on National Health and Nutrition Examination Survey (NHANES) III data, 42% of patients aged 80 to 84 would be expected to have a T score below −2.5. Thus, approximately 50% of the risedronate patients over age 80 would be expected to have osteoporosis. The combination of injurious falls in group 2 patients, and the likelihood that only 50% might have T scores below −2.5 may have accounted for the nonsignificant 20% reduction in hip fractures.

Risedronate was evaluated in patients recently started on steroids (42) and on steroids chronically (43). A pooled analysis of the two groups demonstrated a reduction in vertebral fracture of 70% at 1 year (44).

## Other Bisphosphonates

Tiludronate is a nonnitrogen-containing bisphosphonate approved for the treatment of Paget's disease at a dose of 400 mg per day for 6 months. The pivotal trial for osteoporosis used 50 mg and 200 mg orally for 7 days a month for 36 months and failed to show vertebral fracture reduction (45).

Clodronate is another nonnitrogen-containing bisphosphonate that has been shown to increase bone mass to a similar degree compared to other agents. The studies, however, were not powered to show fracture reduction (46).

Although not approved for osteoporosis, intravenous bisphosphonates are used in patients who are unable to tolerate oral agents because of gastrointestinal (GI) side effects. Pamidronate is approved for Paget's disease and hypercalcemia of malignancy. Its oral form is associated with significant GI toxicity (47). Pamidronate response was studied in a small trial of 20 patients given 30 mg every 3 months. Bone density was stable or increased in 84% of patients in the spine and 73% in the femoral neck (48). These nonresponse rates appear to be slightly greater than those reported with oral bisphosphonates.

Ibandronate is approved for postmenopausal osteoporosis orally in doses of 2.5 mg per day and in alternative intermittent dosing regimens—20 mg every other day for 12 doses every 3 months and 20 mg given weekly are being evaluated (49–52). A large MN trial of 2,946 patients (combined European and North American arms and daily and intermittent dosing) showed an increase in spine and hip density and decrease in vertebral fractures of 62% in the daily dosing and 50% in the intermittent dosing group. A large trial of intravenous ibandronate given 1 mg every 3 months did not significantly reduce vertebral fractures (53,54). Turnover markers were reduced but returned toward baseline before the next dose leading to the hypothesis that a more continuous suppression of turnover markers rather than this "seesaw" effect on turnover markers is required to reduce fractures. A trial using 2 mg of ibandronate every 3 months in 115 men and women on steroid treatment showed a significant reduction in vertebral fracture over 36 months compared to an alfacalcidol control group (55). This is the only trial showing fracture reduction with an intravenous bisphosphonate.

Zoledronic acid is approved for hypercalcemia of malignancy and has been studied in osteoporosis trials including ongoing studies to evaluate fracture reduction. In a trial evaluating doses of 0.25 mg, 0.5 mg, or 1 mg given at 3-month intervals, 2 mg at 6-month intervals, and one 4-mg dose, bone mass increases were significant and turnover markers were suppressed equally in all groups at 12 months (56). Because bone density increases in the 0.25-mg dose at 3-month intervals was the same as the 4-mg dose, it is possible that a one-time, 1-mg dose would be an effective dosing regimen. At 12 months there was no trend for recovery of the markers, and because the group was not followed beyond 12 months, the appropriate dose and interval for optimal effect is not known. The routine use of this drug cannot be recommended until additional dosing and fracture studies are published; however, its use (along with pamidronate) in patients who cannot tolerate oral agents and parathyroid hormone should be considered.

## SIDE EFFECTS

Shortly after the release of alendronate, numerous reports of severe GI side effects were reported, primarily esophageal erosions and stricture (57,58). Many of these cases were related to an under appreciation of the proper dosing to reduce the risk for this toxicity. Pill esophagitis can occur with many different medications. Patients with esophageal motility disorders and esophageal stricture are at greater risk for toxicity. In clinical trials between 20% to 40% of patients report GI side effects, but the rate is generally equal to that seen in the placebo group. Endoscopic studies of alendronate and risedronate have shown short-term effects on gastric mucosa, but the clinical relevance of these endoscopic findings and the risk of serious GI adverse events is not known. Those studies are similar to the experience with short-term endoscopic studies with nonsteroidal antiinflammatory agents. Rechallenge studies with alendronate show no difference in alendronate or placebo for GI symptoms. Endoscopic studies using 30 mg risedronate and 40 mg alendronate show no significant differences in GI toxicity between the two drugs (59). Although our clinical impression is that GI toxicity is frequent, the highest level of evidence, randomized controlled trials, suggest little or no increase in risk of upper GI tract problems if bisphosphonates are administered properly. Upper GI tract symptoms have a high background incidence in patients with osteoporosis making a causal relationship to therapy difficult to ascertain (60). The effect of acid and a protective effect of proton pump inhibitors on GI toxicity is unclear. The concomitant use of nonsteroidal antiinflammatory drugs does not seem to increase the risk of serious GI side effects.

With intravenous bisphosphonates, an influenza-like illness may occur for 24 to 48 hours after infusion with fever (15%), myalgia (15%), arthralgia (5%), and nausea (10%) (46,52) the most commonly reported side effects. Rapid infusion of pamidronate has been reported to cause renal failure.

Skeletal side effects include impaired mineralization with etidronate but not with alendronate or risedronate. Some patients complain of bone pain with bisphosphonates that may be is related to the small decrease in serum calcium and subsequent rise in PTH values. Impaired fracture healing in dogs has been reported with continuous dosing of etidronate but not with alendronate or risedronate. Although therapy of up to 10 years appears safe, long-term safety concerns include osteomalacia, retention of drug in bone, low turnover with impaired repair, accumulation of microdamage, and increased fracture risk.

## SPECIAL SITUATIONS

Intravenous pamidronate has been used in children with osteogenesis imperfecta (OI) without deleterious effects

(61,62). However, osteopetrosis in a child who received 4 to 5 times the OI dose has been reported (4). Cartilaginous islands entrapped in trabecular bone, the hallmark of osteopetrosis, represent failure of osteoclasts to resorb spongiosa, are seen in children with OI treated with prolonged intravenous pamidronate. Healing of fractures is not impaired with pamidronate, and there is no inhibition of linear growth in children with OI. Delayed mineralization of surgical osteotomy sites has been reported.

Small studies of oral bisphosphonates have been published in children treated with steroids (63,64). The effect of bisphosphonates on premenopausal women has not been studied. The effect of bisphosphonates in pregnant women has also not been studied. Although the skeletal half-life of bisphosphonates is long, the serum levels fall quickly with discontinuation and the effects of a few years of bisphosphonates retained in the skeleton of a pregnant women on her fetus would likely be minimal. In rats, bisphosphonates have been associated with skeletal abnormalities and fetal growth abnormalities. The only study in patients over the age of 80 is the risedronate hip fracture trial (41). There have been bone mass studies in patients age 85 to 90 that show the expected rise in bone density with these agents (65,66).

Bisphosphonates have been studied in arthritis. There have been seven double-blind, placebo-controlled trials of bisphosphonates in rheumatoid arthritis (RA), four with pamidronate, one with alendronate, one with clondronate, and one with etidronate. No firm conclusions can be drawn, although there appears to be marginal evidence for efficacy when higher doses of pamidronate have been examined (67). Intravenous pamidronate, 60 mg monthly for 6 months, has been examined in patients with ankylosing spondylitis refractory to nonsteroidals. Modest efficacy was demonstrated in those patients with axial inflammation (68). Orally administered agents are unlikely to achieve serum levels that would affect synovitis. Inflammatory arthritides with osteitis may be responsive to intravenous bisphosphonates because transiently high serum levels are attained, which may have effects in subchondral bone. Bisphosphonates have not been examined in large enough trials in RA to evaluate their effect on progression of structural damage in RA. There is some evidence that bisphosphonates may be chondroprotective in some models of animal osteoarthritis. In human osteoarthritis, a 1-year, phase-II trial with 5 and 15 mg of risedronate suggested symptomatic and radiographic improvement, but a larger phase III study failed to confirm these effects (69).

Use of parathyroid hormone (PTH) in patients previously treated with alendronate has been shown to blunt the anabolic response to PTH. (70) Simultaneous alendronate and PTH use also blunts the anabolic response to PTH (71,72). No data is available with risedronate. Raloxifene and estrogen do not appear to blunt the response to PTH. How this blunting of BMD response affects fracture is not known at this time. Whether this blunting effect could be overcome with longer duration of therapy is also unknown.

# REFERENCES

1. Fleisch H. *Bisphosphonates in bone disease: from the laboratory to the patient*, 4th ed. San Diego: Academic Press, 2000.
2. Watts WB. Bisphosphonate treatment of osteoporosis. *Clin Geriatr Med* 2003;395–414.
3. Eastell R, Barton I, Hannon RA, et al. Antifracture efficacy of risedronate prediction by change in bone resorption markers. *J Bone Miner Res* 2001;16(Suppl 1):S163.
4. Whyte MP, Wenkert D, Clements RN, et al. Bisphosphonate-induced osteopetrosis. *N Engl J Med* 2003;349:457–463.
5. Mashiba T, Turner CH, Hirano T, et al. Effects of suppressed bone turnover by bisphosphonates on microdamage accumulation and biochemical properties in clinically relevant site in beagles. *Bone* 2001;28:524–531.
6. Roschger P, Rinnerthaler S, Yates J, et al. Alendronate increases degree and uniformity of mineralization in cancellous bone and decreases the porosity in cortical bone of osteoporotic women. *Bone* 2001;29:185–191.
7. Dufresne TE, Chmielewski MD, Manhart TD, et al. Risedronate preserves bone architecture in early postmenopausal women in 1 year as measured by three-dimensional microcomputed tomography. *Calcif Tissue Int* 2003;73:423–432.
8. McClung MR. Bisphosphonates. *Endocrinol Metab Clin North Am* 2003;32:253–272.
9. Paschalis EP, Verdelis K, Doty SB, et al. Spectroscopic characterization of collagen cross-links in bone. *J Bone Miner Res* 2001;16:1821–1828.
10. Herd RJM, Balena R, Blake GM, et al. The prevention of early postmenopausal bone loss by cyclical etidronate therapy. A 2-year, double-blind, placebo-controlled study. *Am J Med* 1997;103:92–99.
11. Storm T, Thamsborg G, Steiniche T, et al. Effect of intermittent cyclical etidronate therapy on bone mass and fracture rate in women with postmenopausal osteoporosis. *N Engl J Med* 1990;322:1265–1271.
12. Watts JB, Harris ST, Genant HK, et al. Intermittent cyclical etidronate treatment of postmenopausal osteoporosis. *N Engl J Med* 1990;323:73–79.
13. Cranney A, Welch V, Adachi JD, et al. Etidronate for treating and preventing postmenopausal osteoporosis. *Cochrane Database Sys Rev* 2001;4:CD003376.
14. Adachi JD, Bensen WG, Brown J, et al. Intermittent etidronate therapy to prevent corticosteroid-induced osteoporosis. *N Engl J Med* 1997;337:382–387.
15. Liberman UA, Weiss SR, Broll J, et al. Effect of oral alendronate on bone mineral density and the incidence of fractures in postmenopausal osteoporosis. *N Engl J Med* 1995;333:1437–1443.
16. McClung M, Clemmesen B, Daifotis A, et al. Alendronate prevents postmenopausal bone loss in women without osteoporosis. A double-blind, randomized, controlled trial. *Ann Intern Med* 1998;128:253–261.
17. Hosking D, Chilvers CED, Christiansen C, et al. Prevention of bone loss with alendronate in postmenopausal women under 60 years of age. *N Engl J Med* 1998;338:485–492.
18. Schnitzer T, Bone HG, Crepaldi G, et al. Therapeutic equivalence of alendronate 70 mg once-weekly and alendronate 10 mg daily in the treatment of osteoporosis. *Aging (Milano)* 2000;12:1–2.
19. Black DM, Cummings SR, Karpf DB, et al. Randomized trial of effect of alendronate on risk of fracture in women with existing vertebral fractures. *Lancet* 1996;348(9041):1535–1541.
20. Cummings SR, Black DM, Thompson D, et al. Effect of alendronate on risk of fracture in women with low bone density but without vertebral fractures. Results from the Fracture Intervention Trial. *JAMA* 1998;280:2077–2082.

21. Karpf DB, Shapiro DR, Seeman E, et al. Prevention of nonvertebral fractures by alendronate. A meta-analysis. Alendronate Osteoporosis Treatment Study Group. *JAMA* 1997;277:1159–1164.

22. Pols HA, Felsenberg D, Hanley DA, et al. Multinational, placebo-controlled, randomized trial of the effects of alendronate on bone density and fracture risk in postmenopausal women with low bone mass: results of the FOSIT study. *Osteoporosis Int* 1999;9:461–468.

23. Black DM, Thompson DE, Bauer DC, et al. Fracture risk reduction with alendronate in women with osteoporosis: the fracture intervention trial—FIT Research Group. *J Clin Endocrinol Metab* 2000; 85:4118–4124.

24. Black DM, Thompson DE, Bauer DC, et al. Fracture risk reduction with alendronate in women with osteoporosis: the fracture intervention trial. *J Clin Endocrinol Metab* 2999;85:4118–4124.

25. Tonino RP, Meunier PJ, Emkey R, et al. Skeletal benefits of alendronate: 7-year treatment of postmenopausal osteoporotic women. Phase III Osteoporosis Treatment Study Group. *J Clin Endocrinol Metab* 2000;85:3109–3115.

26. Bone HG, Hosking D, Devogelaer JP, et al. Alendronate Phase III Osteoporosis Treatment Study Group. Ten years' experience with alendronate for osteoporosis in postmenopausal women. *N Engl J Med* 2004;350(12):1189–1199.

27. Bagger YZ, Tanko LB, Alexandersen P, et al. Alendronate has a residual effect on bone mass in postmenopausal Danish women up to seven years after treatment withdrawal. *Bone* 2003;33: 301–307.

28. Ensrud K, Santora A, Schwartz A, et al. The fracture intervention trial long term extension (FLEX). *J Bone Miner Res* 2003;18(2): S90.

29. Ravn P, Weiss SR, Rodriguez-Portales JA, et al. Alendronate in early postmenopausal women: effects on bone mass during long-term treatment and after withdrawal. *J Clin Endocrinol Metab* 2000;85:1492–1497.

30. Ascott-Evans BH, Guanabens N, Kivinen S, et al. Alendronate prevents loss of bone associated with discontinuation of hormone replacement therapy: a randomized control trial. *Arch Int Med* 2003;163:789–794.

31. Orwoll E, Ettinger M, Weiss S, et al. Alendronate for the treatment of osteoporosis in men. *N Engl J Med* 2000;343:604–610.

32. Saag KG, Emkey R, Schnitzer TJ, et al. Alendronate for the prevention and treatment of glucocorticoid-induced osteoporosis. *N Engl J Med* 1998;339:292–299.

33. Nevitt MC, Thompson DE, Black DM, et al. Effect of alendronate on limited-activity days and bed-disability days caused by back pain in postmenopausal women with existing vertebral fractures. *Arch Int Med* 2000;160:77–85.

34. Mortensen L, Charles P, Bekker PJ, et al. Risedronate increases bone mass in an early postmenopausal population: two years of treatment plus one year of follow-up. *J Clin Endocrinol Metab* 1998;83:396–402.

35. Fogelman I, Ribot C, Smith R, et al. Risedronate reverses bone loss in postmenopausal women with low bone mass: results from a multinational, double-blind, placebo-controlled trial. *J Clin Endocrinol Metab* 2000;85:1895–1900.

36. Brown JP, Kendler DL, McClung MR, et al. The efficacy and tolerability of risedronate once a week for the treatment of postmenopausal osteoporosis. *Calcif Tissue Int* 202;71:103–111.

37. Harris ST, Watts NB, Genant HK, et al. Effects of risedronate treatment on vertebral and nonvertebral fractures in women with postmenopausal osteoporosis. *JAMA* 1999;282:1344–1352.

38. Reginster J, Minne HW, Sorensen OH, et al. Randomized trial of the effects of risedronate on vertebral fractures in women with established postmenopausal osteoporosis. *Osteoporosis Int* 2000;11:83–91.

39. Watts NB, Adami S, Chesnut C, et al. Risedronate reduces the risk of clinical vertebral fractures in just 6 months. *J Bone Miner Res* 2001;16(1):S407.

40. Sorenson OH, Crawford GM, Mulder H, et al. Long-term efficacy of risedronate: a 5-year placebo-controlled clinical experience. *Bone* 2003;32:120–128.

41. McClung MR, Geusens P, Miller PD, et al. Effect of risedronate on the risk of hip fracture in elderly women. *N Engl J Med* 2001;344:333–340.

42. Cohen S, Levy RM, Keller M, et al. Risedronate therapy prevents corticosteroid-induced bone loss: a twelve-month, multicenter, randomized, double-blind, placebo-controlled, parallel group study. *Arthritis Rheum* 1999;42:2309–2318.

43. Reid DM, Hughes RA, Laan RFJM, et al. Efficacy and safety of daily risedronate in the treatment of corticosteroid-induced osteoporosis in men and women: a randomized trial. *J Bone Miner Res* 2000;15:1006–1013.

44. Wallach S, Cohen S, Reid DM, et al. Effects of risedronate treatment on bone density and vertebral fracture in patients on corticosteroid therapy. *Calcif Tissue Int* 2000;67:277–285.

45. Reginster YJ, Christiansen C, Roux C, et al. Intermittent cyclic tiludronate in the treatment of postmenopausal osteoporosis. *Osteoporos Int* 2001;12:169–177.

46. Kanis JA, McCloskey EV, Beneton MN. Clodronate and osteoporosis. *Maturitas* 1996;23:S81–S86.

47. Lufkin EG, Argueta R, Whitaker MD, et al. Pamidronate: an unrecognized problem in gastrointestinal tolerability. *Osteoporos Int* 1994;4:320–322.

48. Younes H, Farhat G, Fuleihan G, et al. Efficacy and tolerability of cyclical intravenous pamidronate in patients with low bone mass. *J Clin Denistom* 2002;5:143–149.

49. Ravn P, Clemmeson B, Riis BJ, et al. The effect on bone mass and bone markers of different doses of ibandronate: a new biphosphonate for prevention and treatment of postmenopausal osteoporosis. A 1-year, randomized, double-blind, placebo-controlled dose-ranging study. *Bone* 1996;19:527–533.

50. Riis BJ, Ise J, von Stein T, et al. Ibandronate: a comparison of oral daily dosing versus intermittent dosing in postmenopausal osteoporosis. *J Bone Miner Res* 2001;16:1871–1878.

51. Wasnich R, Felsenberg D, Lorenc R, et al. A multinational study demonstrating significant reduction in the incidence of new vertebral fractures with oral and daily and intermittent ibandronate. *J Bone Miner Res* 2003;18(2):S100.

52. Tanko LB, Felsenberg D, Czerwinske E, et al. Oral weekly ibandronate prevents bone loss in postmenopausal women. *J Intern Med* 2003;254:159–167.

53. Thiebaud D, Burckhardt P, Kriegbaum H, et al. Three monthly intravenous injections of ibandronate in the treatment of postmenopausal osteoporosis. *Am J Med* 1997;103:298–307.

54. Recker RR, Stakkestad JA, Felsenberg D, et al. A new treatment paradigm: quarterly injections of ibandronate reduce the risk of fractures in women with postmenopausal osteoporosis (PMO): Results of a 3-year trial. *Osteoporosis Int* 2000;11(Suppl 2): S209.

55. Ringe JD, Dorst A, Farber H, et al. Intermittent intravenous ibandronate injections reduce vertebral fracture risk in corticosteroid-induced osteoporosis: results from a long-term comparative study. *Osteoporos Int* 2003;14:801–807.

56. Reid, IR, Brown, JP, Burckhardt P, et al. Intravenous zoledronic acid in postmenopausal women with low bone mineral density. *N Engl J Med* 2002;346:653–661.

57. De Groen PC, Lubbe DF, Hirsch LJ, et al. Esophagitis associated with the use of alendronate. *N Engl J Med* 1996;335:1016–1021.

58. Levine J, Nelson D. Esophageal stricture associated with alendronate therapy. *Am J Med* 1997;102:489–491.

59. Lanza F, Schwartz H, Sahba B, et al. An endoscopic comparison of the effects of alendronate and risedronate on upper gastrointestinal mucosae. *Am J Gastroenterol* 2000;11:3112–3117.

60. Cryer B, Bauer DC. Oral bisphosphonates and upper gastrointestinal tract problems: what is the evidence. *Mayo Clin Proc* 2002;77:1031–1043.

61. Astrom E, Soderall S. Beneficial effect of long-term intravenous bisphosphonate treatment of osteogenesis imperfecta. *Arch Dis Child* 2002;86:356–364.

62. Glorieux FH, Bishop NJ, Plotkin H, et al. Cyclic administration of pamidronate in children with severe osteogenesis imperfecta. *N Engl J Med* 1998;339:947–952.

63. Bianchi ML, Cimaz R, Bardare M, et al. Efficacy and safety of alendronate for the treatment of osteoporosis in diffuse connective disease in children: a prospective multicenter study. *Arthritis Rheum* 2000;43:1960–1966.

64. Brumsen C, Hamdy NA, Papapoulos SE. Long-term effects of bisphosphonates on the growing skeleton. Studies of young patients

with severe osteoporosis. *Medicine (Baltimore)* 1997;76: 2166–2183.

65. Bone HG, Downs RW, Tucci JR, et al. Dose-response relationships for alendronate treatment in osteoporotic elderly women. *J Clin Endocrinol Metab* 1997;82:265–274.

66. Greenspan SL, Schneider DL, McClung MR, et al. Alendronate improves bone mineral density in elderly women with osteoporosis residing in long-term care facilities. A randomized, double-blind, placebo-controlled trial. *Ann Intern Med* 2002;136: 742–746.

67. Maksymowych WP. Bisphosphonates for arthritis—a confusing rationale. *J Rheumatol* 2003;31:876–888.

68. Maksymowych WP, Lambert R, Jhangri GS, et al. Clinical and radiologic ameliorarion of refractory peripheral spondyloarthropathies by pulse intravenous pamidronate therapy. *J Rheumatol* 2001;28: 144–155.

69. Spector TD, Conaghan P, Buckland-Wright JC, et al. Risedronate produces disease modification and symptomatic benefit in the treatment of knee osteoarthritis: results from the BRISK Study. *Arthritis Rheum* 2003;48(12):3650 (abst).

70. Ettinger B, San Martin J, Crans GG, et al. Response of markers of bone turnover and bone density to teriparatide in postmenopausal women previously treated with an antiresorptive drug. *J Bone Miner Res* 2003;18(suppl 2):S15.

71. Finkelstein JS, Hayes A, Hunzelman JL, et al. The effects of parathyroid hormone, alendronate, or both in men with osteoporosis. *N Engl J Med* 2003;349:1216–1226.

72. Black DM, Greenspan SL, Ensrud KE, et al. The effects of parathyroid hormone alone or in combination in post-menopausal osteoporosis. *N Engl J Med* 2003;349:1207–1215.

# Selective Estrogen Receptor Modulators in the Prevention and Treatment of Osteoporosis

*Michael Maricic    Oscar Gluck*

There are several compounds that exhibit the properties of selective estrogen receptor modulators (SERMs), either in clinical use or in development. Four SERMs are approved for use in the United States: clomifene, tamoxifen, toremifene, and raloxifene. At the present time, only raloxifene is approved for the prevention and treatment of osteoporosis. Although tamoxifen is not approved for either of these indications, there have been a number of clinical trials demonstrating beneficial effects on bone density, and these trials are discussed here. Raloxifene and tamoxifen have not been specifically studied in patients with rheumatic diseases.

## PHARMACOLOGY AND MECHANISM OF ACTION OF SERMs

SERMs are synthetic compounds known to possess tissue-selective estrogen agonist or antagonist properties. Estrogen and SERMs manifest their biological activity through two distinct estrogen receptors, ER-alpha and ER-beta. These receptors have different relative distributions in target tissues but with considerable overlap. Both subtypes are found in the bone, uterus, breast, prostate, and brain

(1). Estrogen receptors have two domains: a ligand binding and a DNA binding domain. After ligand-receptor binding, the receptor bound to the estrogen or SERM dissociates from its heat-shock proteins and unites with coactivator or corepressor molecules before initiating activation of the DNA promoter (2) (Fig. 19.1).

Differential estrogen receptor expression and ligand binding in the presence of corepressors and coactivators explains the actions of the SERMs in a given target tissue (2,3). ER-alpha has two activating regions: AF1 and AF2. When estrogen binds to ER-alpha, helix 12 completes the formation of the receptor AF2 region, exposing several amino acids that are critical for binding specific coactivator proteins. In contrast, when raloxifene binds to the estrogen receptor, helix 12 shifts rightward to block the AF2 site, preventing coactivator binding and subsequent gene transcription (4–7).

Raloxifene, tamoxifen, clomifene, and toremifene have different clinical functions because of these interactions (8). In addition, there is evidence that some of the rapid actions of SERMs or estrogen (vasodilation) may be mediated by nongenomic interactions such as activation of mitogen-activated protein (MAP)-kinase signal transduction pathways (9).

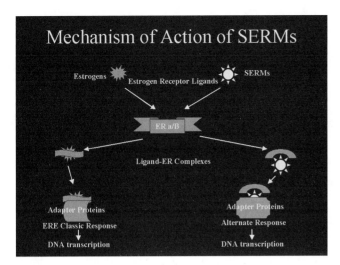

**Figure 19.1**   Mechanism of action of SERMs

## SERMs EFFECT ON BONE

### Tamoxifen

Tamoxifen is a triphenylethyleme derivative, approved in the United States for the reduction of the risk of breast cancer in women at high risk and as adjuvant therapy for the treatment of breast cancer. In a breast cancer chemoprevention trial (10), 54 women were assigned to receive tamoxifen 20 mg every day or placebo for 2 years. Small, but significant beneficial differences in both hip and spine bone mineral density (BMD) were seen in the postmenopausal tamoxifen-treated group. However, in the premenopausal women, tamoxifen treatment led to a significant decrease in spine and hip BMD density compared to placebo. Thus, it appears that the effects of tamoxifen on bone are complex. As a partial estrogen agonist, it has a positive effect on bone density in postmenopausal women; however, tamoxifen's effect on BMD in premenopausal women is negative, perhaps because of competition for estrogen-receptor binding sites.

Two studies to date have examined the effects of tamoxifen on fracture risk. In the Danish Breast Cancer Cooperative Group (11), 1,716 women were randomized to placebo or tamoxifen. There was no difference in hip fractures after 1 year of treatment. Other fractures were not examined. The National Surgical Adjuvant Breast and Bowel Project (NSABP) breast cancer prevention trial (12) was a randomized prospective study of tamoxifen versus placebo in 13,388 pre- and postmenopausal women at high risk for development of breast cancer. A secondary outcome in this trial was fracture reduction. At the end of 36 months, there was no difference in total fractures between the tamoxifen (472 fractures) and placebo (483) groups. However, when fragility fractures (clinically symptomatic vertebral fractures, hip, and radial fractures) were examined separately, there was a 19% reduction in relative risk in the tamoxifen-treated group [confidence intervals (CI): 0.63–1.05]. The reduction in risk was greater in the group of women over the age of 50 [relative risk (RR): 0.75, CI: 0.60–1.05] than in women less than 50 years old (RR: 0.88, CI: 0.46–1.68). Therefore, there is no evidence of skeletal benefit with tamoxifen in premenopausal women.

### Raloxifene

In a randomized, placebo-controlled, 2-year study of 601 healthy Caucasian early postmenopausal women (13), raloxifene increased BMD significantly in the lumbar spine, total hip, femoral neck, and total body compared to women given placebo (all groups were given calcium and vitamin-D supplements). The differences in BMD between the placebo and 60 mg/day (currently approved dosage) group at 24 months were 2.4% at the lumbar spine, 2.4% at the total hip, and 2% at the total body ($p < 0.001$ at all sites).

The Multiple Outcomes of Raloxifene Evaluation (MORE) trial (14) was a randomized, double-blind, placebo-controlled study of raloxifene 60 or 120 mg/day versus placebo (all women received calcium 500 mg and vitamin D 400 IU/day) in 7,705 postmenopausal women. The study was conducted for 36 months. The primary end point of MORE was the reduction in the percentage of women taking raloxifene who had at least one new vertebral fracture compared to the control group. Secondary end points were reductions in the relative risk of nonvertebral fractures, breast cancer, and cardiovascular events. Approximately one-third of the women had prevalent vertebral fractures at baseline and the other two-thirds did not. The average age was 65 years in those without and 69 years in those with prevalent fractures.

In the women with prevalent vertebral fractures at baseline, raloxifene reduced the relative risk of patients with at least one new radiological vertebral fracture by 30%. In those women without prevalent fractures, the relative risk reduction was 50%. The number needed to treat (NNT) for 3 years to prevent one vertebral fracture was 46 in those without prevalent vertebral fracture and 16 in those with at least one prevalent vertebral fracture. Although the relative risk reduction was higher (50%) in the women without baseline fractures than in the group with baseline fractures (30%), the absolute risk reduction is higher and the NNT lower in the group with baseline fractures because of their higher fracture incidence during the trial. Raloxifene reduced the number of women with multiple new vertebral fractures by 93%.

When the MORE trial was designed, each manufacturer's normative reference database was used for calculating T scores for the hip and spine. In 1995, NHANES III (National Health and Nutritional Examination Survey) published a database that has since become the standard for calculating hip T scores (15). As the Hologic database for young normal hip bone density had a higher BMD than NHANES III, the effect of substituting the lower NHANES III femoral neck, young normal database resulted in less of these subjects having a T score above −2.5. It is now apparent that a subset of patients in MORE had osteopenia and not osteoporosis. In postmenopausal women with osteopenia in the MORE trial, raloxifene decreased the risk of new radiographic vertebral fractures by 47% and new clinical vertebral fractures by 75% (16). Although the study was not designed to investigate fracture reduction in patients with osteopenia, because of the problem mentioned above with the manufacturer's normative database, this study is one of the first to suggest that fracture reduction may be possible in women who are osteopenic and not yet osteoporotic.

The relative risk of new clinical vertebral fractures in the MORE study has also been reported (17). At 1 year, raloxifene 60 mg/day decreased the risk of new clinical vertebral fractures by 68% (95% CI: 20–87%) compared with placebo. The risk with raloxifene was decreased by 46% (95% CI: 14–66%) at 2 years and by 41% (95% CI: 17–59%) at 3 years. This early 1-year relative risk reduction in clinical vertebral fractures is similar to that reported with other antiresorptive agents.

Although not a primary end point of the MORE study (14), there was no significant difference in the overall risk of nonvertebral fractures at 3 years (9.3% versus 8.5% for the placebo and pooled raloxifene groups, respectively) (RR = 0.9, CI: 0.8–1.1). There were 18 hip fractures in the placebo group (0.7%) and 40 hip fractures in the pooled raloxifene groups (0.8%) (RR = 1.1, 95% CI: 0.6–1.9).

A logistical regression model suggested that percentage changes in BMD could only account for 4% of the observed vertebral fracture risk reduction as a result of raloxifene. The other 96% of the risk reduction is unexplained by BMD. Another small percentage is probably due to changes in bone turnover; however, the exact contributions of factors reducing the risk of vertebral fractures are unknown. Biochemical markers of bone turnover including serum osteocalcin and urinary C-telopeptide demonstrated significant reductions compared with placebo throughout the study. Raloxifene maintains normal bone quality, including the absence of woven bone, marrow fibrosis, and mineralization defects.

The combined effects of raloxifene and other antiresorptive medications, specifically bisphosphonates, on bone density and biochemical markers have been studied (18). Combined raloxifene and alendronate reduced bone turnover and increased BMD more than either drug alone. It is not yet known whether this will result in better fracture risk reduction because there have not yet been any fracture-risk-assessment studies with combination antiresorptive therapy.

Bone density changes upon withdrawal of raloxifene after 5 years of treatment in postmenopausal women have also been assessed (19). Five years of treatment with raloxifene did not protect against bone loss after 1 year from withdrawal of this therapy, and the rate of bone loss was not significantly different from that of placebo-treated women, indicating that continuous raloxifene therapy is necessary for continued BMD preservation and probably for continued fracture reduction.

## NONSKELETAL EFFECTS OF RALOXIFENE

The MORE trial was not specifically conducted in women at high risk for breast cancer; however, raloxifene at a dose of 60 or 120 mg/day reduced the risk of invasive breast cancer by 76% (20). At present, raloxifene is not recommended for use as adjuvant therapy for breast cancer outside of a clinical trial.

## RALOXIFENE CARDIOVASCULAR EFFECTS

It is well known that patients with rheumatic disease are at increased risk for cardiovascular morbidity and mortality (21,22). In the MORE trial, raloxifene therapy did not significantly affect the risk of cardiovascular events in the overall cohort. A *post hoc* analysis revealed a reduction in the risk of vascular events in the subset of women with increased cardiovascular risk at baseline (23).

## RALOXIFENE SAFETY AND TOLERABILITY

The most common adverse effects associated with raloxifene during clinical trials were hot flashes and leg cramps (14). Hot flashes were more commonly reported in the prevention trials of early postmenopausal women (13). Similar to estrogen, raloxifene has been associated with a threefold increase in the risk for venous thromboembolic events, including deep vein thrombosis, pulmonary embolism, and retinal vein thrombosis (14). The use of raloxifene, including the antiphospholipids, in patients with hypercoagulability should be undertaken with great caution.

## SUMMARY

Raloxifene is effective in preventing and treating postmenopausal osteoporosis. Vertebral fracture reduction in osteoporotic women is comparable to other antiresorptive agents, including bisphosphonates. Because clinical trials have not yet demonstrated hip fracture reduction, raloxifene may be most useful at this time for the prevention of osteoporosis and for women with predominantly spinal osteoporosis. Over the next few years, results for additional large-scale raloxifene trials will add to our knowledge of the potential cardiovascular and breast cancer prevention efficacy of this drug. As knowledge of how different ligands modulate the estrogen receptor grows, a number of other SERMs are likely to be designed targeted to selective clinical applications.

# REFERENCES

1. Kuiper JGM, Carlsson B, Grandien K, et al. Comparison of the ligand binding specificity and transcript tissue distribution of estrogen receptors α and β. *Endocrinology* 1997;138:863–870.
2. Riggs BL, Hartmann LC. Selective estrogen-receptor modulators—mechanisms of action and application to clinical practice. *N Engl J Med* 2003;348:618–629.
3. Webb P, Nguyen P, Kushner P, et al. Differential SERM effects on co-repressor binding dictates ER-alpha activity. *J Biol Chem* 2003;278(9):6912–6920.
4. Bryant HU. Mechanism of action and preclinical profile of raloxifene, a selective estrogen receptor modulator. *Rev Endo Metabol Dis* 2001;2:129–138.
5. Wijayaratne AL, Nagel SC, Paige LA, et al. Comparative analysis of mechanistic differences among antiestrogens. *Endocrinology* 1999;140:5828–5840.
6. Diamanti-Kandarakis E, Sykiotis GP, Papavassiliou AG. Selective modulation of postmenopausal women: cutting the Gordian knot of hormone replacement therapy with breast carcinoma. *Cancer* 2003;97:12–20.
7. McDonnell DP, Wijayaratne A, Chang C, Norris JD. Elucidation of the molecular mechanism of action of selective estrogen receptor modulators. *Am J Cardiol* 2002;90(suppl):35F–43F.
8. Plouffe L. Selective estrogen receptor modulators (SERMs) in clinical practice. *J Soc Gynecol Invest* 2000;7:S38–S46.
9. Chen Z, Yuhanna IS, Galcheva-Gargova Z, et al. Estrogen receptor alpha mediates the nongenomic activation of endothelial nitric oxide synthase by estrogen. *J Clin Invest* 1999;103:401–406.
10. Powles TJ, Hickish T, Kanis JA, et al. Effect of tamoxifen on bone mineral density measured by dual energy x-ray absorptiometry in health premenopausal and postmenopausal women. *J Clin Oncol* 1996;14:78–84.
11. Kristensen B, Ejlertsen B, Mouridsen HT, et al. Femoral fractures in postmenopausal breast cancer patients treated with adjuvant tamoxifen. *Breast Cancer Res Treat* 1996;39:321–326.
12. Fisher B, Constantino JP, Wickerham DL, et al. Tamoxifen for prevention of breast cancer: report of the National Surgical Adjuvant Breast and Bowel Project P-1 Study. *J Natl Cancer Inst* 1998;90:1371–1388.
13. Delmas PD, Bjarnason NH, Mitlak BH, et al. Effects of raloxifene on bone mineral density, serum cholesterol concentration and uterine endometrium in postmenopausal women. *N Engl J Med* 1997;337:1641–1647.
14. Ettinger B, Black DM, Mitlak BH, et al. Reduction of vertebral risk in postmenopausal women with osteoporosis treated with raloxifene. Results from a 3-year randomized clinical trial. *JAMA* 1999;282:637–645.
15. Looker AC, Wahner HW, Dunn WL, et al. Updated data on proximal femur bone mineral levels of US adults. *Osteoporosis Int* 1998;8:468–489.
16. Kanis JA, Johnell O, Black DM, et al. Effect of raloxifene on the risk of new vertebral fracture in postmenopausal women with osteopenia or osteoporosis: a reanalysis of the Multiple Outcomes of Raloxifene Evaluation trial. *Bone* 2003;33:293–300.
17. Maricic M, Adachi J, Meunier P, et al. Early effects of Raloxifene on clinical vertebral fractures at 12 months in postmenopausal women with osteoporosis. *Arch Int Med* 2002;162:1140–1143.
18. Johnell O, Scheele WH, Lu Y, et al. Additive Effects of Raloxifene and Alendronate on Bone Density and Biochemical Markers of Bone Remodeling in Postmenopausal Women with Osteoporosis. *J Clin Endocrinol Metab* 2002;87(3):985–992.
19. Neele SJM, Evertz R, De Valk-de Roo G, et al. Effect of 1 year discontinuation of raloxifene or estrogen therapy on bone mineral density after 5 years of treatment in healthy postmenopausal women. *Bone* 2002;30:599–603.
20. Cummings S, Eckert S, Krueper K, et al. The Effect of Raloxifene or Risk of Breast Cancer in Post-Menopausal Women. Results from the MORE randomized trial. *JAMA* 1999;281:2189–2197.
21. Solomon Dh, Karlsson EW, Rimm EB, et al. *Circulation* 2003;10(9):1303–1307.
22. Salmon JE, Roman MJ. Accelerated atherosclerosis in systemic lupus erythematosus: implications for patient management. *Curr Opin Rheum* 2001;13(5):341–344.
23. Barrett-Conner E, Grady D, Sashegui A, et al. Raloxifene and cardiovascular events in osteoporotic postmenopausal women. *JAMA* 2002;287:847–856.

# The Use of Androgens and Dehydroepiandrosterone in Rheumatic Bone Disease

## 20

Tim A. Bongartz   Jürgen Schölmerich   Rainer H. Straub

## ANDROGENS AND DEHYDROEPIANDROSTERONE IN THE TREATMENT OF OSTEOPOROSIS

Bone is a vital dynamic tissue undergoing a continuous process of resorption and formation, influenced by numerous factors. A disbalance within this process favoring resorption leads to bone loss, which appears as generalized and localized forms. Androgens have important effects on bone development and homeostasis (Table 20.1). Observations on the morbidity attributable to osteoporosis in men receiving antiandrogenic treatment for prostate cancer or suffering from chronic inflammatory disorders have stimulated considerable interest in the mechanisms by which androgens act on bone.

Androgen receptors can be found in all three bone cells: osteoblasts, osteoclasts, and osteocytes (1). Binding of androgens to receptors on these cells leads to an active ligand-receptor complex that binds to DNA and influences the transcription of target genes (2). Although testosterone is the major circulating androgen, there is evidence that its skeletal effects are at least partially mediated by metabolites produced by enzymes present in bone. The expression in bone, therefore, has been reported for two important enzymes participating in androgen metabolism: 5-alpha reductase, which reduces testosterone to dehydrotestosterone (DHT) (3), and aromatase, which converts testosterone to estradiol and androstendione to estrone (4). Case reports of patients with aromatase deficiency emphasize the importance of the peripheral androgen metabolism. In a man with a homozygous mutation and severe aromatase deficiency, the phenotype is characterized by tall stature, delayed skeletal maturation, and osteopenia. Manifestations of aromatase deficiency in women include pubertal failure and delayed bone age (5). Effects of androgens on osteoblastic cells have been demonstrated both *in vitro* and *in vivo*. The proliferation of osteoblasts is stimulated by androgens, but, conversely, prolonged exposure to androgens under experimental conditions may inhibit osteoblast proliferation significantly (6). Of interest, it is not known whether intermittent androgen therapy improves bone mineral density (BMD) in women to a greater degree than does continuous therapy. Androgens also appear to have an important influence on bone matrix production and organization. Exposure of osteoblasts to testosterone or dehydroepiandrosterone (DHEA) enhances cell differentiation and the synthesis of extracellular matrix proteins such as type-I collagen, osteocalcin, and osteonectin (7–9). Both testosterone and DHT upregulate tumor growth factor (TGF)-βsynthesis, which is one of the most potent osteoblast mitogens (10). Other growth factors influenced by androgens include fibroblast growth factor and

**TABLE 20.1**

**EFFECTS OF ANDROGENS ON BONE CELLS**

| Reference | Cell type | Effect |
|---|---|---|
| Kasperk C 1989 | Osteoblasts | Stimulation of proliferation |
| Kasperk C 1990 | Osteoblasts | Increased expression of TGF beta, increased responsiveness to IGF II and FGF |
| Gray C 1992 | Osteoblasts | Inhibition of cAMP response to PTH |
| Bellido T 1995 | Osteoclasts | Inhibition of osteoclastogenesis by reduction of IL-6 production in stroma cells |
| Benz DJ 1991 | Osteoblast-like sarcoma cells | Increased production of type I collagen |
| Pilbeam CC 1990 | Osteoblasts | Inhibition of IL-1 and PTH-stimulated PGE2 production |

TGF beta = tissue growth factor beta; IGF II = insulin-like growth factor II; FGF = fibroblast growth factor; PTH = parathyroid hormone; PGE2 = prostaglandin E2; IL = interleukin.

insulin-like growth factor (11). Androgens also decrease formation of osteoclasts by inhibiting the production of interleukin (IL)-6 in bone marrow (12). In addition, they reduce osteoclast activity by inhibition of parathyroid hormone and IL-1-stimulated prostaglandin E2 (PGE2) production (13).

The continuously increasing evidence for the important role of androgens in bone homeostasis has promoted clinical research addressing the possible benefit of androgen therapy in different forms of osteoporosis. So far, research has focused on androgen replacement in hypoandrogenic men and postmenopausal women.

## OSTEOPOROSIS IN HYPOANDROGENIC MEN

In men, hypogonadism is an important risk factor of osteoporosis and osteoporosis-related fractures (14,15). Several studies have demonstrated an association between low serum testosterone levels and decreased BMD (16–19). Androgen deprivation therapy has been reported to increase fracture risk in men with prostate cancer (20–23). The prevalence of hypogonadism was reported to be increased fivefold in elderly men with hip fractures (15). There is increasing evidence that androgen replacement therapy can prevent bone loss in elderly hypogonadal men (24–30). Besides a significant increase of BMD, a decline in markers of bone resorption may be demonstrated in these studies (Table 20.2). No beneficial effects of androgen treatment were seen in men with normal pretreatment serum testosterone (29).

However, no study so far has shown that testosterone replacement decreases fracture risk in these patients. As a consequence, testosterone is not approved by the Food and Drug Administration (FDA) for treatment or prevention of osteoporosis in hypoandrogenic men. Nevertheless,

hypogonadal men are candidates for testosterone treatment to correct other problems of hypogonadism such as loss of libido, erectile dysfunction, fatigue, and poor sense of well-being. Increase of BMD under testosterone treatment can be seen as a secondary benefit, which is proved by the numerous studies previously mentioned.

Safety issues associated with long-term testosterone treatment have not been thoroughly studied. It is contraindicated in men with prostate cancer, and an elevated prostate specific antigen (PSA) during testosterone treatment has been reported (31).

## OSTEOPOROSIS IN POSTMENOPAUSAL WOMEN

In women, menopause induces accelerated bone loss. The rate of bone loss is influenced by estrogen deficiency and can be prevented with estrogen replacement therapy, as proved by placebo-controlled trials (32,33). The role of androgens in postmenopausal osteoporosis and the efficacy of androgen replacement therapy in this setting is less clear. Decreased levels of androgens in postmenopausal women are associated with an increased risk of fractures of the spine and hip (34,35). In women affected by androgen insensitivity syndrome, low BMD is a frequent finding even in those treated with long-term estrogen therapy (36). This observation underlines an estrogen-independent influence of androgens on BMD in women. The possible advantage of combined therapy with estrogen and androgen compared to estrogen alone is revealed in a recent clinical study in postmenopausal women. Treatment for 9 weeks with a daily combination of estrogen and testosterone or estrogen alone showed similar decreases in the urinary excretion of bone resorption markers, but estrogen- and -androgen-treated women had a significant increase in serum bone formation markers (37). These

**TABLE 20.2**

**INFLUENCE OF ANDROGEN REPLACEMENT ON BONE MINERAL DENSITY AND PARAMETERS OF BONE METABOLISM IN HYPOANDROGENIC MEN**

| Reference | Study design | Treatment | Patients | Outcome |
| --- | --- | --- | --- | --- |
| Katznelson L 1996 | Cross-sectional. Follow up for 18 months | Testosterone enanthate 100 mg weekly | 36 men with primary and secondary hypogonadism | Increase in bone and muscle mass, decline in parameters of bone resorption |
| Tenover JS 1992 | Randomized, placebo-controlled. Follow up for 3 months | Testosterone enanthate, 100 mg weekly i.m. | 13 older hypoandrogenic men | Decline in parameters of bone resorption |
| Leifke E 1998 | Single arm. Follow up for 1–7 years | Testosterone enanthate 250 mg i.m. every 2–4 weeks | 32 male patients with hypogonadotropic hypogonadism | Significant increase in BMD of the spine. Increase in paraspinal muscle mass |
| Behre HM 1997 | Cross-sectional. Follow up for 16 years | Testosterone enanthate 250 mg i.m. every 2–4 weeks | 75 male patients with primary and secondary hypogonadism | Normalization of BMD and maintenance within the normal range |
| Snyder PJ 1999 | Randomized, placebo-controlled. Follow up for 36 months | Testosterone patch | 108 men > 65 yrs | Significant effect on BMD of lumbar spine in men with low pretreatment serum testosterone. No effect on BMD in men with normal pretreatment testosterone |
| Zacharin MR 2003 | Cross-sectional. Follow up for 6.6 years | Subcutaneous testosterone implant 600–800 mg every 6 months | 37 male patients with primary and secondary hypogonadism | Maintenance of normal BMD |

I.M. = intramuscularly, BMD = bone mineral density.

findings support the rationale that the anabolic bone-building potential of androgens should be considered especially when nonresponse to adequate estrogen therapy is observed.

This idea is supported by a second study that investigated the bone-building effect of androgen treatment. Postmenopausal women on estrogen therapy were separated into two groups, one remaining on daily oral estrogen, the other changing to subcutaneous hormone implants consisting of estrogen and testosterone. One year later, BMD increased significantly in the women on combination therapy (38).

The beneficial effect of combined estrogen and androgen treatment could also be demonstrated in appropriately designed, randomized, placebo-controlled studies. Surgically induced menopausal women were treated for 2 years with daily doses of either esterified estrogen or esterified estrogen and methyltestosterone. Both treatment regimens prevented bone loss at the spine and hip, but only combination therapy was able to significantly increase spinal BMD compared to baseline values (39).

The correlation of low DHEA levels with the risk of osteoporotic fractures has led to the investigation of DHEA treatment and its effects on BMD in clinical trials. In summary, bone resorption decreased and bone formation increased with DHEA treatment, especially in elderly postmenopausal women (40-42). The increase of BMD under DHEA treatment was only modest compared to the effects

of combined estrogen and androgen treatment, and no conclusion can be drawn concerning the effects on fracture risk (Table 20.3).

Unfortunately, androgen therapy in postmenopausal women can have negative side effects such as acne and hair disorders (39). Furthermore, there is no data addressing the effect on the frequency of osteoporotic fractures. Consequently, androgen treatment for osteoporosis should be the subject of controlled long-term trials with the number of osteoporotic fractures as a parameter.

## ANDROGENS AND DHEA IN THE TREATMENT OF RHEUMATOID ARTHRITIS

In rheumatoid arthritis (RA), effects on bone structure are manifest in three different ways: first, as juxtaarticular osteoporosis, second as generalized osteoporosis, and third as bone erosion of individual joints. Generalized and periarticular osteoporosis leads to an increased risk of both vertebral and nonvertebral fractures. Fracture risk in patients with RA is increased twofold compared to healthy controls (43,44).

The pathophysiologic mechanisms of the three bony manifestations of RA have largely been thought to be separate (45). Recent studies, however, are challenging this concept and suggest a common pathophysiologic

## TABLE 20.3

## INFLUENCE OF ANDROGEN THERAPY ON BONE MINERAL DENSITY AND PARAMETERS OF BONE METABOLISM IN POSTMENOPAUSAL WOMEN

| Reference | Study design | Patients | Treatment | Outcome |
|---|---|---|---|---|
| Raisz LG 1996 | Randomized-controlled trial. Follow up for 9 weeks | 86 postmenopausal women | Conjugated equine estrogen vs. esterified estrogen/ methyltestosterone combination | Estrogen/androgen combination led to a significant increase in markers of bone formation |
| Savvas M 1992 | Crossover. Follow up for 1 year | 20 postmenopausal women | Oral conjugated equine estrogen vs. estradiol/testosterone implants | Only estradiol/testosterone combination led to a significant increase in bone formation |
| Watts NB 1995 | Randomized, placebo-controlled. Follow up for 2 years | 66 surgically post-menopausal women | Oral esterified estrogen vs.estrogen/ methyltestosterone therapy | Significant increase in BMD in the estrogen/methyltestosterone group |
| Barrett-Connor E 1999 | Randomized, placebo-controlled. Follow up for 2 years | 311 postmenopausal women | Estrogen vs. esterified estrogen plus methyl-testosterone | Only combination therapy significantly increased BMD |
| Davis SR 1995 | Randomized, controlled. Follow up for 2 years | 34 postmenopausal women | Estradiol vs. estradiol/testosterone | BMD increased in both treatment groups but to a greater degree in the estradiol/testosterone group |
| Labrie F 1997 | Single arm. Follow up for 12 months | 14 postmenopausal women | Percutaneous DHEA | Significant increase of hip BMD, nonsignificant increase of spine BMD. Decrease in markers of bone resorption |
| Villareal DT 2000 | Nonrandomized, matched controls. Follow up for 6 months | 10 postmenopausal women | Oral DHEA | Significant increase of spine BMD |
| Baulieu EE 2000 | Randomized, double blind placebo-controlled. Follow up for 12 months | 280 men and women, 60–79 yrs old | Oral DHEA vs. placebo | Significant increases in BMD at the femoral neck and Ward's triangle in women aged 60–69 and at the proximal radius in the women aged 70–79 |

DHEA = dehydroepiandrosterone, BMD = bone mineral density.

background. Tumor necrosis factor (TNF) and IL-1, which play a central role in the pathogenesis of synovitis in RA, are found to be regulators of osteoclastic bone resorption. Inflammatory cells infiltrating the joint and synovial fibroblasts express the receptor activator of nuclear factor-κB ligand (RANKL), which appears to be responsible for mediating osteoclast differentiation and activation (46,47). This pathway provides a link between all three bony manifestations of RA and the inflammatory disease process itself.

Osteoporosis in RA is characterized by relatively preserved bone mass in the axial bone (lumbar spine) and marked loss in peripheral bones. Long disease duration and disease activity could be strong risk factors for generalized osteoporosis, giving further evidence for a close link between inflammation and bone loss (48). Consequently, efficient suppression of disease activity by disease-modifying antirheumatic drugs not only retards progression of joint erosions but also decreases the reduction of BMD over time.

Because loss of BMD in RA occurs early in the disease, osteoporosis management should be considered very early (49). The ideal strategy, therefore, seems to include measures that lead to complete inflammation control and modulation of osteoclast activity.

Androgens such as testosterone or DHEA exert immunosuppressive effects in different *in vitro* and *in vivo* experiments: Testosterone inhibits IL-1βsecretion by PBMC of RA patients (50) and decreases IL-1 syntheses in primary cultures of human synovial macrophages (51). Biologically active androgen has demonstrated inhibition of human IL-6 gene promotor activity in human fibroblasts (52). In the collagen-induced arthritis model, intraarticular application of testosterone reduces the extent and severity of synovial hyperplasia significantly more than intraarticular dexamethasone (53). An osteoprotective role of systemic testosterone in adjuvant-induced arthritis could also be demonstrated (54). In systemic lupus erythematosus (SLE), DHEA has already proved its beneficial effects on disease activity in large controlled clinical trials (55,56). In addition, adjuvant DHEA treatment in SLE was able to maintain BMD while at the same time there was a significant reduction of lumbosacral spine BMD in the control group (56). The DHEA effects may be mediated by its IL-6 inhibiting capacities (57).

In RA, sex-hormone levels have frequently been found to be altered especially in men and postmenopausal women (58). Low levels of androgens in RA patients lead to a significantly elevated ratio of free estrogens and free androgens especially in synovial fluid, which favors the local predominance of proinflammatory estrogens relative to antiinflammatory androgens (59).

Although BMD in rheumatic patients does not correlate with testosterone levels (49), androgen adjuvant therapy has been proposed for rheumatoid arthritis treatment because of its immunosuppressive actions. Furthermore, testosterone replacement in hypoandrogenic men has clearly demonstrated a beneficial effect on different markers of bone resorption and BMD. Androgens, therefore, are interesting adjuncts to counteract both inflammation and bone resorption in RA.

Treatment of male RA patients with androgens, however, showed conflicting results (Table 20.4). Cutolo, et al. (60) treated seven biochemically hypogonadal men with 120 mg testosterone undecanoate daily in an uncontrolled study. None of the patients received disease-modifying antirheumatic drug (DMARD) therapy. After 6 months, there was a significant decrease in the joint tenderness count and

daily NSAID intake. However, in a larger placebo-controlled trial with 35 male RA patients, no significant changes in parameters of disease activity were achieved by adjunct therapy with 250 mg testosterone enanthate every 4 weeks for 9 months. Furthermore, no beneficial effect on the decrease of BMD could be observed after this time period. Of interest, the 5 patients who showed a flare in disease activity were all receiving testosterone treatment (61).

A randomized, placebo-controlled study of postmenopausal women with RA osteoporosis was able to demonstrate significant effects on disease activity and general well-being by adding 50 mg testosterone proprionate and 2 mg progesterone to standard treatment with DMARDs. Parameters of general well-being like pain scale and general health assessment showed a statistically significant improvement. Erythrocyte sedimentation rate (ESR) and tender joint count failed to show a significant decrease, but American College of Rheumatology (ACR)-20 response was achieved by 12 patients (of 57) in the treatment group and only 2 patients (of 50) in the placebo group after 12 months (62).

The only clinical trial using DHEA as an adjunctive treatment in RA was published by Giltay, et al. (63). Eleven male and female postmenopausal RA patients were treated with DHEA 200 mg/day for 16 weeks. None of the median values of the efficacy parameters like tender and swollen joint count, pain visual analog scale (VAS), health assessment questionnaire (HAQ), C-reactive protein, or European League Against Rheumatism (ESR) changed signifi-

---

### TABLE 20.4

### EFFECTS OF ANDROGEN TREATMENT IN RHEUMATOID ARTHRITIS

| Reference | Study design | Patients | Study Medication | Outcome |
|---|---|---|---|---|
| Hall GM 1996 | Randomized, placebo-controlled. Follow up at 9 months | 35 male RA | Testosterone enanthate | No significant change in disease activity parameters |
| Booij A 1996 | Randomized, placebo-controlled. Follow up at 1 year | 107 female post-menopausal | Testosterone proprionate | No significant decrease of tender and swollen joint count. Significant reduction of ESR, pain, and HAQ |
| Cutolo 1991 | Single arm. Follow up at 6 months | 7 male patients | Testosterone undecanoate | Significant decrease of tender joint count and daily NSAID dosage |
| Giltay EJ | Single arm. Follow up at 16 weeks | 11 men and post-menopausal women | DHEA | No significant effect on tender and swollen joint count, HAQ, pain, ESR, CRP, and patients assessment of well-being |

RA = rheumatoid arthritis, DHEA = dehydroepiandrosterone, ESR = erythrocyte sedimentation rate, HAQ = health assessment questionnaire, NSAID = nonsteroidal antiinflammatory drug.

cantly over time. Two female patients responded to the ACR-20 and EULAR response criteria.

For the divergence between the strong antiinflammatory effects of androgens in different *in vitro* experiments and the mild beneficial effects observed in clinical studies, an intriguing explanation was recently presented (59). Inflammatory cytokines such as TNF, IL-1β, and IL-6 have been found to stimulate the local activity of aromatase, resulting in accelerated conversion of antiinflammatory androgens to proinflammatory estrogens. This shift might imprint the proinflammatory situation in the joint.

In summary, testosterone or DHEA treatment failed to demonstrate a strong influence on disease activity in RA. The study of Booji, et al. (62) suggests, however, that concomitant androgen therapy in postmenopausal women with RA might result in positive general well-being. Parallel use of an aromatase inhibitor to prevent local conversion of androgens to proinflammatory estrogens in the inflamed tissue may lead to new therapeutic options. As for now, routine use of androgens in RA cannot be recommended.

# REFERENCES

1. Abu EO, Horner A, Kusec V, et al. The localization of androgen receptors in human bone. *J Clin Endocrinol Metab* 1997;82: 3493–3497.
2. McKenna NJ, Lanz RB, O'Malley BW. Nuclear receptor coregulators: cellular and molecular biology. *Endocr Rev* 1999;20:321–344.
3. Schweikert HU, Totzauer P, Rohr HP, Bartsch G. Correlated biochemical and stereological studies on testosterone metabolism in the stromal and epithelial compartment of human benign prostatic hyperplasia. *J Urol* 1985;134:403–407.
4. Nawata H, Tanaka S, Takayanagi R, et al. Aromatase in bone cell: association with osteoporosis in postmenopausal women. *J Steroid Biochem Mol Biol* 1995;53:165–174.
5. Morishima A, Grumbach MM, Simpson ER, et al. Aromatase deficiency in male and female siblings caused by a novel mutation and the physiological role of estrogens. *J Clin Endocrinol Metab* 1995;80:3689–3698.
6. Kasperk CH, Wakley GK, Hierl T, Ziegler R. Gonadal and adrenal androgens are potent regulators of human bone cell metabolism in vitro. *J Bone Miner Res* 1997;12:464–471.
7. Kasperk CH, Wergedal JE, Farley JR, et al. Androgens directly stimulate proliferation of bone cells in vitro. *Endocrinology* 1989;124:1576–1578.
8. Benz DJ, Haussler MR, Thomas MA, et al. High-affinity androgen binding and androgenic regulation of alpha 1(I)-procollagen and transforming growth factor-beta steady state messenger ribonucleic acid levels in human osteoblast-like osteosarcoma cells. *Endocrinology* 1991;128:2723–2730.
9. Bodo M, Venti Donti G, Becchetti E, et al. Effects of steroids on human normal and otosclerotic osteoblastic cells: influence on thymidine and leucine uptake and incorporation. *Cell Mol Biol* 1991;37:597–606.
10. Centrella M, Horowitz MC, Wozney JM, McCarthy TL. Transforming growth factor-beta gene family members and bone. *Endocr Rev* 1994;15:27–39.
11. Kasperk C, Fitzsimmons R, Strong D, et al. Studies of the mechanism by which androgens enhance mitogenesis and differentiation in bone cells. *J Clin Endocrinol Metab* 1990;71:1322–1329.
12. Bellido T, Jilka RL, Boyce BF, et al. Regulation of interleukin-6, osteoclastogenesis, and bone mass by androgens. The role of the androgen receptor. *J Clin Invest* 1995;95:2886–2895.
13. Pilbeam CC, Raisz LG. Effects of androgens on parathyroid hormone and interleukin-1-stimulated prostaglandin production in

14. cultured neonatal mouse calvariae. *J Bone Miner Res* 1990;5: 1183–1188.
14. Seeman E, Melton LJ 3rd, O'Fallon WM, Riggs BL. Risk factors for spinal osteoporosis in men. *Am J Med* 1983;75:977–983.
15. Stanley HL, Schmitt BP, Poses RM, Deiss WP. Does hypogonadism contribute to the occurrence of a minimal trauma hip fracture in elderly men? *J Am Geriatr Soc* 1991;39:766–771.
16. Clarke BL, Ebeling PR, Jones JD, et al. Changes in quantitative bone histomorphometry in aging healthy men. *J Clin Endocrinol Metab* 1996;81:2264–2270.
17. Murphy S, Khaw KT, Cassidy A, Compston JE. Sex hormones and bone mineral density in elderly men. *Bone Miner* 1993;20: 133–140.
18. Greendale GA, Edelstein S, Barrett-Connor E. Endogenous sex steroids and bone mineral density in older women and men: the Rancho Bernardo Study. *J Bone Miner Res* 1997;12:1833–1843.
19. Khosla S, Melton LJ 3rd, Atkinson EJ, et al. Relationship of serum sex steroid levels and bone turnover markers with bone mineral density in men and women: a key role for bioavailable estrogen. *J Clin Endocrinol Metab* 1998;83:2266–2274.
20. Daniell HW. Osteoporosis after orchiectomy for prostate cancer. *J Urol* 1997;157:439–444.
21. Townsend MF, Sanders WH, Northway RO, Graham SD Jr. Bone fractures associated with luteinizing hormone-releasing hormone agonists used in the treatment of prostate carcinoma. *Cancer* 1997;79:545–550.
22. Hatano T, Oishi Y, Furuta A, et al. Incidence of bone fracture in patients receiving luteinizing hormone-releasing hormone agonists for prostate cancer. *BJU Int* 2000;86:449–452.
23. Oefelein MG, Ricchuiti V, Conrad W, et al. Skeletal fracture associated with androgen suppression induced osteoporosis: the clinical incidence and risk factors for patients with prostate cancer. *J Urol* 2001;166:1724–1728.
24. Katznelson L, Finkelstein JS, Schoenfeld DA, et al. Increase in bone density and lean body mass during testosterone administration in men with acquired hypogonadism. *J Clin Endocrinol Metab* 1996;81:4358–4365.
25. Tenover JS. Effects of testosterone supplementation in the aging male. *J Clin Endocrinol Metab* 1992;75:1092–1098.
26. Morley JE, Perry HM 3rd, Kaiser FE, et al. Effects of testosterone replacement therapy in old hypogonadal males: a preliminary study. *J Am Geriatr Soc* 1993;41:149–152.
27. Leifke E, Korner HC, Link TM, et al. Effects of testosterone replacement therapy on cortical and trabecular bone mineral density, vertebral body area and paraspinal muscle area in hypogonadal men. *Eur J Endocrinol* 1998;138:51–58.
28. Zacharin MR, Pua J, Kanumakala S. Bone mineral density outcomes following long-term treatment with subcutaneous testosterone pellet implants in male hypogonadism. *Clin Endocrinol (Oxf)* 2003;58:691–695.
29. Snyder PJ, Peachey H, Hannoush P, et al. Effect of testosterone treatment on bone mineral density in men over 65 years of age. *J Clin Endocrinol Metab* 1999;84:1966–1972.
30. Behre HM, Kliesch S, Leifke E, et al. Long-term effect of testosterone therapy on bone mineral density in hypogonadal men. *J Clin Endocrinol Metab* 1997;82:2386–2390.
31. Gerstenbluth RE, Maniam PN, Corty EW, Seftel AD. Prostate-specific antigen changes in hypogonadal men treated with testosterone replacement. *J Androl* 2002;23:922–926.
32. Quigley ME, Martin PL, Burnier AM, Brooks P. Estrogen therapy arrests bone loss in elderly women. *Am J Obstet Gynecol* 1987;156:1516–1523.
33. Harris ST, Genant HK, Baylink DJ, et al. The effects of estrone (Ogen) on spinal bone density of postmenopausal women. *Arch Intern Med* 1991;151:1980–1984.
34. Longcope C, Baker RS, Hui SL, Johnston CC Jr. Androgen and estrogen dynamics in women with vertebral crush fractures. *Maturitas* 1984;6:309–318.
35. Davidson BJ, Ross RK, Paganini-Hill A, et al. Total and free estrogens and androgens in postmenopausal women with hip fractures. *J Clin Endocrinol Metab* 1982;54:115–120.
36. Soule SG, Conway G, Prelevic GM, et al. Osteopenia as a feature of the androgen insensitivity syndrome. *Clin Endocrinol (Oxf)* 1995;43:671–675.

37. Raisz LG, Wiita B, Artis A, et al. Comparison of the effects of estrogen alone and estrogen plus androgen on biochemical markers of bone formation and resorption in postmenopausal women. *J Clin Endocrinol Metab* 1996;81:37–43.

38. Savvas M, Studd JW, Norman S, et al. Increase in bone mass after one year of percutaneous oestradiol and testosterone implants in post-menopausal women who have previously received long-term oral oestrogens. *Br J Obstet Gynaecol* 1992;99:757–760.

39. Watts NB, Notelovitz M, Timmons MC, et al. Comparison of oral estrogens and estrogens plus androgen on bone mineral density, menopausal symptoms, and lipid-lipoprotein profiles in surgical menopause. *Obstet Gynecol* 1995;85:529–537.

40. Labrie F, Diamond P, Cusan L, et al. Effect of 12-month dehydroepiandrosterone replacement therapy on bone, vagina, and endometrium in postmenopausal women. *J Clin Endocrinol Metab* 1997;82:3498–3505.

41. Villareal DT, Holloszy JO, Kohrt WM. Effects of DHEA replacement on bone mineral density and body composition in elderly women and men. *Clin Endocrinol (Oxf)* 2000;53:561–568.

42. Baulieu EE, Thomas G, Legrain S, et al. Dehydroepiandrosterone (DHEA), DHEA sulfate, and aging: contribution of the DHEAge Study to a sociobiomedical issue. *Proc Natl Acad Sci U S A* 2000;97:4279–4284.

43. Cooper C, Coupland C, Mitchell M. Rheumatoid arthritis, corticosteroid therapy and hip fracture. *Ann Rheum Dis* 1995;54:49–52.

44. Hooyman JR, Melton LJ 3rd, Nelson AM, et al. Fractures after rheumatoid arthritis. A population-based study. *Arthritis Rheum* 1984;27:1353–1361.

45. Sambrook PN. The skeleton in rheumatoid arthritis: common mechanisms for bone erosion and osteoporosis? *J Rheumatol* 2000;27:2541–2542.

46. Goldring SR, Gravallese EM. Pathogenesis of bone lesions in rheumatoid arthritis. *Curr Rheumatol Rep* 2002;4:226–231.

47. Jones DH, Kong YY, Penninger JM. Role of RANKL and RANK in bone loss and arthritis. *Ann Rheum Dis* 2002;61(Suppl 2):32–39.

48. Shibuya K, Hagino H, Morio Y, Teshima R. Cross-sectional and longitudinal study of osteoporosis in patients with rheumatoid arthritis. *Clin Rheumatol* 2002;21:150–158.

49. Tengstrand B, Hafstrom I. Bone mineral density in men with rheumatoid arthritis is associated with erosive disease and sulfasalazine treatment but not with sex hormones. *J Rheumatol* 2002;29:2299–2305.

50. Li ZG, Danis VA, Brooks PM. Effect of gonadal steroids on the production of IL-1 and IL-6 by blood mononuclear cells in vitro. *Clin Exp Rheumatol* 1993;11:157–162.

51. Cutolo M, Sulli A, Barone A, et al. Macrophages, synovial tissue and rheumatoid arthritis. *Clin Exp Rheumatol* 1993;11:331–339.

52. Keller ET, Chang C, Ershler WB. Inhibition of NFkappaB activity through maintenance of IkappaBalpha levels contributes to dihydrotestosterone-mediated repression of the interleukin-6 promoter. *J Biol Chem* 1996;271:26267–26275.

53. Steward A, Bayley DL. Effects of androgens in models of rheumatoid arthritis. *Agents Actions* 1992;35:268–272.

54. Harbuz MS, Perveen-Gill Z, Lightman SL, Jessop DS. A protective role for testosterone in adjuvant-induced arthritis. *Br J Rheumatol* 1995;34:1117–1122.

55. Chang DM, Lan JL, Lin HY, et al. Dehydroepiandrosterone treatment of women with mild-to-moderate systemic lupus erythematosus: a multicenter randomized, double-blind, placebo-controlled trial. *Arthritis Rheum* 2002;46:2924–2927.

56. van Vollenhoven RF, Park JL, Genovese MC, et al. A double-blind, placebo-controlled, clinical trial of dehydroepiandrosterone in severe systemic lupus erythematosus. *Lupus* 1999;8:181–187.

57. Straub RH, Konecna L, Hrach S, et al. Serum dehydroepiandrosterone (DHEA) and DHEA sulfate are negatively correlated with serum interleukin-6 (IL-6), and DHEA inhibits IL-6 secretion from mononuclear cells in man in vitro: possible link between endocrinosenescence and immunosenescence. *J Clin Endocrinol Metab* 1998;83:2012–2017.

58. Masi AT. Sex hormones and rheumatoid arthritis: cause or effect relationships in a complex pathophysiology? *Clin Exp Rheumatol* 1995;13:227–240.

59. Castagnetta LA, Carruba G, Granata OM, et al. Increased estrogen formation and estrogen to androgen ratio in the synovial fluid of patients with rheumatoid arthritis. *J Rheumatol* 2003;30:2597–2605.

60. Cutolo M, Balleari E, Giusti M, et al. Androgen replacement therapy in male patients with rheumatoid arthritis. *Arthritis Rheum* 1991;34:1–5.

61. Hall GM, Larbre JP, Spector TD, et al. A randomized trial of testosterone therapy in males with rheumatoid arthritis. *Br J Rheumatol* 1996;35:568–573.

62. Booji A, Biewenga-Booji CM, Huber-Bruning O, et al. Androgens as adjuvant treatment in postmenopausal female patients with rheumatoid arthritis. *Ann Rheum Dis* 1996;55:811–815.

63. Giltay EJ, van Schaardenburg D, Gooren LJ, et al. Effects of dehydroepiandrosterone administration on disease activity in patients with rheumatoid arthritis. *Br J Rheumatol* 1998;37:705–706.

# The Use of Parathyroid Hormone in Patients with Rheumatic Diseases

## 21

*Robin Dore*

A significant number of patients in a rheumatology practice present with primary or secondary osteoporosis because they are older or suffer from an inflammatory condition that causes bone loss or requires therapy that has adverse effects on bone tissue (1). Rheumatologists frequently take primary responsibility for fracture risk reduction in these patients and initiate therapy for osteoporosis prevention or treatment.

Until recently all medications indicated for the treatment of osteoporosis were antiresorptive. These therapies reduce the rate of remodeling and possibly prolong the lifespan of osteocytes (2). As a result of reduction in osteoclast activity, reversible remodeling space is filled with osteoid that undergoes primary, then secondary, mineralization. While increases in bone mineral density (BMD), a positive response to antiresorptive therapy, may occur to a greater or lesser degree with various agents, these agents provide similar fracture-risk reduction, at least regarding vertebral fractures. Reductions in excessive bone turnover contribute significantly to bone strength, and it should no longer be considered a "paradox" that small changes in BMD may be associated with large changes in fracture risk reduction. Consistent with this realization, the definition of osteoporosis was redefined as a condition of "compromised bone strength"; bone strength comes from bone density and bone quality, the latter including turnover, mineralization, damage accumulation, and architecture (3).

Despite antiresorptive therapy, patients may suffer an osteoporotic fracture or may experience significant decreases in BMD, both of which increase their risk of future fracture. There are some patients who are unable to tolerate any of the antiresorptive therapies or have contraindications such as severe gastroesophageal reflux disorder, deep vein thromboses, or chronic nasal congestion. For patients who are either unwilling or unable to use available antiresorptive therapy, or whose osteoporosis has not responded optimally to antiresorptive therapy, recombinant human parathyroid hormone (1-34), or rhPTH (1-34), at a dose of 20 µg/ day has been approved in the United States and other countries as a bone formation agent for the treatment of osteoporosis. Teriparatide is the generic name for the 34 amino acid, N-terminal fragment of the parathyroid hormone (PTH) molecule.

## PTH OVERVIEW

The use of parathyroid hormone to treat osteoporosis seems to be another "paradox" as hyperparathyroidism is a cause of bone loss. One can expect, then, that continuous infusions of parathyroid hormone stimulate receptor activator of nuclear factor-κB (RANK) ligand and suppress osteoprotegerin (OPG) resulting in increased osteoclastogenesis followed by bone resorption having a catabolic effect on bone.

Intermittent infusion of PTH also leads to an increase in osteoclast activity; however, it also causes an increase in the number and function of osteoblasts that have been attributed to an increase in number of preosteoblasts, decreased osteoblast apoptosis, and renewed bone synthesizing ability of bone lining cells. Bone formation by osteoblasts exceeds the resorption from increased osteoclast activity, and intermittent PTH treatment therefore has an anabolic effect on bone tissue (4).

The effects of PTH on osteoblasts are mediated via binding of PTH to the seven membrane-spanning, G protein–coupled receptor (PTH/PTHrP), which has been localized to bone forming osteoblasts and their precursors. This binding initiates a complex biologic response (4) that may generate different signals and cause different results in bone depending on the time that the serum concentration of PTH is above a certain threshold (5). In a rat model, the same amount of teriparatide that is anabolic when given as a daily single dose is catabolic when given in six divided doses over 6 hours. Thus, duration of elevated serum concentration of PTH determines the bone effect. A 20-µg teriparatide subcutaneous injection in human beings reaches its peak serum concentrations in approximately 30 minutes, has a half-life of 1 hour, and declines to nonquantifiable concentrations within 3 hours (6). This brief exposure accounts for the increase in bone formation over resorption.

Preclinical studies in rats suggest that the initial increases in osteoblast number and bone formation after PTH therapy in large part result from transformation of bone lining cells (quiescent osteoblasts) into cells capable of bone matrix synthesis (7). A review of the effect of intermittent PTH on human bone architecture suggests that there must be a direct transformation of a quiescent bone surface to one capable of bone formation, a process that has been termed *renewed modeling*, and postulates that intermittent PTH renews modeling and postpones osteoblast apoptosis on both the periosteal and endocortical surface of bone, with renewed modeling more important on the periosteal surface (because it increases diameter and bone strength) and the postponement of apoptosis more important on the endocortical surface (8).

PTH therapy is therefore very different from antiresorptive therapy. Antiresorptive therapy can be viewed as "static," preserving and strengthening the status quo. PTH is a dynamic therapy that takes advantage of the body's ability to synthesize bone and offers an opportunity to rebuild the skeleton.

## CLINICAL STUDIES

### Postmenopausal Women

The clinical benefit of increased bone formation by teriparatide was established in the Fracture Prevention Trial published by Neer et al. (9). In this study 1,637 postmenopausal women with prior nontraumatic vertebral fractures were treated with placebo, teriparatide 20 µg/day or teriparatide 40 µg/day by once daily subcutaneous injection. Calcium 1,000 mg/day and vitamin D 400 to 1,200 IU/day supplementation were given to all participants. The planned duration of therapy was 36 months. The actual duration of therapy was up to 2 years with a median of 19 months as the study was terminated prematurely because of the unexpected findings of osteosarcoma in a concurrent rat toxicology study.

Subjects were ambulatory women 5 or more years postmenopausal with either two or more moderate vertebral fractures, two or more mild vertebral fractures and spine or hip BMD T score of less than or equal to −1, or one moderate vertebral fracture and hip or spine BMD T score of less than or equal to −1. BMD was measured by dual-energy x-ray absorptiometry (DXA). Mean spine BMD was in the osteoporotic range, approximately 60% of the patients had two or more vertebral fractures, and only 13% to 16% had received prior osteoporosis therapy. (The therapies available at that time were etidronate, calcitonin and estrogen; patients were required to taper off these before entering the clinical trial.) In the women in the teriparatide 20- and 40-µg groups who had one or more vertebral fractures, the relative risk of new vertebral fractures was reduced by 65% and 69%, respectively, relative risk of moderate and severe new vertebral fractures was reduced by 90% and 78%, respectively, and relative risk of multiple new vertebral fractures was reduced by 77% and 86%, respectively; the absolute risk reduction (ARR) for new vertebral fractures was 9.3% and 9.9%, respectively. The relative risk reduction for vertebral fractures was similar regardless of age, baseline BMD, and the number of prevalent vertebral fractures (10).

Associated with the reduction in vertebral fractures was a reduction in the incidence of new or worsening back pain, with 17% of the patients in the 20-µg group complaining of new or worsening back pain compared with 23% in the placebo group (p = 0.007). In patients with incident vertebral fractures, mean height loss was 0.2 cm in the teriparatide 20-µg group compared with 1.1 cm height loss in patients assigned to placebo (p < 0.002). These data suggest that even in those women who did have vertebral fractures, the fractures were less severe in those assigned to teriparatide. In a smaller study comparing teriparatide 40 µg/day to alendronate 10 mg/day having BMD increase as a primary outcome, complaints of new or increased back pain were 5.5% in the teriparatide-treated group compared to 19.2% in the alendronate-treated group (p = 0.012); none of the patients suffered a vertebral fracture during the study (11).

In the teriparatide 20- and 40-µg groups of the Fracture Prevention Trial, relative risk of nonvertebral fragility fractures was reduced by 53% and 54% and ARR was 2.9% and 3%, respectively. The time to nonvertebral fragility fracture reduction was approximately 9 months. Although data from this trial have shown beneficial effects of teriparatide on the structural geometry of the hip consistent with increased axial and bending strength (12), teriparatide's efficacy in decreasing hip fractures was not demonstrated in this trial, most likely because of small sample size and low incidence of hip fragility fractures (placebo = 4, teriparatide 20 μg = 1, teriparatide 40 μg = 3).

## Adverse Events

Women who received teriparatide in the Fracture Prevention Trial had slightly higher rates of leg cramps, nausea, dizziness, and irritation at the injection sites. Hypercalcemia was absent or mild and transient (normalizing by 24 hours after the dose). However, because teriparatide was not studied in patients with preexisting hypercalcemia, patients with this condition should not be prescribed teriparatide.

Mean 24-hour urine calcium increased 0.75 millimols per day and mean serum uric acid concentrations increased 13% to 25%. No clinical adverse events were associated with these increases in urinary calcium or serum uric acid. These changes reversed after teriparatide withdrawal. There was no effect on blood pressure, heart rate, or creatinine clearance, no increase in the incidence of cardiovascular disease, mortality, or life threatening illness, and no increase in the incidence of cancer, urolithiasis, peptic ulcer, or renal insufficiency. Teriparatide's effect on serum calcium begins at 2 hours and is maximal at 4 to 6 hours. If a patient develops hypercalcemia on teriparatide, he or she should reduce oral calcium intake by 50% (13). The prescribing information does not recommend routine monitoring of serum calcium (6).

## RAT OSTEOSARCOMA

Fischer 344 rats given 3 to 60 times the human dose of 20 μg/day in a toxicology study of teriparatide showed a dose-dependent increase in osteosarcomas. Forty-five percent of the rats given the highest dose of teriparatide (75 μg/kg/day) developed osteosarcomas. These osteosarcomas were found at multiple skeletal sites and were frequently metastatic. Exaggerated skeletal response to teriparatide and marrow obliteration occurred at the higher doses. The spontaneous rate of osteosarcoma in Fischer 344 rats is 1 to 3 per 1000. In contrast, the spontaneous rate in human beings is 4.5 in 1,000,000. In a 70-kg patient, a dose of 20 μg/day is equal to 0.3 μg/kg, whereas the rats were given doses of 0, 5, 30 and 75μg/kg/day (14).

A follow-up carcinogenicity study in female Fischer 344 rats evaluated the effects of dose, duration of therapy and initiation age using doses of 0, 5, and 30 μg/kg of teriparatide injected subcutaneously daily (15). Ages of initiation were 2 months (skeletally immature rats) or 6 months

(skeletally mature). Duration of therapy was 6 months, 20 months, or 24 months. Dose and duration of treatment appeared to be primary factors in the development of the rat bone tumors; the role of age at initiation of therapy was not conclusive. No neoplasms were found when teriparatide 5 μg/kg was initiated at 6 months of age and continued for either 6 or 20 months despite a 47% increase in bone mineral content (BMC) and significant reduction of bone marrow space in rats treated for 20 months. One osteoma and one osteosarcoma were found when teriparatide 5 μg/kg was initiated at 2 months of age and continued for 6 months, but incidences were not statistically different from one osteosarcoma found in the control group. Compared to women given teriparatide at a dose of 20 μg/day for 24 months, the rats treated at 5 μg/kg/day were exposed to three times greater serum level of teriparatide; based on the percentage of lifespan, they were treated approximately 23 times longer than human beings would be.

No osteosarcomas were reported in the more than 2,000 patients treated with teriparatide in clinical trials. As the relevance of the rat findings to human beings is uncertain, United States regulatory approval required a "black boxed" warning in the prescribing information (6) disclosing an increased incidence of osteosarcoma in rat studies and stating teriparatide should not be prescribed for patients who are at increased baseline risk for osteosarcoma (including those with Paget's disease of bone, unexplained elevations of alkaline phosphatase, open epiphyses, or prior radiation therapy involving the skeleton). Similarly, patients with bone metastases, a history of skeletal malignancies, or metabolic bone diseases other than osteoporosis should be excluded from treatment with teriparatide.

## MALE OSTEOPOROSIS

Another study assessed the effects of teriparatide on BMD as measured by DXA in 437 men with spine or hip BMD T score less than −2 (male reference) (16). The men were a mean age of 59 years, 59% had prior nonvertebral fractures, and 49% had low free-serum testosterone levels at baseline. Randomized assignment was either to placebo, teriparatide 20 μg/day, or teriparatide 40 μg/day self-administered by once daily subcutaneous injection. Enrollment was stratified by type of osteoporosis (idiopathic or hypogonadal); men with other causes of osteoporosis were excluded from the study. The median study drug exposure was 11 months because the study was terminated early due to the rat osteosarcoma data. Lumbar spine BMD increased 5.9% and 9.0% in the 20 and 40 μg groups, respectively, versus a 0.5% increase in the placebo group (p < 0.001). BMD also increased at the femoral neck and the total hip. BMD improved regardless of free serum testosterone levels or estradiol levels.

## RECOMBINANT HUMAN PTH

Full-length (1–84) recombinant human PTH (rhPTH[1–84]) is currently in phase-III clinical trials to determine if it reduces fracture risk in postmenopausal women with established osteoporosis. Phase-II data suggest that this is another promising anabolic agent, with increases of 7.8% in lumbar spine BMD after 12 months (measured by DXA) at the highest dose of therapy (100 μg/day self administered by once-daily subcutaneous injection) (17).

## IMPROVEMENT IN BONE STRENGTH

Because teriparatide decreases the risk of vertebral and nonvertebral fractures in women, it must preserve or increase bone strength in cortical as well as trabecular bone. By forming bone, PTH is changing the architecture of the bone. External changes may increase bone diameter by adding bone to the periosteal surface of cortical bone, which adds significant strength (2). Internally, the volume of bone may increase, trabeculae may be thickened, more connections between trabeculae may be established, or the cortex may thicken. Changes in trabecular size may result in changes in shape, converting weak rod-like trabeculae to stronger, plate-like structures. As direct measures of bone strength cannot be made (except with cadavers), other tools must be used for this type of analysis. Imaging and biopsy data from the Fracture Prevention Trial provide evidence that teriparatide improves bone strength at the femoral neck, distal radius, and other sites. The clinical results of this study and such data should allay concerns that PTH might improve trabecular bone at the expense of cortical bone (18).

DXA hip scans from a subset of the Fracture Prevention Trial (placebo n = 189, teriparatide 20 μg n = 186, and teriparatide 40 μg n = 183) were analyzed to derive structural geometry (12). A Hip Structure Analysis program (19) measured BMD and the geometric properties of cortical bone within narrow regions across the femoral neck, intertrochanter, and femoral shaft from the scan images. Using baseline values as covariates, linear models assessed the effects of teriparatide treatment on bone structure.

In the teriparatide 20-μg group, compared to placebo, the mean increase [95% confidence interval (CI)] in BMD was 4.2% (2.4% to 6.0%). The mean difference in axial strength (bone cross-sectional area) was 3.5% (1.8% to 5.3%) and in bending strength (section modulus) was 3.6% (1.4% to 5.8%). The mean increase in cortical thickness was 4.5% (2.6% to 6.4%), while buckling ratio decreased by 5.5% (3.5% to 7.5%). The buckling ratio is an estimate of relative cortical thickness (subperiosteal radius/cortical thickness)—a decrease in the buckling ratio reflects a thicker cortical shell, which is more protective against hip fracture. Increases were also seen in the teri-

paratide 40-μg group. Changes at the intertrochanteric region were comparable to those at the narrow neck, but treatment effects did not reach significance at the cortical shaft.

A primate study, which allows quantitative analyses that cannot be captured in clinical trials, supports this conclusion that teriparatide increases bone strength in the proximal femur. Sato, et al. (20) mechanically tested the proximal femurs from sacrificed monkeys treated with teriparatide. They hypothesized that teriparatide increased cortical area and cortical thickness, which more than compensated for any increased cortical porosity that may have occurred. Teriparatide also increased trabecular bone volume and trabecular number and reduced trabecular spacing in the femoral neck. They concluded that these changes in trabecular volume and connectivity were important contributors to hip strength in addition to the changes in cortical bone properties.

Bone biopsies provided additional evidence of bone strength. Jiang, et al. (21) evaluated paired iliac crest biopsies from patients in the Fracture Prevention Trial. Biopsies were performed at baseline and after 12 to 24 months of therapy on a small subset of placebo (n = 19), teriparatide 20 μg/day (n = 18), and teriparatide 40 μg/day (n = 14) patients. Teriparatide groups were pooled for analysis because of the small sample size. Three-dimensional (3-D) parameters were measured using a Scanco micro computed tomograph (CT) with an isotropic resolution of 17 μm³.

Significant increases were seen compared to placebo in trabecular bone volume ($p < 0.001$), connectivity density, a 3-D measure of trabecular connectivity ($p < 0.05$), and cortical thickness ($p < 0.05$). Structure model index decreased significantly ($p < 0.05$), reflecting improved trabecular morphology with a shift from rod-like trabeculae to a more plate-like structure.

No woven bone, mineralization defects, hypercellularity, or abnormal architecture were observed. No increase in cortical porosity was seen in the teriparatide 20-μg/day group. In the teriparatide 40-μg/day group, increased cortical porosity was seen at 12 months but was resolved by 21 months. Given the apparent transient nature of the cortical porosity, and the fact that there was no difference between the clinical efficacy observed in the teriparatide 20-μg and 40-μg groups in terms of nonvertebral fragility fracture risk reduction, increased cortical porosity does not appear to be a practical concern. Coupled with this information are observations by Zanchetta, et al. (22) that at the predominantly cortical distal radius site treatment with teriparatide resulted in improved bone strength, as measured by changes in cortical bone geometry, due to increased periosteal mineral apposition—and despite endocortical resorption.

In the teriparatide 20-μg day arm of the Fracture Prevention Trial, lumbar spine BMD increased significantly at 18 months by 9.7% with 96% of the patients having an increase in BMD. Nevertheless, DXA may underestimate the increases in bone mass seen with teriparatide. DXA measures density as mass per unit area, whereas quantitative computed tomography (QCT) measures mass per unit volume. In a comparison of teriparatide and alendronate (23), patients treated for 6 months with teriparatide 20 µg/day or alendronate 10 mg/day had rapid increases in BMD as measured by DXA of 4.7% and 3.2%, respectively. When measured by QCT, however, the increase in bone mass was 14.6% with teriparatide and 2.9% with alendronate. This rapid increase in volumetric bone mass is consistent with a substantial increase in bone formation.

Small increases in vertebral size could be responsible for increased bone strength and decreased fracture risk. Rehman, et al. (24) evaluated postmenopausal women treated with glucocorticoids and hormone replacement therapy. The women were given hPTH (1-34) or placebo for 1 year. At baseline, vertebral cross-sectional area (VCSA) was measured on QCT scans and spine BMD was measured by DXA and QCT. The control group had no change in VCSA. VCSA increased in the hPTH (1-34)–treatment group by 4.8% after 1 year and was still 2.6% higher than baseline 1 year after hPTH (1-34) was discontinued. These increases were felt to be related to increased cortical bone width as a result of periosteal bone apposition.

Compressive bone strength is a function of BMD squared and cross-sectional area. A significant increase in BMD was observed in this group at 2 years (DXA: approximately 12.6%; QCT: approximately 38%) and estimated vertebral compressive strength increased by almost 200%. While this is largely a result of increased BMD, increased size is a contributing factor. The authors speculate that the increase in size may contribute to bone strength, which in turn contributes to the vertebral fracture risk reduction observed with PTH.

## CLINICAL PRACTICE

Teriparatide is indicated for postmenopausal women with osteoporosis and for men with primary osteoporosis or osteoporosis associated with hypogonadism who, in the opinion of their physicians, are at high risk for fracture, including those with a history of osteoporotic fracture, who have multiple risk factors for fracture, who failed previous osteoporosis therapy, or who are intolerant to previous osteoporosis therapy. Recommended duration of use is 2 years given the limited length of the pivotal trials.

Teriparatide use is not restricted to patients who have had multiple fractures or who have tried and failed available osteoporosis treatment. While initiating teriparatide in an osteoporosis treatment naive patient may be an unusual case, a clinician may be presented with an elderly, frail patient at high risk for fracture with extremely low BMD, one or more fragility fractures, and/or high risk of falling. It may be reasonable to prescribe an antiresorptive agent or teriparatide for this patient.

## SEQUENTIAL AND COMBINATION THERAPY

There is no evidence that suggests that if a decision is made to initiate teriparatide treatment in a treatment-naive patient, the patient should be pretreated with antiresorptive therapy before receiving teriparatide.

There is not yet evidence to suggest that concurrently initiating PTH and antiresorptive therapy will have an additive effect. A short study, results of which are as yet unavailable, has been conducted in postmenopausal women comparing effects of initiating teriparatide alone to initiating teriparatide plus raloxifene. Hormone replacement therapy (HRT) initiated concurrently with teriparatide 40 µg/day in postmenopausal women resulted in a 16.9% increase in lumbar spine BMD (measured by DXA) compared to a 4.6% BMD increase in the de novo HRT alone user group ($p < 0.001$) (25). There was no teriparatide alone arm, so it unknown if this substantial increase in BMD seen with teriparatide was the result in part of the HRT therapy. On the other hand, studies of PTH in combination with alendronate suggest that PTH should not be administered concurrently with alendronate (26).

Concurrent initiation of an investigational PTH agent and alendronate therapy was evaluated by Black, et al. (27) in the PaTH Study. Because PTH and antiresorptive therapies have different mechanisms of action, and both have been shown to increase bone density and reduce fracture risk, it was hoped that concurrent administration of the two agents would increase bone density more than the use of either agent alone. The PaTH trial enrolled 238 postmenopausal women 55 to 85 years of age with a BMD T score (at the femoral neck, total hip, or spine) of less than −2.5 or less than −2.0 with a risk factor. Patients were only allowed minimal prior use of bisphosphonates. Patients were randomized for 1 year to rhPTH (1-84) 100 µg/day alone (n = 119), rhPTH (1-84) 100 µg/day plus alendronate 10 mg/day (n = 59), or alendronate 10 mg/day alone (n = 60). PTH was self-administered by subcutaneous injection. All patients received 500 mg of calcium and 400 units of vitamin D per day. After the first year, the PTH monotherapy arm was stopped and patients were assigned to placebo or alendronate 10 mg/day; the PTH plus alendronate arm stopped PTH and continued solely on alendronate 10 mg/day; and the alendronate monotherapy arm continued on alendronate 10 mg/day. Key end points were DXA BMD of the spine, hip and radius, QCT BMD of the spine and hip measuring both cortical and trabecular density and geometry, and bone turnover markers (bone-specific alkaline phosphatase, BSAP; N-propeptide of type-I procollagen, PINP, and serum C-terminal telopeptide of type-1 collagen, CTX). Safety and adverse events were also evaluated.

The 12-month results do not support concurrent initiation of PTH and alendronate. BMD of the lumbar spine measured by DXA increased in all treatment groups, with no significant difference between the PTH monotherapy (6.3%) and PTH combination (6.1%) groups. BMD of the total hip and femoral neck, measured by DXA in the PTH monotherapy group, was unchanged but increased in the combination therapy group and the alendronate monotherapy group. Trabecular BMD of the lumbar spine, measured by QCT, increased almost 2-fold in the PTH monotherapy group (25.5%) compared to the value for the combination therapy group (12.9%) and alendronate monotherapy group (10.5%). Trabecular hip BMD increased in all treatment groups, similar to changes in the spine, but not significantly different from each other. The pattern of change in the cortical bone measurements was different from that observed in the trabecular bone. Volumetric density of the cortical bone at the total hip and femoral neck decreased significantly in the PTH monotherapy group, remained stable in the combination group, and increased in the alendronate monotherapy group. Cortical volume at the total hip and femoral neck increased significantly in the PTH monotherapy group alone. Bone formation markers increased significantly in the PTH monotherapy group alone. Bone resorption increased in the PTH monotherapy group and decreased in the other groups.

In another study of PTH and alendronate, no advantage was seen when synthetic human PTH (1-34) was added to alendronate after 6 months of alendronate pretreatment and the two were thereafter taken together for 2 years (28). This 30-month trial studied 83 men ages 46 to 85 years old with osteoporosis who were randomly assigned to combination therapy (n = 28) receiving alendronate 10 mg/day alone for 6 months followed by 24 months treatment with alendronate plus PTH 40 μg/day; alendronate monotherapy (n = 28) for 30 months; or PTH monotherapy (n = 27) for 24 months (therapy starting 6 months after the other groups began therapy). The primary endpoint was rate of change in BMD at the posterioranterior (PA) spine. BMD was measured by DXA every 6 months and by QCT at baseline and month 30. Serum alkaline phosphatase levels were measured every 6 months.

PA spine BMD increased significantly more in men treated with PTH alone (18.1%) than in those in the other groups (alendronate, 7.9%; combination, 14.8%; $p < 0.001$). Femoral neck BMD increased significantly more in the PTH group (9.7%) than in the alendronate group (3.2%; $p < 0.001$) or in the combination therapy group (6.2%; $p = 0.01$). At 12 months, changes in bone specific alkaline phosphatase were greater in the PTH group than in the alendronate group or the combination therapy group ($p < 0.001$). Consistent with the PaTH Trial, alendronate was found to impair the ability of PTH to increase BMD at the lumbar spine and femoral neck in males.

An additional study in which PTH was compared to PTH plus another agent involved a sequential combination study (29). This study compared 3-month cycles of PTH for 28 days followed by calcitonin for 42 days followed by 20 days of no therapy (sequential combination therapy) to

3-month cycles of PTH for 28 days followed by 62 days of no therapy. Sequential combination therapy was no better than PTH alone. Other studies have combined PTH and estrogen therapy (ERT), but because they did not have a PTH-alone active control, it is not possible to determine if PTH plus ERT was better than PTH alone with regards to BMD changes. Results of the alendronate and calcitonin combination studies suggest that PTH will likely be given as monotherapy. It is possible, however, that a post-menopausal woman who has had an osteoporotic fracture on estrogen therapy might wish to continue on estrogen for "nonbone" reasons and add PTH for treatment of her severe osteoporosis. Cosman, et al. (30) randomized post-menopausal women who had been on hormone replacement therapy for 2 or more years to remain on hormone replacement therapy alone (n = 25) or to add PTH (1-34) 400 units (25 μg) subcutaneously daily (n = 27). Patients received PTH plus HRT or HRT alone for 3 years. At 3 years, BMD increased in the PTH plus HRT group by 13.4% in the spine, 4.4% in the hip, and 3.7% in the total body. While lacking a PTH-only arm, this study suggests that estrogen, unlike alendronate, does not blunt the effect of PTH when given before and then concurrently with PTH.

Except for the occasional case of a woman continuing estrogen, most patients who start teriparatide therapy stop antiresorptive therapy, and a substantial number of those patients take alendronate. Because alendronate continues to have an effect on bone even after it is discontinued (31), and combination of PTH and alendronate blunted the effect of PTH, it is important to know how patients discontinuing alendronate or other antiresorptive therapy might respond to PTH therapy.

Ettinger, et al. (32) explored this question in a study enrolling postmenopausal women who were taking raloxifene (n = 26) or alendronate (n = 33) because of a history of osteoporosis (lumbar spine or total hip T score less than −2.5 measured by DXA). These women had a baseline T score less than or equal to −2 when they agreed to stop their respective therapies and participate in this open label study and receive teriparatide 20 μg/day by self-administered subcutaneous injection for 18 months (12-month study plus 6-month extension). Change in BMD at 12 months was the primary outcome; secondary outcomes included 12-month change in bone turnover markers and hip BMD and 12-month and 18-month comparisons of outcome variables between pretreatment groups.

While the pretreatment groups were otherwise evenly matched in baseline characteristics, baseline serum osteo-calcin, BSAP, PINP, and N-telopeptide of collagen (NTX) values were all significantly higher in the raloxifene-pretreated patients. This was expected because alendronate decreases markers of bone remodeling to a greater degree than raloxifene.

Mean lumbar spine BMD for the raloxifene-pretreated group increased by 7.7% and 10.2% after 12 and

18 months, respectively; BMD in the alendronate group increased 2.5% and 4.1% for these periods. During the first 6 months, lumbar spine BMD increased 0.7% in the alendronate pretreated group, essentially unchanged from baseline, while the raloxifene-pretreated group's BMD increased by 5.7%. During the next 12 months, increases in BMD were similar between groups; between 6 and 18 months, the raloxifene-pretreated patients' BMD increased by about 4.5% to 10.2% and the alendronate pretreated group's BMD increased by about 3.4% to 4.1%. At six months, total hip BMD increased 0.5% in the raloxifene-pretreated group and decreased 1.6% in the alendronate-pretreated group. Once again, however, between 6 and 18 months, both groups had similar (about 1.5%) mean hip BMD increases. By 18 months the total hip BMD had increased 1.8% in the raloxifene-pretreated group and had essentially returned to baseline in the alendronate-pretreated group. Thus, while initially there was a limited or negative BMD response in alendronate-pretreated patients, BMD increased in both groups at a similar rate after 6 months of teriparatide treatment.

Teriparatide increased bone turnover in both groups. Raloxifene-pretreated patients' bone formation turnover markers increased more quickly at month 1, but changes in bone turnover markers were similar between the groups thereafter and reached a plateau at 6 to 12 months. Because of the early increase in bone turnover markers, raloxifene-pretreated patients' markers remained higher than the alendronate-pretreated patients' markers throughout the study.

The response to teriparatide was limited by prior alendronate therapy. Given the low rate of remodeling present after treatment with alendronate, fewer osteoblasts would be available to be stimulated by teriparatide. Furthermore, alendronate produces highly mineralized bone with very little resorption space. Teriparatide opens a large new resorption space and replaces the highly mineralized bone with new bone that is less mineralized. This distinction is not appreciated by DXA, and one or both are plausible explanations why hip BMD increased only slightly over 18 months in the alendronate-pretreated group.

Prior raloxifene therapy did not appear to alter the teriparatide response as BMD gains were consistent with those observed in the Fracture Prevention Study. This was expected. Since significant BMD increases were observed when PTH was added to ongoing estrogen therapy (25,30). Also, raloxifene, like estrogen, does not remain in bone after it is discontinued.

From a clinical standpoint, this study is encouraging, as a teriparatide response is observed despite alendronate pretreatment. It is likely that a similar, if not greater, teriparatide response would be observed with risedronate, which does not reduce bone turnover to the extent of alendronate. A few words of caution are in order. The patient population in this study was not a "treatment failure" population—would a treatment failure population have a

better response or worse response to PTH? Also, the maximum duration of alendronate therapy was 3 years; would longer prior exposure to this bisphosphonate lead to a different result?

Less (if at all) problematic for the clinician is how to treat the patient following PTH therapy, because BMD decreased following cessation of PTH therapy in the Fracture Prevention Trial. Antiresorptive therapy is prescribed unless contraindicated or the patient is intolerant to such therapy.

There is evidence that following PTH with alendronate therapy will maintain BMD gains achieved with PTH therapy. Rittmaster, et al. (33) showed that after 1 year of daily subcutaneous injections of rhPTH (1-84), alendronate 10-mg/day therapy led to further increases in BMD over those obtained after 1 year of rhPTH (1-84). The PaTH Study will provide additional information because a treatment group that received rhPTH (1-84) in the first year was divided into groups that receive alendronate or placebo during the second year of the study.

Evidence also suggests that estrogen maintains BMD gains from PTH. Patients in the study by Cosman, et al. (30) received PTH plus HRT or HRT alone for 3 years. All continued on HRT alone for a fourth year. BMD gains in the first 3 years were maintained during the fourth year (30). Lane, et al. (34,35) followed 1 year of PTH plus estrogen treatment with 1 year of estrogen alone in postmenopausal women with glucocorticoid-induced osteoporosis. BMD continued to increase in the spine and femoral neck during the second year.

More important than BMD preservation following PTH therapy is maintenance of bone strength as shown by continued fracture risk reduction. When the Fracture Prevention Trial was abruptly terminated, the decision whether to begin antiresorptive therapy in the study patients, most of whom had severe osteoporosis at study entry, was left to the investigator or the provider treating the patient. An observational study protocol was subsequently approved, and 1,262 of the patients who participated in the Fracture Prevention Trial enrolled in a follow-up observational study (FPT follow-up study), of whom 1,043 had lateral spine radiographs at the end of the Fracture Prevention Trial and 18 months later. By 6 and 30 months after discontinuing teriparatide treatment, approximately 25% and 60%, respectively, of patients across all treatment groups in the Fracture Prevention Trial who were participating in the FPT follow-up study had taken one or more doses of antiresorptive therapy. Such balanced use of poststudy therapy offers a basis to compare outcomes during the FPT follow-up study.

Patients who were in the teriparatide treatment groups (which were pooled for purpose of this analysis) appeared to have continued protection against vertebral fractures during the FPT follow-up study. More vertebral fractures occurred in the FPT follow-up study in the placebo group than in the pooled teriparatide group (19.5% vs. 11.2%, $p < 0.001$).

Patients in the placebo group who suffered a vertebral fracture during the Fracture Prevention Trial had more vertebral fractures during the FPT follow-up study than patients in the placebo group who had not suffered a vertebral fracture during the Fracture Prevention Trial (44.7% vs. 15.8%, $p < 0.001$, Fisher's exact test). This is expected because those who suffer vertebral fractures are at higher risk for future vertebral fractures (36). However, this was not true for the pooled teriparatide-treated patients. Those who had vertebral fractures during the Fracture Prevention Trial were not more likely to suffer a vertebral fracture during the FPT follow-up study compared to those who had not suffered a vertebral fracture during the Fracture Prevention Trial (13.3% vs. 11.3%, $p = 0.453$) (37). This suggests that a positive effect on bone strength persisted for 18 months following discontinuation of teriparatide treatment despite a slight decrease in lumbar spine BMD during that time period.

Nonvertebral fracture incidence was evaluated at the end of the FPT follow-up study, 31 months following discontinuation of teriparatide and 50 months after the baseline visit of the Fracture Prevention Trial. By this time, approximately 60% of all participants had at least one dose of antiresorptive therapy during the follow-up study. At 50 months after baseline, the relative risk reduction in nonvertebral fragility fractures in the teriparatide 20-µg group was 33% ($p < 0.03$) and the ARR was 4.8% compared to placebo (38).

### Glucocorticoid-Induced Osteoporosis and PTH

Because many patients with rheumatic diseases are treated with glucocorticoids (GCs), the adverse effects of GCs, including glucocorticoid-induced osteoporosis (GIO), are well known to rheumatologists and need not be reviewed here. Alendronate and risedronate are approved for treatment of GIO in the United States, and risedronate has a prevention indication. Both have been shown to reduce the incidence of vertebral fractures in small studies (39,40).

While many theories were articulated to explain bone loss caused by GCs (41), studies by Weinstein, et al. (42) and others demonstrated the considerable negative effect of GCs on bone formation that leads to GIO and fractures. GCs cause decreased osteoblastogenesis, increased osteoblast and osteocyte apoptosis, decreased number of cancellous osteoblasts, and decreased bone formation.

Because PTH has a positive effect on osteoblasts, it seems intuitive that it would be an effective treatment for GIO. Studies by Lane, et al. (34,35) evaluated postmenopausal women who were receiving GCs and HRT with one arm receiving hPTH (1-34) plus HRT versus HRT alone. Those patients treated with either HRT or PTH plus HRT showed increases in bone density by 12 months although the PTH-treated group improved approximately 13% from baseline compared to 1% for the HRT alone group suggesting that hPTH (1-34) is a successful therapy for improving BMD while patients were taking GCs and estrogen. There is, however, no fracture data. A clinical trial is currently being performed comparing alendronate 10 mg/day to teriparatide in patients treated with GCs.

Teriparatide is indicated for patients who are at high risk for fracture. It does not have an indication for treating GIO, but patients taking GCs may be at high risk for fracture because of the GCs or due to primary or other secondary causes of osteoporosis, or they may be at high risk of fracture from falling as a result of myopathy caused by GCs. It is anticipated that PTH will be an effective GIO fracture prevention agent, and it is being offered to patients as an alternative to bisphosphonate therapy when there is a lack of efficacy or intolerance (43).

## SUMMARY AND CONCLUSION

Osteoporosis treatment options in the last decade have gone from few to many and from preserving existing bone using antiresorptive therapy to creating new bone by bone-forming agents. Ideally, future efforts to prevent bone loss through diet, exercise, appropriate social behavior, and better control of the rheumatic disease causing the bone loss—using antiresorptive therapy only if necessary—will eliminate the need to use anabolic agents in all but a few individuals. For now, too many individuals have moved down the continuum of bone loss to fracture, and some of these individuals need options other than antiresorptive therapy.

Teriparatide is a therapeutic option for osteoporosis that is quite different from antiresorptive therapy: It forms new bone. It increases cortical thickness and bone size and trabecular thickness, number and connectivity, resulting in increased biomechanical competence, and, most important, significantly reduces vertebral and nonvertebral fractures. For our rheumatology patients with osteoporosis as a result of aging, inflammatory cytokines, or other causes such as glucocorticoids—or resulting from all of these causes—this new anabolic agent offers a means of restoring skeletal strength and, as such, is an important advance in the treatment of osteoporosis.

## REFERENCES

1. Orstavik RE, Haugeberg G, Mowinckel P, et al. Vertebral deformities in rheumatoid arthritis: a comparison with population-based controls. *Arch Intern Med* 2004;164:420–425.
2. Dempster DW. The impact of bone turnover and bone-active agents on bone quality: focus on the hip. *Osteoporos Int* 2002;13:349–352.
3. NIH Consensus Conference. Osteoporosis prevention, diagnosis, and therapy. *JAMA* 2001;285:785–795.
4. Whitfield JF. How to grow bone and treat osteoporosis and mend fractures. *Curr Osteopor Rep* 2003;1:32–40.

5. Frolik CA, Black EC, Cain RL, et al. Anabolic and catabolic bone effects of human parathyroid hormone (1-34) are predicted by duration of human exposure. *Bone* 2003;33:372–379.
6. Forteo prescribing information. Eli Lilly and Company 2002.
7. Dobnig H, Turner RT. Evidence that intermittent treatment with parathyroid hormone increases bone formation in adult rats by activation of bone lining cells. *Endocrinology* 1995;126: 3632–3638.
8. Parfitt AM. Parathyroid hormone and periosteal bone expansion. *J Bone Miner Res* 2002;17:1741–1743.
9. Neer RM, Arnaud CD, Zanchetta JR, et al. Effect of parathyroid hormone (1-34) on fractures and bone mineral density in postmenopausal women with osteoporosis. *N Engl J Med* 2001;344: 1434–1441.
10. Marcus R, Wang O, Satterwhite J, et al. The skeletal response to teriparatide is largely independent of age, initial bone mineral density, and prevalent vertebral fractures in postmenopausal women with osteoporosis. *J Bone Miner Res* 2003;18:18–23.
11. Body JJ, Gaich GA, Scheele WH, et al. A randomized double-blind trial to compare the efficacy of teriparatide [recombinant human parathyroid hormone (1-34)] with alendronate in postmenopausal women with osteoporosis. *J Clin Endocrinol Metab* 2002;87:4528–4535.
12. Semanick LM, Uusi-Rasi K, Zanchetta JR, et al. Teriparatide (rhPTH [1-34]) treatment improves the structure of the proximal femur in women with osteoporosis. *J Bone Miner Res* 2003;18(Suppl);540.
13. Deal C, Gideon J. Recombinant human PTH 1-34 (Forteo): an anabolic drug for osteoporosis. *Cleve Clin J Med* 2003;70: 585–594.
14. Vahle JL, Sato M, Long GG, et al. Skeletal changes in rats given daily subcutaneous injections of recombinant human parathyroid hormone (1-34) for 2 years and relevance to human safety. *Toxicol Pathol* 2002;30(3):312–321.
15. Vahle JL, Long GG, Sandusky G, Westmore M, May YL, Sato M. Bone neoplasms in F344 rats given teriparatide [rhPTH(1-34)] are dependent on duration of treatment and dose. *Toxicol Pathol* 2004;426–438.
16. Orwoll ES, Scheele WH, Paul S, et al. The effect of teriparatide [human parathyroid hormone (1-34)] therapy on bone density in men with osteoporosis. *J Bone Miner Res* 2003;18(1):9–17.
17. Hodsman AB, Hanley DA, Ettinger MP, et al. Efficacy and safety of human parathyroid hormone-(1-84) in increasing bone mineral density in postmenopausal osteoporosis. *J Clin Endocrinol Metab* 2003;88:5212–5220.
18. Horwitz M, Stewart A, Greenspan SL. Editorial: Sequential parathyroid hormone/alendronate therapy for osteoporosis— Robbing peter to pay paul? *J Clin Endocrino Metab* 2000;85: 2127–2128.
19. Beck TJ, Looker AC, Ruff CB, et al. Structural trends in the aging femoral neck and proximal shaft: analysis of the Third National Health and Nutrition Examination Survey dual-energy X-ray absorptiometry data. *J Bone Miner Res* 2000;15:2297–2304.
20. Sato M, Westmore M, Ma L, et al. Teriparatide [PTH (1-34)] strengthens the proximal femur of ovariectomized nonhuman primates despite increasing porosity. *J Bone Miner Res* Published online January 12, 2004; doi:10.1359/JBMR.040112.
21. Jiang Y, Zhao J, Mitlak B et al. Recombinant human parathyroid hormone (1-34)[teriparatide] improves both cortical and cancellous bone structure. *J Bone Miner Res* 2003;18(11):1932–1941.
22. Zanchetta JR, Bogado CE, Ferretti JL, et al. Effects of teriparatide [recombinant human parathyroid hormone (1-34)] on cortical bone in postmenopausal women with osteoporosis. *J Bone Miner Res* 2003; 18:539–543.
23. McClung M, Miller P, Civitelli R, et al. Differential effects of teriparatide and alendronate on markers of bone remodeling and areal and volumetric bone density in women with osteoporosis. *J Bone Miner Res* 2003;18(Suppl):S40.
24. Rehman Q, Lang TF, Arnaud CD, et al. Daily treatment with parathyroid hormone is associated with an increase in vertebral cross-sectional area in postmenopausal women with glucocorticoid-induced osteoporosis. *Osteoporos Int* 2003;14:77–81.
25. St Marie LG, Scheele WH, Jasqui S, et al. Effect of LY333334 [recombinant human parathyroid hormone (1-34), rhPTH (1-34)] on bone density when given to postmenopausal women receiving hormone replacement therapy (HRT). Program and Abstracts the Endocrine Society 84th Annual Meeting June 2001.
26. Khosla S. Parathyroid hormone plus alendronate—a combination that does not add up. *N Engl J Med* 2003;349:1277–1279.
27. Black D, Greenspan S, Ensrud K, et al. The effects of parathyroid hormone and alendronate alone or in combination in postmenopausal osteoporosis. *N Engl J Med* 2003;349:1207–1215.
28. Finkelstein J, Hayes A, Hunzelman J, et al. The effects of parathyroid hormone, alendronate, or both in men with osteoporosis. *N Engl J Med* 2003;349;1216–1226.
29. Hodsman AB, et al. A randomized controlled trial to compare the efficacy of cyclical parathyroid hormone versus cyclical parathyroid hormone and sequential calcitonin to improve bone mass in postmenopausal women with osteoporosis. *J Clin Endocrinol Metab* 1997;82:620–628.
30. Cosman F, Nieves J, Woelfert L, et al. Parathyroid hormone added to established hormone therapy: effects on vertebral fracture and maintenance of bone mass after parathyroid hormone withdrawal. *J Bone Miner Res* 2001;16:925–931.
31. Tonino RP, Meunier PJ, Emkey R, et al. Skeletal benefits of alendronate: 7-year treatment of postmenopausal osteoporotic women. *J Clin Endocrinol Metab* 2000;85:3109–3115.
32. Ettinger B, San Martin J, Crans G, et al. Differential effects of teriparatide on bone mineral density following treatment with raloxifene or alendronate. *J Bone Miner Res* Published online January 19, 2004; doi:10.1359/JBMR.040117.
33. Rittmaster RS, Bolognese M, Ettinger MP, et al. Enhancement of bone mass in osteoporotic women with parathyroid hormone followed by alendronate. *J Clin Endocrinol Metab* 2000;85: 2129–2134.
34. Lane NE, Sanchez S, Modin GW, et al. Parathyroid hormone treatment can reverse corticosteroid-induced osteoporosis. *J Clin Invest* 1998;102:1627–1633.
35. Lane NE, Sanchez S, Modin GW, et al. Bone mass continues to increase at the hip after parathyroid hormone treatment is discontinued in glucocorticoid-induced osteoporosis: results of a randomized controlled clinical trial. *J Bone Miner Res* 2000;15: 944–951.
36. Lindsay R, Silverman SL, Cooper C, et al. Risk of new vertebral fracture in the year following a fracture. *N Eng J Med* 2001;285: 320–323.
37. Lindsay R, Scheele WH, Clancy AD, et al. The reduced risk of new vertebral fracture persists for up to 18 months following treatment of postmenopausal osteoporosis with recombinant human parathyroid hormone (1-34). Presented at the Annual Meeting of the American College of Rheumatology, November 2001.
38. Lindsay R, Scheele WH, Clancy AD, et al. Reduction in nonvertebral fragility fractures and increase in spinal bone density is maintained 31 months after discontinuation of recombinant human parathyroid hormone (1-34) in postmenopausal women with osteoporosis. Program and Abstracts, the Endocrine Society 84th Annual Meeting June 19–22, 2002; #OR35-6, p. 113.
39. Reid DM, Hughes RA, Laan RFJM, et al. Efficacy and safety of daily risedronate in the treatment of corticosteroid-induced osteoporosis in men and women: a randomized trial. *J Bone Miner Res* 2000;15:1006–1013.
40. Adachi JD, Saag KG, Delmas PD, et al. Two-year effects of alendronate on bone mineral density and vertebral fracture in patients receiving glucocorticoids. *Arthritis Rheum* 2001;44:202–211.
41. Canalis E, Bilezikian JP, Angeli A, et al. Perspectives on glucocorticoid-induced osteoporosis. *Bone* 2004;34:593–598.
42. Weinstein RS, Jilka RL Parfitt AM, et al. Inhibition of osteoblastogenesis and promotion of apoptosis of osteoblasts and osteocytes by glucocorticoids. *J Clin Invest* 1998;102:274–282.
43. Adler RA, Hochberg MC. Suggested guidelines for evaluation and treatment of glucocorticoid-induced osteoporosis for the Department of Veterans Affairs. *Arch Intern Med* 2003;163(21): 2619–2624.

# Potential New Biological Therapies for Bone Loss

*Reina Armamento-Villareal*    *Roberto Civitelli*

## OSTEOPROTEGERIN

A variety of local factors, cytokines, as well as an intracellular signaling system are involved in the control of bone remodeling. Many of these factors or pathways have been targeted for development of new pharmaceutical agents that could be used either to inhibit bone resorption or to stimulate bone formation, with different degrees of success. Osteoprotegerin (OPG), also known as osteoclast inhibitory factor (OCIF), was originally identified as a secreted protein from a fetal rat intestine cDNA screen and found to regulate exquisitely bone resorption (1). Produced by osteoblasts/stromal cells, OPG is member of the tumor necrosis factor (TNF) superfamily, and can selectively block osteoclast formation *in vitro* and bone resorption *in vivo*. Its inhibitory action occurs primarily during the differentiation of osteoclast precursors into mature osteoclasts. Thus, OPG can block osteoclastogenesis induced by known physiologic stimulators, that is, cytokines, 1,25(OH)2D3, or parathyroid hormone as well as osteoclast formation in cultured giant cell tumors (2).

The importance of OPG in modulation of bone remodeling has been suggested since the initial seminal study that reported its identification. Transgenic overexpression or parenteral administration of OPG in mice resulted in a nonlethal form of osteopetrosis with profound inhibition of osteoclast formation and function (1). Accordingly, targeted ablation of the gene that codes for OPG in mice results in severe osteoporosis with increased bone resorption (3). Interestingly, homozygous loss-of-function mutation of the *TNFRSF 11 B* gene, the human homolog of the OPG gene, has not been described as associated with osteoporosis as it would be expected but rather with a juvenile form of Paget's bone disease (4). Bone histology of OPG deficient mice, however, revealed that aside from the osteoporosis, which affects both the trabecular and cortical envelopes, there was an increased number of blood vessels, increased osteoclast and osteoblast numbers, and a pattern of primarily woven bone on polarized microscopy, all features characteristic of Paget's bone disease (5). Thus, although the phenotype caused by OPG gene deletion may vary between species, the pathophysiological abnormalities are similar, that is, increased bone turnover, leading to exaggerated woven bone formation.

Shortly after the discovery of OPG, its binding partner was rapidly identified as a membrane-associated TNF ligand, which had already been cloned and given different names—receptor activator of nuclear factor-κB ligand (RANKL); TNF-related, activation-induced cytokine (TRANCE), and osteoclast differentiation factor (ODF). Present on the surface of osteoblasts/stromal cells, RANKL is the most important known stimulator of osteoclast formation and function. For this action, RANKL binds to its receptor, RANK, which is also a membrane-linked factor expressed by osteoclast precursors, chondrocytes, and mature osteoclasts, and this binding initiates osteoclast maturation and activity (6).

Survival of mature osteoclasts is dependent on the presence of RANKL (7) and interleukin (IL)-1 (8), and, in the absence of these factors, mature osteoclasts have been found to undergo apoptosis (9). Therefore, the OPG-RANKL-RANK system constitutes a mechanism by which osteoclast development and function can be finely regulated and in which OPG functions as a decoy receptor for

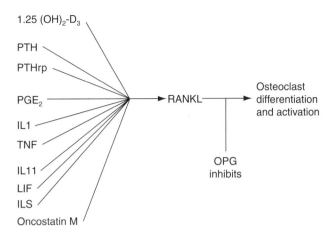

**Figure 22.1** Osteoprotegerin (OPG) inhibits osteoclastogenesis by functioning as a decoy receptor for receptor activator of nuclear factor-κB (RANK), thus, preventing RANK ligand (RANKL) binding to its receptor. OPG is a downstream modulator of many osteoclastogenic factors. (Adapted from *Ann Rheum Dis* 2001;60:iii81–iii84, figure 1.)

RANKL, blocking RANK-RANKL interaction and resulting in inhibition of osteoclast differentiation and activation (1). Thus, the balance between RANKL and OPG dictates the degree of bone resorption (10).

## RANKL AND OPG IN BONE HOMEOSTASIS

Although RANKL is primarily a membrane-associated ligand, a soluble form is present in the circulation, presumably reflecting its abundance in cells and, therefore, its biologic activity. Circulating RANKL has been found to inversely correlate with serum 17–β-estradiol levels, and RANKL abundance in bone marrow cells is upregulated in states of estrogen deficiency (11). Following the increase in biochemical and histological markers of bone resorption, RANKL increases at the time of menopause (11), and both RANKL levels and bone resorption are decreased by estrogen therapy (12).

Likewise, circulating OPG slowly rises after natural menopause (13) and rapidly increases following treatment with gonadotropin-releasing hormone (GnRH) agonists in women with endometriosis (14). Similar to RANKL, OPG levels also directly correlate with the levels of urinary pyridinoline and deoxypyridinoline (DPD) and serum alkaline phosphatase (15), which are also increased with estrogen deficiency. In addition, OPG levels inversely correlate with bone mineral density (BMD) (13), and they are higher in postmenopausal women with osteopenia and osteoporosis relative to age-matched controls with normal BMD (15). Furthermore, levels of OPG are also higher in healthy postmenopausal women with high rate of bone turnover (15). Although an inverse correlation between OPG and bone mass may seem counterintuitive based on

OPG's inhibitory action on osteoclast-mediated bone resorption, an increase of OPG in conditions of accelerated bone turnover represents a compensatory response to the concomitant increase in RANKL-mediated osteoclastic resorption. Similar to RANKL, OPG can also be suppressed by hormone therapy (16) and bisphosphonates (17).

OPG levels are altered in conditions associated with arthritis, such as rheumatoid arthritis, osteoarthritis, and spondyloarthropathies (18). Interestingly, circulating OPG levels are reduced in patients with multiple myeloma especially in those with osteolytic bone disease (19). This unbalance in the OPG/RANKL system may be part of the pathogenesis of increased bone resorption in multiple myeloma. OPG administration inhibits osteolytic lesions associated with multiple myeloma (20).

## THERAPEUTIC POTENTIAL OF OPG: ANIMAL STUDIES

The earliest evidence of the potential of OPG as a therapeutic agent was provided in a demonstration that recombinant OPG at the dose of 5 mg/kg/day had a similar effect as pamidronate in preventing trabecular bone loss and in reducing the number of osteoclasts in ovariectomized rats (1). An antiresorptive effect was observed even at smaller doses. *In vivo*, estrogen-deficient mice given the much lower dose of 0.3 mg/kg/day of recombinant OPG were protected from trabecular bone loss (21). This dose also prevented tail suspension–induced bone loss (22) in rodents.

OPG was also shown to prevent bone loss in animal models of chronic inflammation such as that developing in transgenic mice expressing human TNF-α. This bone loss was not prevented by bisphosphonates or anti-TNF α treatment (23). Furthermore, in mice with established myeloma, administration of recombinant OPG not only prevented the development of osteolytic bone lesions (20) but also decreased tumor growth (24). Thus, OPG may represent a useful agent in preventing bone loss not only from estrogen deficiency but also from chronic inflammatory disorders and malignant bone marrow diseases.

There is also a suggestion of a potential additive effect on BMD when OPG is given in combination with an anabolic agent, such as parathyroid hormone PTH (1-34). Ovariectomized rats given PTH (1-34) in combination with OPG experienced significantly greater lumbar spine and femur BMD relative to the individual PTH (1-34) or OPG therapy (25).

## OPG AS A THERAPEUTIC AGENT: CLINICAL DATA

In a study on 52 healthy postmenopausal women, OPG given subcutaneously at doses of 0.1, 0.3, 1.0, and 3.0 mg/kg as a single dose resulted in a significant decrease in urinary N-telopeptide levels from baseline (26). This effect was seen as early as 12 hours after injection, maximal at around 4 to 5 days, and persisted 85 days after the injection. The magnitude of reduction was the highest for those receiving the highest dose. Decreases of lesser magnitude in urinary DPD were also observed with different doses of OPG and again the greatest decrease was seen at day 5 with the highest dose. Bone specific alkaline phosphatase, an index of bone formation, also decreased but not to the same extent as the indices of bone resorption. This short study demonstrates a clear biologic response to parenteral OPG in terms of rapid, dose-dependent, substantive reduction of bone resorption. However, no long-term data on bone density are yet available.

## ANTI-RANK LIGAND ANTIBODY

RANKL is the most potent known stimulator of osteoclastogenesis and osteoclastic activity. An alternative approach to the inhibition of RANKL by OPG is the utilization of antibodies to RANKL. A fully human monoclonal antibody against RANKL has been developed. This antibody, administered subcutaneously one time, was able to suppress bone resorption for periods of up to 6 months in a human phase-I trial (27). Clinical studies are ongoing to determine efficacy and safety.

## OTHER POTENTIAL BIOLOGICAL THERAPIES

Other potential targets for pharmacological intervention in osteoporosis include cathepsin K, $\alpha v$ $\beta 3$ integrin receptors, Src tyrosine kinase, and peroxisome-proliferator-activated receptor gamma. Cathepsin K is a cysteine proteinase synthesized by osteoclasts and an essential component of osteoclast-medicated bone resorption (28). Cathepsin K is secreted into the extracellular compartment at the attachment site and degrades type-I collagen of bone.

Osteoclasts must first adhere to bone to promote bone resorption. $\alpha v$ $\beta 3$ integrin is a heterodimeric vitronectin receptor on osteoclasts required to make a tight seal around resorption lacunae in bone. Disruption of this adhesion should decrease bone resorption (29).

The SRC protein is a tyrosine kinase enzyme that allows RANK-mediated signaling and osteoclastic activation (30).

Clinically, the decreased bone mass in age-related osteoporosis is accompanied by increased bone marrow fat. Peroxisome-proliferator-activated receptor gamma (PPARγ) is a key transcription factor and dominant regulator of adipogenesis (31). PPARγ drives the differentiation of multipotent mesenchymal progenitor cells toward adipocytes over osteoblasts. Homozygous deficient PPARγ cells fail to differentiate into adipocytes and spontaneously differentiate into osteoblasts, thus increasing bone mass in animal models.

Increasing knowledge of basic biology of osteoclasts, osteoblasts, and osteocytes should continue to provide new insights into potential targets for pharmacological intervention in metabolic bone disease.

## REFERENCES

1. Simonet WS, Lacey DL, Dunstan CR, et al. Osteoprotegerin: a novel secreted protein involved in the regulation of bone density. *Cell* 1997;89(2):309–319.
2. Atkins GJ, Bouralexis S, Haynes DR, et al. Osteoprotegerin inhibits osteoclast formation and bone resorbing activity in giant cell tumors of bone. *Bone* 2001;28(4):370–377.
3. Mizuno A, Amizuka N, Irie K, et al. Severe osteoporosis in mice lacking osteoclastogenesis inhibitory factor/osteoprotegerin. *Biochem Biophys Res Commun* 1998;247(3):610–615.
4. Whyte MP, Obrecht SE, Finnegan PM, et al. Osteoprotegerin deficiency and juvenile Paget's disease. *N Engl J Med* 2002;347(3): 175–184.
5. Bucay N, Sarosi I, Dunstan CR, et al. Osteoprotegerin-deficient mice develop early onset osteoporosis and arterial calcification. *Genes Dev* 1998;12(9):1260–1268.
6. Hsu H, Lacey DL, Dunstan CR, et al. Tumor necrosis factor receptor family member RANK mediates osteoclast differentiation and activation induced by osteoprotegerin ligand. *Proc Natl Acad Sci USA* 1999;96(7):3540–3545.
7. Fuller K, Wong B, Fox S, et al. TRANCE is necessary and sufficient for osteoblast-mediated activation of bone resorption in osteoclasts. *J Exp Med* 1998;188(5):997–1001.
8. Fox SW, Fuller K, Chambers TJ. Activation of osteoclasts by interleukin-1: divergent responsiveness in osteoclasts formed in vivo and in vitro. *J Cell Physiol* 2000;184(3):334–340.
9. Lacey DL, Timms E, Tan HL, et al. Osteoprotegerin ligand is a cytokine that regulates osteoclast differentiation and activation. *Cell* 1998;93(2):165–176.
10. Boyle WJ, Simonet WS, Lacey DL. Osteoclast differentiation and activation. *Nature* 2003;423(6937):337–342.
11. Eghbali-Fatourechi G, Khosla S, Sanyal A, et al. Role of RANK ligand in mediating increased bone resorption in early postmenopausal women. *J Clin Invest* 2003;111(8):1221–1230.
12. Crisafulli A, Altavilla D, Squadrito G, et al. Effects of the phytoestrogen genistein on the circulating soluble receptor activator of nuclear factor kappa B ligand-osteoprotegerin system in early postmenopausal women. *J Clin Endocrinol Metab* 2004;89(1): 188–192.
13. Ueland T, Brixen K, Mosekilde L, et al. Age-related changes in cortical bone content of insulin-like growth factor binding protein (IGFBP)-3, IGFBP-5, osteoprotegerin, and calcium in postmenopausal osteoporosis: a cross-sectional study. *J Clin Endocrinol Metab* 2003;88(3):1014–1018.
14. Uemura H, Yasui T, Umino Y, et al. Circulating osteoprotegerin in women during GnRH-agonist treatment and their relationships with mineral components and biomarkers of bone turnover. *Bone* 2003;33(5):860–866.
15. Yano K, Tsuda E, Washida N, et al. Immunological characterization of circulating osteoprotegerin/osteoclastogenesis inhibitory factor: increased serum concentrations in postmenopausal women with osteoporosis. *J Bone Miner Res* 1999;14(4):518–527.
16. Kang Y, Han K, Kim J, et al. The changes of circulating osteoprotegerin after hormone replacement therapy in postmenopausal women and their relationship with estrogen responsiveness in bone. *J Bone Miner Res* 2003;18(S2):S163.
17. Sankaralingam S, Frost M, Fogelman L, Hampson G. Early changes in serum osteoprotegerin (OPG) correlates with changes in bone mineral density following treatment with risedronate in postmenopausal women with osteoporosis. *J Bone Miner Res* 2003;18(S2):S158.
18. Haynes DR, Barg E, Crotti TN, et al. Osteoprotegerin expression in synovial tissue from patients with rheumatoid arthritis, spondyloarthropathies and osteoarthritis and normal controls. *Rheumatology (Oxf)* 2003;42(1):123–134.

19. Seidel C, Hjertner O, Abildgaard N, et al. Serum osteoprotegerin levels are reduced in patients with multiple myeloma with lytic bone disease. *Blood* 2001;98(7):2269–2271.
20. Croucher PI, Shipman CM, Lippitt J, et al. Osteoprotegerin inhibits the development of osteolytic bone disease in multiple myeloma. *Blood* 2001;98(13):3534–3540.
21. Sasaki N, Kusano E, Ando Y, et al. Changes in osteoprotegerin and markers of bone metabolism during glucocorticoid treatment in patients with chronic glomerulonephritis. *Bone* 2002;30(6):853–858.
22. Bateman TA, Dunstan CR, Ferguson VL, et al. Osteoprotegerin mitigates tail suspension-induced osteopenia. *Bone* 2000;26(5):443–449.
23. Schett G, Redlich K, Hayer S, et al. Osteoprotegerin protects against generalized bone loss in tumor necrosis factor-transgenic mice. *Arthritis Rheum* 2003;48(7):2042–2051.
24. Vanderkerken K, De Leenheer E, Shipman C, et al. Recombinant osteoprotegerin decreases tumor burden and increases survival in a murine model of multiple myeloma. *Cancer Res* 2003;63(2):287–289.
25. Kostenuik PJ, Capparelli C, Morony S, et al. OPG and PTH-(1-34) have additive effects on bone density and mechanical strength in osteopenic ovariectomized rats. *Endocrinology* 2001;142(10):4295–4304.
26. Bekker PJ, Holloway D, Nakanishi A, et al. The effect of a single dose of osteoprotegerin in postmenopausal women. *J Bone Miner Res* 2001;16(2):348–360.
27. Bekker PJ, Holloway DL, Rasmussen AS, et al. A rapid and profound 6 month suppression of bone turnover is seen with a single SC dose of AMG 162 in postmenopausal women. *J Bone Miner Res* 2003;18(2):S31.
28. Garnero P, Borel O, Byrjalsen I, et al. The collagenolytic activity of cathepsin K is unique among mammalian proteinases. *J Biol Chem* 1998;273:32347–32352.
29. Lark MW, Stoup GB, Hwang SM, et al. Design and characterization of orally active Arg-Gly-Asp peptidomimetic vitronectin receptor antagonist SB265123 for prevention of bone loss in osteoporosis. *J Pharmacol Exp Ther* 1999;291:612–617.
30. Wong BR, Besser D, Kim N, et al. TRANCE, a TNF family member, activates Akt/PKB through a signaling complex involving TRAF6 and c-Src. *Molecular Cell* 1999;4(6):1041–1049.
31. Akune T, Ohba S, Kamekura S, et al. PPARγ insufficiency enhances osteogenesis through osteoblast formation from bone marrow progenitors. *J Clin Invest* 2004;113;147–214.

# Other Bone Disorders

# Paget's Disease of Bone

**23**

*Roy D. Altman*

Paget's disease of bone, initially called osteitis deformans, is a chronic skeletal disorder in which localized areas of the adult bone undergo increased resorption and deposition with resultant replacement of the normal bony matrix with a softened and enlarged bone. The initial event involves activation of osteoclasts with large and numerous areas of osteoclastic bony resorption. The repair of bone involves numerous, nearly normal-appearing osteoblasts and a disorganized bony structure that is interspersed with areas of fibrosis. Although Paget's disease is a localized bone disease, there may be widespread distribution.

## EPIDEMIOLOGY

The most commonly affected bones are the pelvis, femur, skull, tibia, vertebrae, clavicle, and humerus. However, virtually any bone may be affected.

The prevalence of Paget's disease of bone is estimated to be approximately 1% of the population over the age of 40 in the United States (1). There is a direct relation between prevalence and age, with the highest prevalence in the older population. There are several hints that the disease is decreasing in frequency (2). There is a slight male predominance ratio of 2:1 men to women. There are differences in the distribution of Paget's disease throughout the world with a higher prevalence in Europe (excluding Scandinavia), Australia, and New Zealand than in the Americas, Africa, and Asia. It appears particularly common in some areas of the United Kingdom.

The cause of Paget's disease is unknown. There is a higher frequency in first generation relatives. Recent research has identified several suspected genes, labeled PD1 to PD7 (3), the most suspicious is the Sequestrim gene that effects NFKβ activation of osteoclasts (3a). Additionally, there is strong evidence that a virus may be a trigger (such as one from the paramyxovirus family) (4). There are isolated cases of consanguineous Paget's disease, suggesting that the disorder is not contagious. There are no animal models of Paget's disease.

## SYMPTOMS

Paget's disease uncommonly produces symptoms; however, bone pain, bony enlargement, or deformity of bones may occur. Rheumatic manifestations are the most common presentation (5). Quality of life may be altered with reduced instrumental activities of daily living (IADL) such as using a telephone or even regular activities of daily living (ADL). Total disability, however, rarely occurs. Complications and their likely pathophysiology are reflected in Table 23.1.

When present, bone pain is often deep, aching, and occasionally severe and may be worse at night. Pain may be accentuated by compressed nerves from enlarging bones. Paget's disease is often associated with painful osteoarthritis. Occasionally, stiff joints and fatigue may develop.

Paget's disease may result in skull enlargement. Frontal bossing, platybasia, and compression of the fourth ventricle may occur. The patient may report requiring a larger-sized hat. Hearing loss, initially felt to be eighth nerve compression, is now felt to be caused by pagetic invasion of the petrous ridge and the cochlea (6). Patients may complain of headaches, dizziness, and spinning sensations. There may be associated bulging scalp veins.

Long bones bow from weight and muscle pull. This often results in an abnormal gait and/or contractures. The involved long bone has a tendency to fracture. Fractures can be incomplete (stress) or complete.

The spine is frequently involved. Vertebrae may enlarge, weaken, and fracture, resulting in an accentuated dorsal kyphosis and loss of lumbar lordosis with a decrease of body height. Bony enlargement may compress nerves, resulting in pain, dysesthesias, weakness, paraparesis, or paraplegia (7).

| TABLE 23.1 | |
| :--- | :--- |
| **CLINICAL COMPLICATIONS AND THEIR CAUSES IN PAGET'S DISEASE OF BONE** | |

| Complication | Cause of the Complication |
| :--- | :--- |
| Bone pain | Periosteal, ischemic bone; unmineralized osteoid |
| Deformity of bone | Softened bone bending to gravity or muscular pull |
| Fracture | Transverse or compression fracture of structurally weakened bone, osteolysis, long-bone microfracture |
| Osteoarthritis | Related to juxtaarticular Paget's disease, change in joint congruity, altered gait dynamics |
| Increased cardiac output | Highly metabolic bone with increased blood flow |
| Malignancy | Sarcomatous degeneration of pagetic bone, metastatic disease from other malignancies |
| Reduced auditory acuity | Pagetic bony invasion of the cochlea |
| Altered mental status | Platybasia with high-pressure hydrocephalus |
| Paraparesis/paraplegia | Spinal cord ischemia, cord compression |
| Low back pain | Vertebral enlargement with altered spinal dynamics, vertebral and facet osteoarthritis, spinal stenosis, active spinal Paget's disease, unrelated osteoarthritis |
| Hypercalcemia | Primary or secondary hyperparathyroidism, active Paget's with immobilization or postfracture |
| Altered visual acuity | Rupture of angioid streak, optic nerve entrapment |

The demand of the bone for blood occasionally results in high-output cardiac failure when there is extensive bony involvement. Malignant degeneration occurs in less than 1% of those with Paget's disease. Hypercalcemia can occur in bedridden elderly people with Paget's disease or anyone with severe Paget's disease who becomes immobilized. Hypercalcemia can result in hypertension, weakness, urinary lithiasis, or mild bowel disturbances. Except with pagetic sarcoma, the prognosis is generally good.

## DIAGNOSIS

Paget's disease is most often discovered as part of a workup when x-rays or laboratory tests are performed for other reasons. Paget's disease may be suspected on the basis of symptoms and deformity found on physical examination. Confirmation of the diagnosis is most often from the characteristic findings on x-ray.

With any degree of activity of Paget's disease, new bone activity can be detected by an increase in serum alkaline phosphatase. Bone breakdown can be determined from urine markers of collagen breakdown, detected by collagen crosslink assays, which are uncommonly needed in the management of patients with Paget's disease. When there is normal serum alkaline phosphatase, or when there is concern the alkaline phosphatase is of hepatic origin, a bone-specific alkaline phosphatase is available.

One can determine the extent of skeletal involvement from a pertechnitate radionuclide bone scan. Bone biopsy is rarely needed and should be limited to those patients for whom there is concern for malignant deterioration of the pagetic lesion or metastatic disease to the pagetic site.

## THERAPY

There are now potent and reasonably safe suppressive agents for Paget's disease therapy. Suppressive therapy now appears warranted for anyone with evidence of active Paget's disease (8) including the asymptomatic patient with a serum alkaline phosphatase twice the upper limits of normal. This therapeutic principle is based on the hypothesis that suppressive therapy prevents or retards progression of complications of the pagetic process. Suppressive therapies, however, are not expected to correct existing hearing loss, deformity, or osteoarthritis.

All of the bisphosphonates have been shown to be effective suppressive agents in Paget's disease of bone. They are particularly useful before surgery to reduce bleeding from the involved bone. They are also given to treat pain caused by Paget's disease, to prevent or slow the progression of weakness or paralysis in people who cannot have surgery, and to attempt to prevent arthritis, prevent further hearing loss, or retard further deformity. Other agents such as parenteral calcitonin and plicamycin are still occasionally of value. Several bisphosphonates are discussed here.

### Alendronate

Alendronate (Fosamax) is a potent nitrogen-containing bisphosphonate. Benefit has been demonstrated in several clinical trials without evidence of abnormal mineralization in bone biopsy (9,10). Oral alendronate 40 mg/day for 6 months was effective in normalizing the serum alkaline phosphatase in 27 patients with Paget's disease. Improvement was seen regardless of prior therapy, and there was radiological improvement in osteolysis in

48%. Alendronate was compared to disodium etidronate in a double-blind, multicenter trial of 89 patients. Serum alkaline phosphatase normalized in 63% of the alendronate patients and 17% of the disodium etidronate patients. Alendronate was similarly more effective in the overall reduction in serum alkaline phosphatase and urinary deoxypyridinoline.

Alendronate should be administered as 40 mg/day for 6 months. It should be taken in the early morning with 6 to 8 ounces of water, and the patient should remain upright and not eat for at least 30 minutes. Alendronate should not be taken for more than 3 months if the alkaline phosphatase has normalized at that time.

Oral alendronate is well tolerated with esophageal and gastric ulceration the major adverse effect. The incidence of these gastrointestinal adverse events is not known for the dose of alendronate used in Paget's disease.

## Disodium Etidronate

The first of the bisphosphonates to be used in Paget's disease was disodium etidronate (Didronel). Short- and long-term clinical and chemical suppression of Paget's disease has been demonstrated (11). Clinical improvement may occur after the first month of therapy, yet it is often not apparent for 3 to 6 months. Sometimes benefit is not achieved until after therapy has been discontinued. The duration of response correlates inversely with the pretreatment level of serum alkaline phosphatase. The response to repeated therapy with disodium etidronate is variable and there is increasing resistance to repeated retreatment. Despite concern for delayed calcification, there is prompt bone healing after fracture or surgery with calcified callus during disodium etidronate therapy.

The usual dose of disodium etidronate for Paget's disease is 5 mg/kg per day or 400 mg daily for a 40-kg (88-lb) to 80-kg (176-lb) patient. The drug is supplied in 200- and 400-mg tablets. The entire disodium etidronate dose should be administered at one time, in the early morning, midway between breakfast and lunch, or at bedtime. Adverse reactions to disodium etidronate include abdominal cramps, diarrhea, hyperphosphatemia, increasing bone pain, and a possible increase in fractures. Esophagitis is uncommon.

## Pamidronate

Pamidronate (Aredia) is a potent inhibitor of bone resorption. It appears to be 100 times more potent than disodium etidronate in its effect on osteoclasts. Pamidronate most often produces rapid and dramatic biochemical responses in Paget's disease (12). A single intravenous infusion of 60 mg was effective in 10 of 11 patients at 1 year, the exception having extremely active disease. Weekly intravenous infusions of 30 mg for 6 weeks led to a clinical improvement in 83% of 30 patients. There was a normal serum alkaline phosphatase at 6 months in 53%, with an average reduction of 68%; at 2 years, 51% still had normal values.

Pamidronate should be administered intravenously in 60- to 90-mg infusions with normal saline or dextrose water. A variety of regimens have been used effectively, including daily infusions for 3 to 5 days, once weekly for 3 to 5 weeks, once with reevaluation monthly, etc.

Adverse reactions to pamidronate include transient fever (usually less than 39.2°C), transient lymphopenia, mild and transient nausea, and uveitis. Oral pamidronate has been associated with erosive esophagitis and is, therefore, not available.

## Risedronate

Risedronate (Actonel) is a potent tertiary nitrogen containing bisphosphonate with demonstrated efficacy as an oral agent in Paget's disease (13,14). Risedronate 30 mg/day for 84 days was tested in an open-label study of 162 patients with a mean serum alkaline phosphatase level of seven times the upper limits of the normal range. Four months after completing the risedronate, the alkaline phosphatase was normal in 54% with an average reduction of 66%. Half the patients were retreated for a second cycle if the alkaline phosphatase did not achieve normal values or rose from the nadir. Of this latter group, 39% normalized their serum alkaline phosphatase with a reduction of 69% in the values.

A double-blind study compared risedronate 30 mg/day for 2 months to disodium etidronate 400 mg/day for 6 months with monitoring for 12 to 18 months. Serum alkaline phosphatase normalized in 73% of the risedronate group and 15% of the disodium etidronate patients at month 12. The median time to normalization was 3 months for risedronate and over a year for disodium etidronate. Normal values continued at 18 months in 53% of the risedronate and 14% of the disodium etidronate groups.

Risedronate should be administered orally as 30 mg/day for 2 months. As a precaution, it should be taken in the early morning with 6 to 8 ounces of water at least 30 minutes before eating. The patient should not lie down after taking the medication.

There are few reports of esophageal or other gastrointestinal problems with risedronate.

## Tiludronate

Tiludronate (Skelid) is a nitrogen-containing bisphosphonate. Tiludronate should be administered as 400 mg/day for 3 months. The major adverse event is esophagitis.

## Calcitonin

Calcitonin is not commonly used because of the effectiveness and safety of the new bisphosphonates (15). Most studies of calcitonin have been with the parenteral form. Nasal spray calcitonin is not FDA approved for use in Paget's disease. Salmon calcitonin analgesia appears independent of the calcitonin effects on bone turnover.

The proposed initial dose of synthetic salmon calcitonin is 100 Medical Research Council (MRC) units or 0.5 mL of salmon calcitonin subcutaneously or intramuscularly daily for the first month. The dose can be decreased or the interval between doses increased depending on the severity of disease and response to therapy. Salmon calcitonin should be refrigerated. It is supplied as 400 units per 2-mL vial.

The most important adverse reactions to parenteral calcitonin are gastrointestinal (nausea, vomiting, diarrhea, abdominal cramps) and vascular (flushing of face, tingling of hands and feet), with local reactions at the injection sites and other reactions such as urinary frequency, rash, unpleasant metallic taste, and occasional angioedema. Most symptoms occur within several minutes of injection and last about 1 hour. Adverse reactions are most common during the initial period of therapy.

## Plicamycin

The first agent effectively used in Paget's disease was plicamycin (Mithramycin). Because of its potential adverse reactions, plicamycin has been relegated to a backup role in the treatment of Paget's disease.

## REFERENCES

1. Altman RD, Bloch DA, Hochberg MC, et al. Prevalence of pelvic Paget's disease in the United States. *J Bone Miner Res* 2000;15: 461–465.
2. Cooper C, Schafheutle K, Dennison E, et al. The epidemiology of Paget's disease in Britain: is the prevalence decreasing? *J Bone Miner Res* 1999;14:192–197.
3. Van Hul W. The genetics of Paget's disease [Abstract]. *Calcif Tissue Int* 2003;72:770.
3a. Johnson-Pais TL, Wisdom JH, Weldon KS, et al. Three novel mutations in SQSTM1 identified in familial Paget's disease of bone.. *J Bone Miner Res* 2003;18:1748–1756.
4. Roodman GD. Potential role of paramyxoviruses in Paget's disease [Abstract]. *Calcif Tissue Int* 2003;72:770.
5. Altman RD, Collins B. Musculoskeletal manifestations of Paget's disease of bone. *Arthritis Rheum* 1980;23:1121–1127.
6. Monsell EM. Emerging concepts of hearing loss in Paget's disease of bone. *Clin Rev Bone Mineral Metab* 2002;1:145–147.
7. McCloskey EV, Kanis JA. Neurological complications of Paget's disease. *Clin Rev Bone Mineral Metab* 2002;1:135–143.
8. Lyles KW, Siris ES, Singer FR, Meunier PJ. A clinical approach to diagnosis and management of Paget's disease of bone. *J Bone Miner Res* 2001;16:1379–1387.
9. Khan SA, Vasikaran S, McCloskey EV, et al. Alendronate in the treatment of Paget's disease of bone. *Bone* 1997;20:263–271.
10. Siris E, Weinstein RS, Altman R, et al. Comparative study of alendronate versus etidronate for the treatment of Paget's disease of bone. *J Clin Endocrinol Metab* 1996;81:961–967.
11. Altman RD. Long-term follow-up therapy with intermittent etidronate disodium in Paget's disease of bone. *Am J Med* 1985;79: 583–590.
12. Mazieres B, Ahmed I, Moulinier L, et al. Pamidronate infusions for the treatment of Paget's disease of bone. *Rev Rhum* (English edition) 1996;63:36–43.
13. Miller PD, Brown JP, Siris ES, et al., for the Paget's Risedronate/ Etidronate Study Group. A randomized, double-blind comparison of risedronate and etidronate in the treatment of Paget's disease of bone. *Am J Med* 1999;106:513–520.
14. Brown JP, Hosking DJ, Ste-Marie L, et al. Risedronate, a highly effective, short-term oral treatment for Paget's disease: a dose response study. *Calcif Tissue Int* 1999;64:93–99.
15. MacIntyre I, Evans IMA, Hobitz HHG. Chemistry, physiology, and therapeutic applications of calcitonin. *Arthritis Rheum* 1980;23: 1139–1147.

# Osteomalacia

**24**

*Mihail Moroianu    Dana Fletcher    Michael Kleerekoper*

Severe osteomalacia and rickets are uncommon in developed countries. However, many patients with measured low bone mineral density (BMD) are found to have levels of 25 hydroxyvitamin D that are inadequate to maintain optimal bone health.

Abnormalities of vitamin D and/or its metabolites are one of the more common causes of osteomalacia (Table 24.1). Various disorders leading to phosphate deficiency or inhibitors of bone mineralization may also result in this syndrome.

This chapter reviews the diagnosis and management of bone diseases that result in defective mineralization, the hallmark of osteomalacia and rickets.

## CLINICAL MANIFESTATIONS

Osteomalacia may be asymptomatic and present as densitometric low bone mass or radiological osteopenia. When symptomatic, muscle weakness and/or diffuse bone pain and tenderness are characteristic symptoms (1). The bone pain is usually diffuse and symmetrical, is worse with weight bearing, and ranges from dull to severe. This pain is from insufficiency (stress) fractures and is usually most pronounced in the lumbar spine, pelvis, and lower extremities. Muscle weakness is predominantly proximal and symmetrical. Patients may develop a "waddling" gait or a result of hip flexor weakness.

There is a high prevalence of hypovitaminosis D in patients with chronic, nonspecific musculoskeletal pain (2). This was found in younger, nonhousebound and nonimmigrant populations as well as elderly housebound individuals.

## DIAGNOSIS

The diagnosis of osteomalacia from any cause is based on history, physical, laboratory, radiological, and/or histological findings.

## Laboratory Findings

The laboratory findings in osteomalacia may vary according to the cause. Vitamin D deficiency is characterized by elevated parathyroid hormone (PTH), hypophosphatemia, and elevated alkaline phosphatase values (3,4). Serum calcium levels remain normal or near normal until the very late stages of the disease by which time the alkaline phosphatase is elevated several fold. Serum 25-hydroxyvitamin D, 25(OH)D levels are low by laboratory reference ranges, and many are less than 5 ng/ml[2]. Early on in the development of vitamin-D deficiency, 1,25-OH vitamin D levels are typically normal or elevated because of PTH-driven conversion of 25OHD to 1,25OHD. As 25(OH)D, the substrate for 1-25(OH)2D, disappears, however, 1-25(OH)2D levels also decrease. It is at this stage that hypocalcemia is most prevalent.

There is considerable discussion in the literature about what level of 25(OH)D constitutes vitamin-D sufficiency, and to date no level has been agreed upon. In physiologic terms, it is that level of 25(OH)D that is necessary to prevent secondary hyperparathyroidism. Malabanan, et al. (5) demonstrated that a level of greater than or equal to 20 ng/ml is needed to maintain calcium homeostasis and avoid secondary hyperparathyroidism. More recently, Heaney, et al. (6) showed that calcium absorption does not plateau until 25(OH)D levels reach greater than 80 nmol/liter (33 ng/ml). Thus, it is likely that a level somewhere between 20 and 33 ng/ml is adequate to maintain calcium homeostasis.

In patients with primary phosphate wasting disorders, hypophosphatemia and hyperphosphaturia would be expected. The renal phosphate wasting may be an isolated defect or part of a generalized Fanconi syndrome.

The expected laboratory findings in proximal renal tubular acidosis are low serum bicarbonate and phosphate, inappropriately high urinary pH, hypercalciuria, and secondary hyperparathyroidism.

## TABLE 24.1
### CAUSES OF OSTEOMALACIA

**Abnormal Vitamin D Metabolism**

Deficient diet or absorption
  Dietary
  Inadequate sunlight exposure
  Malabsorption
    Status post gastrectomy (s/p)
    Pancreatic insufficiency
    Small bowel disease (sprue)
  Abnormal 25-OH vitamin-D metabolism
    Anticonvulsants
    Biliary cirrhosis
  Defective 1-alpha 25 hydroxylation
  Renal failure
  Vitamin-D dependent rickets type I
Defective target organ response
  Vitamin-D dependent rickets type II

**Phosphate Deficiency**

Decreased absorption (antacids)
Impaired reabsorption
  X-linked hypophosphatemic rickets
  Hereditary hypophosphatemic rickets with hypercalciuria
  Sporadic acquired hypophosphatemic rickets
  Fanconi syndrome
  Renal tubular acidosis
  Oncogenic osteomalacia

**Mineralization Defects**

Abnormal Matrix
  Osteogenesis imperfecta
  Axial osteomalacia
Inhibitors of Mineralization
  Fluoride
  Etidronate
  Aluminum
Enzyme Deficiency
  Hypophosphatasia

## Radiologic Findings

Radiological findings of osteomalacia include those resulting from impaired mineralization and secondary hyperparathyroidism. The most common radiographic feature of osteomalacia in adults is generalized osteopenia (6). This is noted on x-ray and on bone densitometry and is neither specific nor diagnostic. Somewhat more specific are Looser's zones or pseudofractures (Figs. 24.1 and 24.2). Looser's zones may be found at the medial aspect of the femoral neck, pubic rami, ribs, posterior proximal ulna, and axillary margin of the scapula. These thin radiolucent lines that traverse the cortex at a right angle may resemble fractures or arterial pathways. They are often symmetrical and bilateral, and when present in large numbers define Milkman's syndrome (7). Looser's zones are defects in the bone where newly formed osteoid has not yet mineralized. They tend to occur in regions near arteries and may contain

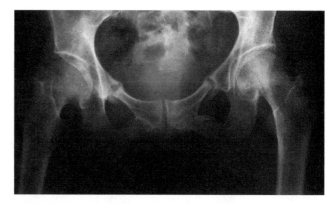

**Figure 24.1** Looser's zones (pseudofractures) in the superior and inferior pubic rami of a 62-year-old woman. When this radiograph was obtained, she had severe vitamin-D deficiency and secondary hyperparathyroidism 15 years after subtotal gastrectomy.

within them small incomplete fractures caused by mechanical stress.

Findings specific to the vertebrae include loss of trabecular pattern, cod fish vertebrae, and occasionally compression fractures. The vertebral trabecular pattern or network of fine radiopaque lines becomes less well defined from lack of osteoid mineralization, and there is blurring of

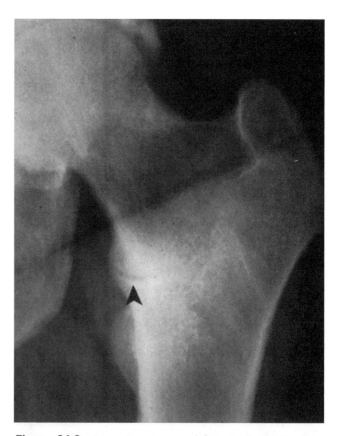

**Figure 24.2** Looser's zones are defects in the bone where newly formed osteoid has not yet mineralized. These thin, radiolucent lines that traverse the cortex at a right angle may resemble fractures or arterial pathways. They are often symmetrical and bilateral.

the corticomedullary junction (6). The term *cod fish verte-brae* describes the appearance of the spine when vertebral bodies soften and become biconcave and the intervertebral discs become biconvex. This is also nonspecific and occurs in osteoporosis. Finally, compression fractures do occur in osteomalacia but much less frequently than in osteoporosis.

Subperiosteal resorption (8) resulting from hyper-parathyroidism is commonly is found on the radial surface of the middle phalanges and the index fingers (9). Periarticular resorption occurs at various locations of the skeleton and may mimic rheumatoid arthritis in the hands (6,10) or ankylosing spondylitis at the sacroiliac joint (6).

Other radiographic techniques such as computed tomography (CT), magnetic resonance imaging (MRI), and bone scan may be necessary to diagnose fractures not detected with x-rays. Pseudofractures appear as areas of increased uptake on bone scan and may be mistaken for metastatic lesions (11). Pseudofractures are typically symmetrical (Fig. 24.3), whereas metastatic lesions typically are not.

### Histological Findings

While most cases of osteomalacia can be diagnosed by history, physical examination, and laboratory results, the most sensitive and specific test to establish the diagnosis of osteomalacia is a tetracycline-labeled bone biopsy. At the interface between mineralized bone and newly deposited, actively mineralizing bone matrix (mineralization front) tetracycline is deposited. When viewed under ultraviolet (UV) illumination, tetracycline fluoresces with different tetracyclines fluorescing as either green or yellow. Two weeks before biopsy, a 3-day course of one tetracycline is given and 10 days later a 3-day course of a second tetracy-cline (with a different flurochrome spectrum) is given. The two bands of fluorescence can be readily identified and the distance between them measured. Knowing the time inter-val between the two labels allows calculation of the bone formation rate.

Early in the development of osteomalacia, secondary hyperparathyroidism predominates and bone formation rate is increased. As the disease progresses and active metabolites of vitamin D become unavailable, mineraliza-tion is inhibited. At that stage, there is abundant unminer-alized osteoid (new matrix) but an absence of tetracycline labeling because there is no longer a mineralization front.

## PREVENTION AND TREATMENT OF VITAMIN-D DEFICIENCY

Prevention of nutritional vitamin-D deficiency has several clinical benefits including prevention of proximal myopa-thy (12–14), reduction of falls in the elderly (15), and a decrease in fractures (16–18). Adequate exposure to the ultraviolet B rays of sunlight during the summer, late spring, and early fall months provides 90% to 100% of vitamin D needs (19). Without this exposure, the diet must be supplemented to prevent deficiency.

The current recommendations for daily intake of Vitamin D are 200 IU/day up to age 50, 400 IU/day for ages 51 to 70, and 800 IU for those above 70 years old or during pregnancy and lactation (20). Regimens of an average of 800 IU/day have had a significant effect on fracture reduc-tion in the elderly (16–18) and are inexpensive and safe.

Replacement of vitamin D is the mainstay of therapy in nutritional deficiency. While both vitamins D2 (calciferol) and D3 (cholecalciferol) raise the 25(OH)D level, D3 has been shown to increase levels by 70% more than D2 (21). Older children and adults may be treated with 5,000 to 15,000 IU/day for 6 to 12 months to replenish stores and normalize PTH, calcium, phosphorus, and alkaline phos-phatase levels. An alternative regimen using an oral dose of 50,000 IU/week (for 6 to 12 months) may have greater compliance (22). After the initial treatment phase, mainte-nance doses of 400 to 800 IU/day should be continued. Doses of greater than 10,000 IU/day increase the risk of toxicity. For this reason, calcium and 25(OH)D levels should be monitored during therapy with high-dose vitamin D3.

In the presence of severe malabsorption, hepatic, dis-ease or renal disease, 1,25(OH)D may provide a better

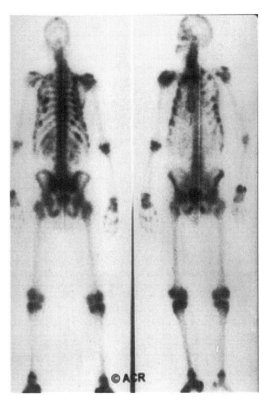

**Figure 24.3**  Total body technetium bone scan in a patient with osteomalacia reveals increased uptake bilaterally in multiple ribs and both inferior pubic rami, corresponding to insufficiency or "pseudofractures." This pattern of uptake in a patient with osteopenia is not usually seen in osteoporosis and should raise sus-picion for osteomalacia. There is also increased uptake in the right lesser trochanter.

therapeutic response than vitamins D2 or D3. Finally, 1 to 3 grams of elemental calcium should be taken with the vitamin D to aid in decreasing PTH levels.

## TUMOR-INDUCED OSTEOMALACIA

Tumor-induced osteomalacia (TIO) is a rare disorder characterized by a proximal myopathy and defective mineralization of bone associated with a tumor (23). Production by the tumor of a substance or substances that affect renal tubular reabsorption of phosphate appears to be the basis of the biochemical and clinical features of this syndrome. Biochemically, patients display significant hypophosphatemia, abnormally low renal tubular maximum resorption for phosphate (hyperphosphaturia), and low or inappropriately normal calcitriol (1,25-dihydroxy vitamin D) levels. Serum 25(OH)D and calcium levels are typically normal while PTH levels may be normal or slightly high. The tumors described have been mainly of mesenchymal origin but have also been described with prostate, lung, and breast carcinoma (23). Because many of the mesenchymal tumors contain receptors for somatostatin, octreotide scanning may be beneficial in localization of the tumor (24).

TIO is most effectively treated by removal of the causative tumor. If this is not possible or the mass cannot be removed in its entirety, medical therapy with phosphorus and calcium supplementation may be beneficial (25).

## HYPOPHOSPHATASIA

Hypophosphatasia is an autosomal dominant disease that may present in adult life because of incomplete penetrance (26,27). Hypophosphatasia is usually diagnosed by the findings of low serum alkaline phosphatase levels adjusted for age. Serum calcium, phosphorus, vitamin D metabolites, and normal PTH levels are all normal in most cases. Pyridoxal 5-phosphate (PLP) tends to accumulate in patients with hypophosphatasia and when elevated may be the most sensitive and specific marker of this disease.

Treatment of adults with hypophosphatasia is limited to placement of load sharing intermedullary rods for treatment and prevention of fractures (28). Dietary phosphate restriction may also be beneficial (29).

## REFERENCES

1. Reginato AJ, Falasca GF, Pappu R, et al. Musculoskeletal manifestations of osteomalacia: report of 26 cases and literature review. *Semin Arthritis Rheum* 1999;28(5):287–304.
2. Plotnikoff GA, Quigley JM. Prevalence of severe hypovitaminosis D in patients with persistent, nonspecific musculoskeletal pain. *Mayo Clin Proc* 2003;78:1463–1470.
3. Mawer BE, Davies M. Vitamin D nutrition and bone disease in adults. *Rev Endocr Metab Disord* 2001;2:153–164.
4. Malabanan A, Veronikis IE, Holick MF. Redefining vitamin D insufficiency. *Lancet* 1998;351:805–806.
5. Heaney RP Dowell MS, Hale CA Bendich A. Calcium absorption varies within the reference range for serum 25-hydroxyvitamin D. *J Am Coll Nutr* 2003;22:142–146.
6. Cooper KL. Radiology of metabolic bone disease. *Endocrinol Metab Clin North Am* 1989;18(4):955–976.
7. Milkman LA. Multiple spontaneous idiopathic symmetrical fractures. *Am J Roentgenol* 1934;32:622–634.
8. Adams J. Dialysis bone disease. *Semin Dial* 2002;15(4):277–289.
9. Pugh D. Roentgenologic manifestations of primary hyperparathyroidism and renal osteodystrophy. *AJR* 1051;66:577–586.
10. Davies M, Stanbury SW. The rheumatic manifestations of metabolic bone disease. *Clin Rheum Dis* 1981;7(3):595–646.
11. Fogelman I, McKillop JA, Bessent RG, et al. The role of bone scanning in osteomalacia. *J Nucl Med* 1978;19:245–248.
12. Glerup H, Mikkelsen K, Poulsen L, et al. Hypovitaminosis D myopathy without biochemical signs of osteomalacic bone involvement. *Calcif Tissue Int* 2000;66:419–424.
13. Russell JA. Osteomalacic myopathy. *Muscle Nerve* 1994;17:578–580.
14. Prabhala A, Garg R, Dandona P. Severe myopathy associated with vitamin D deficiency in western New York. *JAMA* 1000;160:1199–1203.
15. Bischoff HA, Stahelin HB, Dick W, et al. Effects of vitamin D and calcium supplementation on falls: a randomized controlled trial. *J Bone Mineral Res* 2003;18(2):343–351.
16. Trivedi DP, Doll R, Khaw KT. Effect of four monthly oral vitamin D3 (cholecalciferol) supplementation on fractures and mortality in men and women living in the community: randomized double blind controlled trial. *BMJ* 2003;326:469–472.
17. Chapuy MC, Arlot ME, Duboeuf F, et al. Vitamin D3 and calcium to prevent hip fractures in the elderly women. *N Engl J Med* 1992;327:1637–1642.
18. Dawson-Hughes B, Harris SS, Krall EA, Dallal GE. Effect of calcium and vitamin D supplementation on bone density in men and women 65 years of age or older. *N Engl J Med* 1997;337:670–676.
19. Holick MF. Vitamin D: A millennium perspective. *J Cell Biochem* 2003;88(2):296–307.
20. Standing Committee on the Scientific Evaluation of Dietary Reference Intakes, Food and Nutrition Board, Institute of Medicine. Vitamin D. In: *Dietary reference intakes for calcium, phosphorus, magnesium, vitamin D, and fluoride.* Washington, DC: National Academy Press, 1997:250–281.
21. Trang HM, Cole DEC, Rubin LA. Evidence that vitamin D increases serum 25-hydroxyvitamin D more efficiently than does vitamin D2. *Am J Clin Nutr* 1998;68:854–858.
22. Pettior JM. Nutritional and drug-induced rickets and osteomalacia. In: Favus MJ, ed. *Primer on metabolic bone diseases and disorders of mineral metabolism,* 5th ed. Philadelphia: Lippincott-Raven, 2003:399–407.
23. Drezner MK. Tumor-induced osteomalacia. *Rev Endocr Metabol Dis* 2001;2:175–186.
24. Garcia CA, Spencer RP. Bone and In-111 octreotide imaging in oncogenic osteomalacia: a case report. *Clin Nucl Med* 2002;27(8):582–583.
25. Jan de Beur SM. Tumor induced osteomalacia. In: Favus MJ, ed. *Primer on metabolic bone diseases and disorders of mineral metabolism,* 5th ed. Philadelphia: Lippincott-Raven, 2003:418–422.
26. Whyte MP. Hypophosphatasia. In: Scriver CR, Beaudet AL, Sly WS, et al. (eds.) *The metabolic an molecular bases of inherited disease,* 8th ed. New York: McGraw-Hill, 1991:5313–5329.
27. Whyte MP. Hypophosphatasia: Nature's window on alkaline phosphatase function in man. In: Bilezikian J, Raisz L, Rodan G, eds. *Principles of bone biology,* 2nd ed. San Diego: Academic Press, 2002:1229–1248.
28. Coe JD, Murphy WA, Whyte MP. Management of femoral fractures and pseudofractures in adult hypophosphatasia. *J Bone Joint Surg Am* 1986;68:981–990.
29. Wenkert D, Podgornik MN, Cogurn SP, et al. Dietary phosphate restriction therapy for hypophosphatasia: preliminary observations. *J Bone Miner Res* 2002;17:S384.

## 25

# Primary Hyperparathyroidism: Rheumatologic Manifestations and Bone Disease

*Mishaela R. Rubin*    *Shonni J. Silverberg*    *John P. Bilezikian*

The effects of parathyroid hormone (PTH) on its major target organs, the skeleton and the kidneys, brought about the description of primary hyperparathyroidism, when it was first described over 70 years ago, as a disease of bones, stones and groans (1). The classical bone disease, osteitis fibrosa cystica, included degranulation of the skull (so-called salt-and-pepper appearance), distal tapering of the clavicles, subperiosteal bone resorption (seen particularly in the phalanges), brown tumors, and bone cysts. In addition to these skeletal manifestations, rheumatologic symptoms of primary hyperparathyroidism were also commonly described. When patients had elevated serum uric acid concentrations, gout was the result (2). Pseudogout caused by calcium pyrophosphate crystal deposition disease was also known as a classic manifestation of primary hyperparathyroidism (3). In addition, when the disease was overtly symptomatic, patients occasionally developed gout or pseudogout after surgical removal of the offending parathyroid adenoma (4). Patients also not infrequently complained of nonspecific articular symptoms best characterized as arthralgias. A neuromuscular disorder with atrophy of type-II muscle fibers was sometimes a major manifestation of the disease (5). These manifestations of primary hyperparathyroidism were consistent with the traditional idea that excess parathyroid hormone can affect, in

some patients with primary hyperparathyroidism, organ systems besides the skeleton and the kidneys.

This traditional description of primary hyperparathyroidism has been replaced over the past 30 years by one that is primarily asymptomatic. The major reason for this change in clinical phenotype is the widespread use of the multichannel autoanalyzer that includes the serum calcium measurement. Patients, therefore, have their serum calcium concentration measured when the multichannel autoanalyzer test is performed for reasons unrelated to the serum calcium concentration (6).

Most patients with primary hyperparathyroidism are women in their postmenopausal years (7). The serum calcium concentration is typically within 1 mg/dL above the upper limit of normal. The parathyroid hormone concentration is usually 1.5 times above the upper limit of normal (7,8). Hypercalciuria occurs in approximately 40% of patients. Hypophosphatemia, reflecting the physiological actions of PTH to cause phosphaturia, occurs in less than 25% of patients. Overt hyperparathyroid bone disease with specific radiologic findings rarely occurs. The incidence of kidney stone disease has diminished to approximately 15% to 20% of all patients with hyperparathyroidism. Stone disease, however, is still the most common complication of primary hyperparathyroidism (9). Consistent with this modern presentation, patients rarely have overt neuromuscular disease, but they still may complain of vague muscle weakness. Rheumatologic manifestations that can be ascribed specifically to the articular system have become most unusual, but they are reviewed here.

## PRIMARY HYPERPARATHYROIDISM AND GOUT

The incidence of gout appears to be increased in patients with primary hyperparathyroidism who have hyperuricemia (10). Rather dramatic radiologic manifestations can sometimes be seen as in the case report of an individual who presented with a lytic lesion initially assumed to be a brown tumor but was found on joint aspiration to contain urate deposits (11). A possible explanation for the association of gout and primary hyperparathyroidism is the increased levels of serum urate that have been described in some (2), but not all (9), cohorts of patients with primary hyperparathyroidism. In one study of patients with primary hyperparathyroidism that is more active than is commonly seen in the United States today, 53 subjects were compared with age- and sex-matched control subjects. Patients with primary hyperparathyroidism had significantly higher serum urate levels and a reduction in the clearance of urate (2). Serum urate levels were later compared in 26 of the subjects who underwent parathyroidectomy. A significant decrease in serum urate levels was found within 6 months of surgery. Urate levels, however, did not correlate with levels of serum calcium, PTH, or markers of bone turnover, making a direct relationship between the activity of the hyperparathyroid state and hyperuricemia questionable (2).

## PRIMARY HYPERPARATHYROIDISM AND CALCIUM PYROPHOSPHATE CRYSTAL DEPOSITION DISEASE (PSEUDOGOUT)

Primary hyperparathyroidism and calcium pyrophosphate crystal deposition disease (CPPD) have been associated in numerous reports (12–14). As is the case for CPPD in general, older age increases the risk for radiographic evidence of CPPD in primary hyperparathyroidism. General wear and tear on joints as a function of age along with years of chronic hypercalcemia could be a simple explanation for the relationship between age and CPPD. Other mechanisms might be particularly relevant to the process of CPPD in joints of patients with primary hyperparathyroidism. The function of proteoglycans that normally inhibit calcium pyrophosphate crystallization might be impaired by elevated calcium in serum and in joint fluid (14). More recently, it was found that hyperparathyroid patients with CPPD may have abnormal local cartilage metabolism of pyrophosphate (15). The nucleoside triphosphate pyro-

phosphohydrolase (NTPPH) enzymes, which normally catalyze the production of pyrophosphate, appear to be overactive (16). The excess NTPPH activity might promote the formation and ultimate deposition of calcium- and pyrophosphate-containing material (17).

## PRIMARY HYPERPARATHYROIDISM AND PSEUDOGOUT

The clinical event of pseudogout is an uncommon complication of CPPD disease in primary hyperparathyroidism as it is in subjects without primary hyperparathyroidism who have CPPD. Curiously, the more recent literature has described pseudogout in patients with primary hyperparathyroidism after successful parathyroid surgery when the serum calcium has become normal (4,18). This association has yet to be shown to have a pathophysiological basis.

In 1969, Wang, et al. (19) described six patients who had primary hyperparathyroidism and pseudogout, three of whom developed pseudogout at the nadir of serum calcium after curative parathyroidectomy. In a similar report, Bilezikian and colleagues (4) reported four cases of acute arthritis that occurred within 10 days of parathyroidectomy for primary hyperparathyroidism. All had radiographic findings of CPPD, and two had intracellular rhomboidal crystals with weakly positive birefringence in joint fluid. In 1989, 20 patients with primary hyperparathyroidism and pseudogout were described (20); 8 had previously been diagnosed with CPPD, while the remainder were diagnosed after parathyroidectomy. In another report, an attempt to prevent postoperative pseudogout was described in three hyperparathyroid patients with radiographic CPPD, who received immediate, aggressive vitamin-D treatment (21). There was no occurrence of pseudogout after parathyroidectomy, although admittedly, one cannot know whether or not the attacks would have occurred in any event.

A pseudogout attack after parathyroid surgery appears to be triggered by the drop in serum calcium. The fall in serum calcium presumably causes a decrease in calcium concentration in the synovial fluid, making the CPPD crystals more soluble so that they are released from their mold (22) and shed into the synovial space (12). The idea that a rapid reduction in serum calcium is primarily responsible for the attack and not the primary hyperparathyroidism per se comes from other reports in which pseudogout attacks have been reported after medical treatment that precipitates hypocalcemia. One report describes a case of pseudogout in the setting of mithramycin treatment for hypercalcemia (23) and another in the setting of hypocalcemia after pamidronate treatment (24). Similarly, joint injection of hyaluronate can precipitate pseudogout, possibly because the phosphate in the hyaluronate preparation may lower intraarticular calcium concentrations, leading to crystal shedding (25).

# PRIMARY HYPERPARATHYROIDISM AND THE SKELETON: THE CHANGING PROFILE

The evidence reviewed above, although mostly dated and from case reports, is consistent with an adverse effect of excess PTH on joints. These rheumatologic effects are consistent with the "classical" notion that PTH is catabolic at skeletal sites. Our understanding of the skeletal effects of PTH, however, has evolved dramatically along with the changing clinical profile of primary hyperparathyroidism. Since the advent of the multichannel autoanalyzer in the early 1970s, primary hyperparathyroidism has presented more typically in a milder form, often without clinical manifestations of overt bone disease. In fact, the overwhelming majority of patients with primary hyperparathyroidism, in countries where multichannel biochemical screening is routine, has no radiological evidence for bone disease. In the series of Silverberg, et al. (26), fewer than 2% of patients with primary hyperparathyroidism have specific manifestations of hyperparathyroidism on conventional x-ray examination. Along with the rarity of overt skeletal disease in primary hyperparathyroidism, other less common target organs of the primary hyperparathyroid state, including the articular system, have also become rare, modern-day manifestations. The modern profile of primary hyperparathyroidism is reviewed here.

# THE SKELETAL EFFECTS OF MILD PRIMARY HYPERPARATHYROIDISM

With primary hyperparathyroidism now commonly presenting as an asymptomatic disorder, it has been possible to address a far more subtle but critically important question: do patients with asymptomatic primary hyperparathyroidism have evidence for skeletal involvement? With the advent of a technology by which skeletal bone density can be precisely and accurately quantified, this question can be directly addressed. The technology, dual energy x-ray absorptiometry (DXA), has provided important new insights into the skeleton of patients with asymptomatic primary hyperparathyroidism in whom there are no radiological manifestations of disease. Silverberg, et al. (26) have provided evidence that in asymptomatic primary hyperparathyroidism, there is skeletal involvement. At the distal third of the radius, a site of mainly cortical bone, bone density is reduced. The work of Silverberg, et al. (26) has provided additional information by demonstrating that cancellous bone, the other major compositional form of bone, in the lumbar spine is relatively protected in patients with primary hyperparathyroidism. In the cancellous skeleton, bone mass is relatively well-preserved with only small reductions from age and sex-specific norms (26–28). Bone mineral density of the hip region, which contains a more even admixture of cortical and cancellous

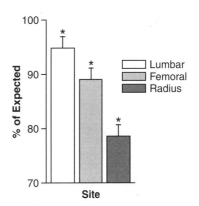

**Figure 25.1**  Bone densitometry in primary hyperparathyroidism. Data are shown in comparison with age- and sex-matched normal subjects. Divergence from expected values is different at each site ($p = 0.0001$). Reprinted with permission from Silverberg SJ, Brown I, Bilezikian JP. Age as a criterion for surgery in primary hyperparathyroidism. *Am J Med* 2002;113(8):681–684. [39]

elements, is intermediate in bone density between cancellous and cortical sites (Fig. 25.1).

The patterns of bone loss in postmenopausal women with primary hyperparathyroidism provide interesting evidence for the anabolic potential of PTH. Preferential cancellous bone loss might be expected in estrogen-deficient women because this site is the most sensitive to the loss of sex steroids. Typically, postmenopausal women who do not take estrogens experience the most rapid period of bone loss at the lumbar spine. However, postmenopausal women with primary hyperparathyroidism demonstrate, in general, well-maintained bone density of the lumbar spine. These observations have helped to fuel interest in the potential anabolic qualities of parathyroid hormone. On the other hand, although a pattern of selective cortical bone loss is most commonly seen in primary hyperparathyroidism (Fig. 25.2), about 15% of patients demonstrate substantial reductions in bone density at the lumbar spine (29–31).

These observations suggest that patients with primary hyperparathyroidism should not be at risk for fractures of the axial skeleton where bone mass is relatively well preserved, whereas they might be expected to show an increase in fracture incidence of the appendicular skeleton where bone mass is preferentially reduced. Unfortunately, there are few studies to confirm this expectation and fracture data are conflicting (32–34). Although Khosla, et al. (35) have reported in a retrospective epidemiological survey an increased risk of fracture at all sites in primary hyperparathyroidism, an increased risk of vertebral fracture is a surprising finding, because most patients have relatively well-preserved vertebral bone density. This observation could be due to surveillance bias because patients with a disorder affecting the skeleton (primary hyperparathyroidism) may be more likely to have vertebral spine x-rays after back pain, allowing more frequent detection. On the other hand, cortical thinning of the vertebral body shell could predispose patients to vertebral fracture even though

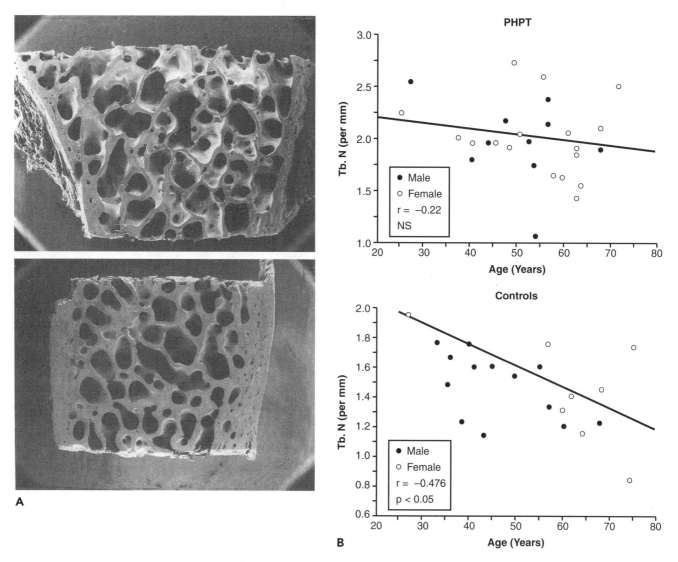

**Figure 25.2    A:** Scanning electron micrographs of iliac crest biopsies of a patient with primary hyperparathyroidism (top) and an age- and sex-matched control subject (bottom). Note the thinning of cortices in the patient with primary hyperparathyroidism as well as the preserved cancellous bone microarchitecture and trabecular connectivity. Reprinted with permission from Parisien M, Silverberg SJ, Shane E, et al. The histomorphometry of bone in primary hyperparathyroidism: preservation of cancellous bone structure. *J Clin Endocrinol Metab* 1990;70(4):930–938.[46]. **(B):** Correlation between age and trabecular number in patients with primary hyperparathyroidism and controls. Note that trabecular number (Tb.N) has less of a decline with age in primary hyperparathyroid patients as compared to controls. Reprinted with permission from Parisien M, Silverberg SJ, Shane E, et al. The histomorphometry of bone in primary hyperparathyroidism: preservation of cancellous bone structure. *J Clin Endocrinol Metab* 1990;70(4):930–938. [46]

their overall lumbar spine bone density is relatively well preserved. An increased incidence of forearm fracture is more consistent with the finding of reduced bone density at this site. Even at this site, however, in the absence of prospective fracture incidence data, this putative increased risk is uncertain. It is now known that exogenous PTH may increase the cross-sectional area of bone and, therefore, strengthen it, even if the bone density appears to be reduced (36). PTH therapy has also been shown to maintain skeletal microarchitecture, another point that might favor fracture protection. The ultimate answer to the question of fracture incidence in primary hyperparathyroidism

must await appropriately powered and controlled prospective clinical studies.

## DIAGNOSIS AND TREATMENT OF PRIMARY HYPERPARATHYROIDISM

The diagnosis of primary hyperparathyroidism is made on the basis of an elevated serum calcium concentration and a PTH level that is either elevated or inappropriately normal (37). When the PTH level is elevated in a patient with hypercalcemia, the differential diagnosis includes thiazide diuretics, lithium, familial hypocalciuric hypercalcemia, and the tertiary hyperparathyroidism associated with end-stage renal disease. Humoral hypercalcemia of malignancy should not be a consideration when the parathyroid hormone level is high, because the hypercalcemic agent in this condition, PTH-related protein, is not detected by the immunoradiometric assay for PTH.

In patients with overt symptoms of classical disease (i.e., kidney stones, osteitis fibrosa cystica), surgery is indicated. In patients with few if any symptoms, guidelines to aid clinical decision making are based on the 2002 NIH Workshop on Asymptomatic Primary Hyperparathyroidism (Table 25.1) (38). Patients who undergo successful parathyroidectomy show rapid normalization of the serum calcium and PTH levels. Improvement in bone mineral density at the spine and hip follows over a 3-to-4-year period after surgery (9). Most patients who are asymptomatic and do not meet surgical criteria do well without evidence for progressive disease (9). However, approximately 25% of patients experience progressive disease. Only age appears to be predictive of progression; patients younger than 50 years of age are approximately three times as likely to experience worsening disease as are patients over 50 (39).

There has been considerable interest in the development of a medical approach to asymptomatic primary hyperparathyroidism. The use of estrogen therapy in postmenopausal women with primary hyperparathyroidism is associated with small reductions in the serum calcium concentration and increases in bone density along with stable parathyroid hormone levels (40). Raloxifene, a selective estrogen receptor modulator, is a potential alternative, with calcium-lowering effects similar to estrogen in postmenopausal women with primary hyperparathyroidism (41). Bisphosphonates have also been considered as a possible medical approach to primary hyperparathyroidism. Recent studies show that alendronate increases lumbar spine bone mineral density in patients with primary hyperparathyroidism ( approximately 4% to 6%) (42,43). Serum calcium and parathyroid hormone levels do not change significantly. The calcimimetic drug, cinacalcet, has been investigated in patients with primary hyperparathyroidism (44) and was recently approved by the Food and Drug Administration (FDA) for use in patients with secondary hyperparathyroidism on dialysis and in patients with parathyroid cancer. This drug binds to the plasma membrane calcium receptor and, thus, increases the affinity of this receptor for its cognate ligand, calcium. The subsequent increase in intracellular calcium leads to a reduction in PTH secretion. With this drug, patients with primary hyperparathyroidism have sustained normalization of serum calcium levels for up to 3 years (45). No improvement in bone density was noted in conjunction with the reduction in calcium.

## PARATHYROID HORMONE THERAPY AND JOINT MANIFESTATIONS

Following leads from the observations previously mentioned, namely that even in a disease like primary hyperparathyroidism, one can find evidence for the anabolic potential of PTH, it has been shown unequivocally that when PTH is given in low dosage as a once daily injection, bone density improves and fracture incidence is reduced. Now that PTH is available to treat osteoporosis in men and in women, it is theoretically possible that adverse rheumatologic effects, formerly seen frequently in primary hyperparathyroidism, will become manifest again in some of these patients. This possibility has not been proved. The incidence of gout or pseudogout in patients treated with recombinant human PTH(1-34) is not increased (Hunter Heath, personal communication), although serum uric acid levels increase slightly. Articular cartilage calcification has not been seen either as an adverse event. Because the dosage used for osteoporosis does not cause hypercalcemia or hypercalciuria, it would be surprising if adverse events in the articular system were to occur.

## CONCLUSIONS

In the past, symptomatic primary hyperparathyroidism was associated with abnormalities of the articular system. Now that primary hyperparathyroidism is generally asymptomatic in the United States and most of the developed world, rheumatologic manifestations are mainly of historical interest only. In patients who present with rheumatologic manifestations along with primary hyperparathyroidism, a search for other conditions should be undertaken before concluding that the patient might be unusually affected in this way by the hyperparathyroid state.

## REFERENCES

1. Cope O. The story of hyperparathyroidism at the Massachusetts General Hospital. *N Engl J Med* 1966;21:1174–1182.

---

## TABLE 25.1

### CRITERIA FOR PARATHYROID SURGERY IN PATIENTS WITH ASYMPTOMATIC PRIMARY HYPERPARATHYROIDISM [38]

| Variable | Guideline |
| --- | --- |
| Serum calcium concentration | 1.0 mg/dl above upper limit of normal |
| 24-hr urinary calcium excretion | >400 mg |
| Reduction in creatinine clearance | 30% |
| Bone mineral density | T score below −2.5 at any site |
| Age | <50 yr |

2. Broulik PD, Stepan JJ, Pacovsky V. Primary hyperparathyroidism and hyperuricaemia are associated but not correlated with indicators of bone turnover. *Clin Chim Acta* 1987;170(2-3): 195-200.

3. Alexander GM, Dieppe PP, Doherty M, Scott DG. Pyrophosphate arthropathy: a study of metabolic associations and laboratory data. *Ann Rheum Dis* 1982;41(4):377-381.

4. Bilezikian JP, Connor TB, Aptekar R, et al. Pseudogout after parathyroidectomy. *Lancet* 1973;1(7801):445-446.

5. Patten BM, Bilezikian JP, Mallette LE, et al. Neuromuscular disease in primary hyperparathyroidism. *Ann Intern Med* 1974;80(2): 182-193.

6. Heath H 3rd, Hodgson SF, Kennedy MA. Primary hyperparathyroidism. Incidence, morbidity, and potential economic impact in a community. *N Engl J Med* 1980;302(4):189-193.

7. Silverberg SJ. Natural history of primary hyperparathyroidism. *Endocrinol Metab Clin North Am* 2000;29(3):451-464.

8. Silverberg SJ, Bilezikian JP. Clinical presentation of primary hyperparathyroidism in the United States. In: Bilezikian JP, Marcus R, Levine M, eds. *The parathyroids*. New York: Academic Press, 2001:349-360.

9. Silverberg SJ, Shane E, Jacobs TP, et al. A 10-year prospective study of primary hyperparathyroidism with or without parathyroid surgery. *N Engl J Med* 1999;341(17):1249-1255.

10. Scott JT, Dixon AS, Bywaters EG. Association of hyperuricaemia and gout with hyperparathyroidism. *BMJ* 1964;5390:1070-1073.

11. Thomas E, Leroux JL, Serre I, et al. Tophaceous gout of the patella with primary hyperparathyroidism. *Clin Exp Rheumatol* 1995;13(2):263-265.

12. McCarty DJ. Calcium pyrophosphate dihydrate crystal deposition disease—1975. *Arthritis Rheum* 1976;19(Suppl 3):275-285.

13. Huaux JP, Geubel A, Koch MC, et al. The arthritis of hemochromatosis. A review of 25 cases with special reference to chondrocalcinosis, and a comparison with patients with primary hyperparathyroidism and controls. *Clin Rheumatol* 1986;5(3):317-324.

14. McGill PE, Grange AT, Royston CS. Chondrocalcinosis in primary hyperparathyroidism. Influence of parathyroid activity and age. *Scand J Rheumatol* 1984;13(1):56-58.

15. Rachow JW, Ryan LM. Adenosine triphosphate pyrophosphohydrolase and neutral inorganic pyrophosphatase in pathologic joint fluids. Elevated pyrophosphohydrolase in calcium pyrophosphate dihydrate crystal deposition disease. *Arthritis Rheum* 1985;28(11):1283-1288.

16. Ryan LM, Wortmann RL, Karas B, McCarty DJ Jr. Cartilage nucleoside triphosphate (NTP) pyrophosphohydrolase. I. Identification as an ecto-enzyme. *Arthritis Rheum* 1984;27(4):404-409.

17. Derfus BA, Rachow JW, Mandel NS, et al. Articular cartilage vesicles generate calcium pyrophosphate dihydrate-like crystals in vitro. *Arthritis Rheum* 1992;35(2):231-240.

18. Kobayashi S, Sugenoya A, Takahashi S, et al. Two cases of acute pseudogout attack following parathyroidectomy. *Endocrinol Jpn* 1991;38(3):309-314.

19. Wang CA, Miller LM, Weber AL, Krane SM. Pseudogout. A diagnostic clue to hyperparathyroidism. *Am J Surg* 1969;117(4): 558-565.

20. Geelhoed GW, Kelly TR. Pseudogout as a clue and complication in primary hyperparathyroidism. *Surgery* 1989;106(6):1036-1041 (discussion 1041-1042.)

21. Yashiro T, Hara H, Ito K, et al. Pseudogout associated with primary hyperparathyroidism: management in the immediate postoperative period for prevention of acute pseudogout attack. *Endocrinol Jpn* 1988;35(4):617-624.

22. Bennett RM, Lehr JR, McCarty DJ. Factors affecting the solubility of calcium pyrophosphate dihydrate crystals. *J Clin Invest* 1975;56(6):1571-1579.

23. Pieters GF, Mol MJ, Boerbooms AM, et al. Pseudogout attacks after successful treatment of hyperparathyroidism. *Neth J Med* 1989; 34(5-6):258-263.

24. Malnick SD, Ariel-Ronen S, Evron E, Sthoeger Z. Acute pseudogout as a complication of pamidronate. *Ann Pharmacother* 1997; 31(4):499-500.

25. Disla E, Infante R, Fahmy A, et al. Recurrent acute calcium pyrophosphate dihydrate arthritis following intraarticular hyaluronate injection. *Arthritis Rheum* 1999;42(6):1302-1303.

26. Silverberg SJ, Shane E, de la Cruz L, et al. Skeletal disease in primary hyperparathyroidism. *J Bone Miner Res* 1989;4(3):283-291.

27. Dempster DW, Cosman F, Parisien M, et al. Anabolic actions of parathyroid hormone on bone. *Endocr Rev* 1993;14(6):690-709.

28. Bilezikian JP, Silverberg SJ, Shane E, et al. Characterization and evaluation of asymptomatic primary hyperparathyroidism. *J Bone Miner Res* 1991;6(Suppl 2):S85-S89 (discussion S121-S124.)

29. Silverberg SJ, Locker FG, Bilezikian JP. Vertebral osteopenia: a new indication for surgery in primary hyperparathyroidism. *J Clin Endocrinol Metab* 1996;81(11):4007-4012.

30. Fuliehan GE, Moore F Jr, LeBoff MS, et al. Longitudinal changes in bone density in hyperparathyroidism. *J Clin Densitom* 1999;2(2): 153-162.

31. Guo CY, Thomas WE, al-Dehaimi AW, et al. Longitudinal changes in bone mineral density and bone turnover in postmenopausal women with primary hyperparathyroidism. *J Clin Endocrinol Metab* 1996;81(10):3487-3491.

32. Kenny AM, MacGillivray DC, Pilbeam CC, et al. Fracture incidence in postmenopausal women with primary hyperparathyroidism. *Surgery* 1995;118(1):109-114.

33. Larsson K, Ljunghall S, Krusemo UB, et al. The risk of hip fractures in patients with primary hyperparathyroidism: a population-based cohort study with a follow-up of 19 years. *J Intern Med* 1993;234(6):585-593.

34. Wilson RJ, Rao S, Ellis B, et al. Mild asymptomatic primary hyperparathyroidism is not a risk factor for vertebral fractures. *Ann Intern Med* 1988;109(12):959-962.

35. Khosla S, Melton LJ 3rd, Wermers RA, et al. Primary hyperparathyroidism and the risk of fracture: a population-based study. *J Bone Miner Res* 1999;14(10):1700-1707.

36. Zanchetta JR, Bogado CE, Ferretti JL, et al. Effects of teriparatide [recombinant human parathyroid hormone (1-34)] on cortical bone in postmenopausal women with osteoporosis. *J Bone Miner Res* 2003;18(3):539-543.

37. Juppner H, Potts JT Jr. Immunoassays for the detection of parathyroid hormone. *J Bone Miner Res* 2002;17(Suppl 2):N81-N86.

38. Bilezikian JP, Potts JT Jr, Fuleihan Gel H, et al. Summary statement from a workshop on asymptomatic primary hyperparathyroidism: a perspective for the 21st century. *J Bone Miner Res* 2002;17(Suppl 2):N2-N11.

39. Silverberg SJ, Brown I, Bilezikian JP. Age as a criterion for surgery in primary hyperparathyroidism. *Am J Med* 2002;113(8):681-684.

40. Marcus R. The role of estrogens and related compounds in the management of primary hyperparathyroidism. *J Bone Miner Res* 2002;17(Suppl 2):N146-N149.

41. Rubin MR, Lee KH, McMahon DJ, Silverberg SJ. Raloxifene lowers serum calcium and markers of bone turnover in postmenopausal women with primary hyperparathyroidism. *J Clin Endocrinol Metab* 2003;88(3):1174-1178.

42. Parker CR, Blackwell PJ, Fairbairn KJ, Hosking DJ. Alendronate in the treatment of primary hyperparathyroid-related osteoporosis: a 2-year study. *J Clin Endocrinol Metab* 2002;87(10):4482-4489.

43. Chow CC, Chan WB, Li JK, et al. Oral alendronate increases bone mineral density in postmenopausal women with primary hyperparathyroidism. *J Clin Endocrinol Metab* 2003;88(2):581-587.

44. Shoback DM, Bilezikian JP, Turner SA, et al. The calcimimetic cinacalcet normalizes serum calcium in subjects with primary hyperparathyroidism. *J Clin Endocrinol Metab* 2003;88(12): 5644-5649.

45. Peacock M, Scumpia S, Bolognese MA, et al. Long-term control of primary hyperparathyroidism with cinacalcet HCl (AMG 073). *J Bone Miner Res* 2003;17(supp 1):1060.

46. Parisien M, Silverberg SJ, Shane E, et al. The histomorphometry of bone in primary hyperparathyroidism: preservation of cancellous bone structure. *J Clin Endocrinol Metab* 1990;70(4):930-938.

# Osteonecrosis

*Eric P. Gall*

Osteonecrosis is a disease characterized by bone cell death leading to skeletal architectural collapse and eventual degenerative arthritis (1). In addition to *osteonecrosis*, this condition has also been variously called *aseptic necrosis*, *ischemic necrosis*, and *avascular necrosis*. Other terms utilized for specific types of osteonecrosis are *osteochondrosis* and *osteochondritis dessicans*. The term, *osteochondrosis*, relates to nontraumatic ischemic necrosis affecting ossification centers. Osteochondritis dessicans is a lesion involving small epiphyseal infarcts near the joint space that cause immediate fracture leading to small dense fragments separating from the bone (Fig. 26.1). This then may appear as a loose body in the joint. The usual location of osteonecrosis is the epiphysis. The term *bone infarct* is used when the same process involves the metaphysis or diaphysis.

An estimated 10,000 to 20,000 cases occur annually in the United States (2). Osteonecrosis most commonly occurs in individuals 20 to 50 years old but may occur at any age. The disease is more common in males than females, except in systemic lupus erythematosus (SLE) (3). An estimated 10% of hip replacements are because of lesions caused by osteonecrosis of the femoral head (4).

## ETIOLOGY AND PATHOGENESIS

The caues of osteonecrosis is related to reduced blood flow (5) or other processes that lead to direct cell death of osteoblasts and osteocytes (6–8). Conditions that interrupt blood supply include traumatic vascular damage, increased viscosity, thrombosis, embolus, or external pressure to the vascular supply.

The following sequence of events is common in most cases of osteonecrosis: (a) reduced blood flow, (b) bone ischemia, which may or may not be associated with increased interosseous pressure, (c) bone infarction and necrosis, (d) collapse of bone, and (e) secondary osteoarthritis of the affected joint.

Table 26.1 lists a variety of disorders that may lead to osteonecrosis. Trauma is the most frequent cause. In the case of femoral neck fracture, the arterial supply from the femoral ligament and limited collateral circulation arising from an extracapsular arterial ring at the base of the femoral neck is disrupted. The ascending cervical branch of the articular ring gives off metaphyseal branches that supply the epiphysis.

Although the overall incidence of osteonecrosis caused by glucocorticoids is low, it is the second most common cause. Prolonged high doses of glucocorticoids convey the greatest risk of developing osteonecrosis; however, patients often have many other risk factors. A theory of the pathogenesis of glucocorticoid-induced osteonecrosis is a disruption of the complex interplay between osteoblasts and osteocytes in the bone remodeling cycle. Glucocorticoid use leads to the inhibition of osteoblastogenesis (the development of osteoblasts) and to accelerated apoptosis of mature osteoblasts (6). Histological studies have indicated that only 20% to 50% of osteoblasts are recovered in glucocorticoid-exposed patients. Apoptosis of osteocytes (lining cells derived from osteoblasts) is also associated with glucocorticoid use (7,8). The function of the osteocytes is to signal detection of microdamage and to initiate the bone remodeling process.

Alcohol induces a shift from hematopoiesis and osteogenesis toward adipogenesis in the bone marrow (9). This results in decreased numbers of osteoblasts and osteocytes that is related to the development to osteonecrosis.

The incidence of clinical osteonecrosis in SLE is 5% to 15%; however, magnetic resonance imaging (MRI) scans of mainly asymptomatic patients have detected lesions in up to 37.5% of SLE patients (10). SLE patients on glucocorticoids are at highest risk. In other patients, small vessel vasculitis and/or antiphospholipid antibodies may contribute to the pathogenesis.

Up to 15% of patients with organ transplants may develop osteonecrosis (11). This appears to be related to glucocorticoid use.

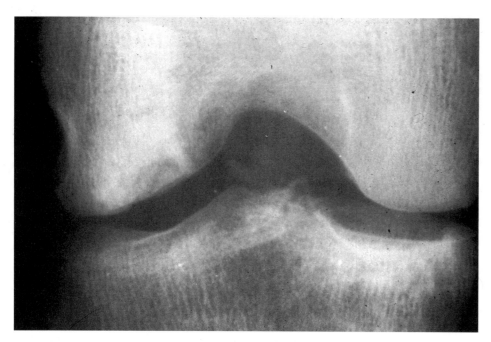

**Figure 26.1** Osteochondritis dessicans is a lesion involving small epiphyseal infarcts near the joint space. Small fragments may separate from the bone and appear as a loose body in the joint.

Increased risk of osteonecrosis with the human immunodeficiency virus (HIV) is associated with glucocorticoid use, hyperlipidemia, alcoholism, and hypercoagulability (12). In a study of 339 asymptomatic HIV-positive adults, compared to 118 age- and sex-matched controls, MRI showed a prevalence of 4.4% of avascular necrosis in the HIV patients.

Evidence for the role of ischemia in the pathogenesis of osteonecrosis includes the association of osteonecrosis with sickle-cell disease, hypercoagulability, thrombophilia, and vasculidities such as lupus and Behcet's disease.

Gaucher's disease, a disorder of glucocerebroside metabolism, leads to accumulation of lipid-laden cells within the bone marrow. External compression of blood vessels within the marrow leads to ischemia and osteonecrosis in 60% of patients with this condition (13).

In children, the prototype of osteonecrosis is Legg-Calvé-Perthes disease (14). In this entity, the capital femoral epiphysis suffers from osteonecrosis. Clinical symptoms usually presents between the ages of 2 and 12 years. The male to female ratio is 4:1; 20% of patients have bilateral disease, and 20% of patients have a family history. The cause is reported to be the result of an interruption of blood flow.

## CLINICAL MANIFESTATIONS

Pain is worst on weight bearing and motion and may be acute or insidious in onset. In the hip, the pain is frequently felt in the groin but may radiate to the buttock, anterior thigh, or the knee. The decreased range of motion and functional compromise may mimic arthritis or a pathologic fracture.

The femoral head is the most commonly involved site. When one hip is involved, up to 72% of the contralateral hips (even though asymptomatic) may also have osteonecrosis on MRI (15,16). Another common bone involved is the humeral head. Pain may be deep seated and radiate to the deltoid tuberosity. Other anatomical sites involved include the femoral condyles, proximal tibia, small bones of the hands and feet, vertebrae, and jaw (17–19).

Three percent of patients with osteonecrosis have multiple bone involvement (16). Most of these patients have been treated with glucocorticoids. Multifocal osteonecrosis is defined as involvement of 3 or more anatomic regions simultaneously. The Collaborative Osteonecrosis Group described sites of involvement in 101 patients with multifocal disease. All 101 patients had compromise of the femoral head. Osteonecrosis was also in the knee (96%), shoulder (80%), and the ankle (44%). Bilateral disease was common, and most lesions were in an early stage.

## DIAGNOSIS

### Plain Radiographic Films

The plain radiograph may be normal initially in osteonecrosis. Early findings are mild changes in subchondral density, followed by sclerosis and cysts formation as the disease progresses. The crescent sign (Fig. 26.2) is felt to be pathognomonic (20). Eventually joint space narrowing and periarticular sclerosis and collapse can occur.

### Radionucleotide Bone Scan

With the advent of MRI, radionucleotide bone scans are seldom performed, although the three-stage bone scan

**TABLE 26.1**
## ETIOLOGY OF OSTEONECROSIS

| Classification | Disease | Mechanism |
|---|---|---|
| Vascular | Pregnancy | |
| | Polycythemia | Hyperviscosity |
| | Lymphoproliferative | Hyperviscosity, tumor mass |
| | Sickle cell (SC) disease | Sludging |
| | Hypercoagulability | |
| | Antiphospholipid syndrome | Thrombosis, embolus |
| | Atherosclerosis | Thrombus |
| | Vasculitis | |
| | Systemic lupus erthematosus (SLE) | Inflammation |
| | Transplantation (allogenic and autologous) | Steroids, vasculitis |
| Infection | Septic emboli | Vascular occlusion |
| | Human immunodeficiency virus (HIV) | |
| Drugs, Toxins | Glucocorticoids | Osteocyte and osteoblast apoptosis |
| | Alcohol | Trauma, other? |
| | Irradiation | Vascular damage |
| | Carbon tetrachloride | Vascular damage |
| | Chemotherapy (vincristine, *cis*-platinum) | Vascular damage |
| Inflammatory and autoimmune | Pancreatitis | Fat emboli |
| | Vasculitis, SLE | Inflammation |
| | Weber Christian disease | |
| | Asthma and rheumatoid arthritis | Steroids, vasculitis |
| Congenital | Gaucher's disease | Increased marrow cellularity |
| | Ehlers Danlos syndrome | Dislocation |
| | Idiopathic familial osteonecrosis | |
| | Hereditary dysostosis | |
| Endocrine/metabolic | Glucocorticoids | Fat embolism, increased interosseous pressure |
| | Cushing's disease | Fat embolism, increased interosseous pressure |
| | Gout | |
| | Osteomalacia | Structural damage |
| | Hyperparathyroidism | Weakened bone |
| | Diabetes | Hyperlipidemia, artherosclerosis |
| | Pregnancy | Marrow edema |
| Trauma | Dislocation | Vascular transection |
| | Fracture | Vascular transection |
| | Dysbaric | Nitrogen emboli |
| | Divers (Caisson's) | Nitrogen bubbles (extravascular) |
| | Irradiation | Vascular damage |
| | Burns | Vascular damage |
| Miscellaneous | Tumor | Vascular pressure |
| | Myeloproliferative disorders | Vascular pressure |
| | Idiopathic | ? |

may be helpful in instances in which MRI is not obtainable (e.g., patients with a pacemaker). Findings depend upon the stage of osteonecrosis. Early, there is decreased uptake in the affected hip as a result of ischemia. Later in the reparative response, the affected hip shows increased uptake because of bone remodeling.

## Computed Tomography

As with bone scintigraphy, computed tomography (CT) scans may have a role in the evaluation of osteonecrosis in patients who have a contraindication to MR imaging. CT can detect subchondral fracture and collapse.

## Magnetic Resonance Imaging

MRI is considered the "gold standard" and the most sensitive method for the diagnosis and classification of osteonecrosis. The early changes on MRI are seen within 6 hours of the initial ischemic event. The most common finding is a low signal intensity area in the subchondral portion of the anterior-superior region of the femoral head, believed to be the area of most vulnerable blood supply. A more specific finding is the "double-line" sign, a low-intensity outer rim and an inner, high-intensity label on spin-spin or transverse relaxation time (T2)-weighted-imaging (Fig. 26.3).

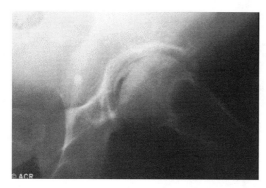

**Figure 26.2**   The joint space is maintained in the hip. The sub-chondral bone of the femoral head has lost its sharp definition, and there is haziness of the underlying trabeculae. The radiolucent crescent line is a plane of cleavage or fracture and is best seen in the abduction position early in the disease. Significant sclerosis is not yet evident. The femoral head is not flattened but may become so later in the disease process.

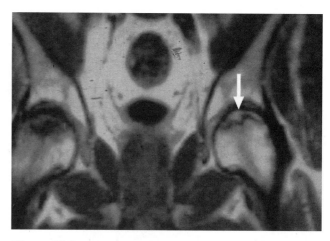

**Figure 26.3**   Serpentine or curvilinear low signal regions in the femoral head with adjacent bands of bright signal (*arrow, the "double line sign"*) are characteristic of avascular necrosis.

The amount of edema seen in the MRI tends to relate to the amount of pain that the patient experiences (21). One should image both the symptomatic and the contralateral asymptomatic joint to look for bilateral disease that is frequently present.

## Staging

There are multiple staging systems for osteonecrosis (22,23). The most recent one is that of the Association for Research on Osseous Circulation (23) (Table 26.2). In stage zero, all diagnostic studies are normal. In stage one, x-rays

are normal, but MRI imaging is positive or the biopsy is positive for necrosis. In stage two, x-rays are positive, but there is no collapse. In stage three, there is flattening and a crescent sign, indicating subchondral collapse. In stage four, in addition to the flattening of the femoral head with joint space narrowing, there is evidence of early osteoarthritis.

## TREATMENT

The treatment for osteonecrosis depends on the stage of the disease, the location of the lesion, and the age of the

## TABLE 26.2

### RADIOGRAPHIC STAGING OF OSTEONECROSIS: INTERNATIONAL CLASSIFICATION OF AVN OF THE FEMORAL HEAD

| Stage | | Findings |
|---|---|---|
| 0 | | Bone biopsy: AVN. All other tests normal |
| I | | Scintigraphic or MRI: positive lesions subdivided based on location (medial, central, and lateral) and percentage of involvement of femoral head |
| | IA | <15% involvement |
| | IB | 15%–30% involvement |
| | IC | >30% involvement |
| II | | Radiographs: osteosclerosis, cystic, osteopenia, or mottled femoral head without collapse or acetabular involvement |
| | | Scintigraphy or MRI: positive lesions subdivided based on location (medial, central, and lateral) and percentage of involvement of femoral head |
| | IIA | <15% involvement |
| | IIB | 15%–30% involvement |
| | IIC | >30% involvement |
| III | | Radiographs: crescent sign, lesions subdivided based on location (medial, central, and lateral) and percentage of involvement of femoral head |
| | IIIA | <15% involvement or <2-mm depression of femoral head |
| | IIIB | 15%–30% involvement or 2- to 4-mm depression of femoral head |
| | IIIC | >30% involvement or >4-mm depression of femoral head |
| IV | | Radiographs: flattened articular surface, joint space narrowing, acetabular changes, osteophytosis |

AVN, avascular necrosis, MRI, magnetic resonance imaging.
From Association for Research on Osseous Circulation. Committee on terminology and classification. *ARCO News* 1992;4:41, with permission.

patient. Analgesics, reduced weight bearing, and exercises to maintain muscle strength and prevent joint contracture are useful. Whether or not reduced weight bearing ultimately has any effect on long-term outcome is unclear.

## Core Decompression of Bone

Core decompression of bone was first described in the femoral head. An approximately 1 cm trochar is inserted into the lateral cortex below the greater trochanter and guided into the necrotic area. Pressure measurements and venography can then be performed. When the bone fragment is removed by the trochar, core decompression has occurred. If this is to be helpful, it must be performed in early stages of the disease before collapse has occurred. Pain relief is usually significant, and there is some contention that this technique may slow progression.

Stulberg, et al. (24) compared core decompression to conservative treatment of patients and found better results in stage-I and stage-II disease. In the conservative group, 80% of patients in stage I and 100% of patients in stage II had clinical progression. A meta-analysis of 22 studies showed success rates for core decompression of 84%, 63%, and 29% for Steinberg stage I, II, and III, respectively. The success rate for core decompression was statistically higher than conservative treatment for stage-I hips only (25). Lieberman (26) has suggested the combination of core decompression with use of osteoinductive and angiogenic medications to improve bone formation and repair.

## Osteotomy

Osteotomy theoretically allows redistribution of weight in more advanced disease. The recovery is long and the results are controversial. Generally, osteotomy is reserved for younger patients when there is reluctance to do total joint implantation.

## Bone Grafts

Corticocancellous bone grafts have been performed using both autologous and allogeneic bone fragments. The anatomic placement of these grafts is critical. These grafts may be vascularized or not. Vascularized grafts are placed with corticocancellous material attached to a vascular pedical. This may be the femoral circumflex artery in the hip and requires precise microvascular surgical techniques. A study of this type of graft in 614 hips for 480 patients who had stage-III and stage-IV disease showed an 89% survival of stage II (99/111) and 81% survival in stage III (405/500). Stage IV was not as successful. Others have shown success with nonvascularized grafts (27).

## Arthroplasty

Osteonecrosis occurs predominantly in patients under age 60, and the initial surgical procedure needs to be considered a first intervention in a lifelong treatment plan. Total joint arthroplasty is usually performed when there is no other option to maintain functional ability. There may be increased prosthetic failure as a result of a weakened bony structure and disuse resulting from the osteonecrosis. Nonetheless, pain relief and good initial results are seen. It is the treatment of choice in advanced disease.

Medical management of the underlying causes of osteonecrosis is obviously necessary. If these causes are not corrected, recurrent disease may well occur. One should be alert to the presence of multiple areas of osteonecrosis that may be asymptomatic as previously mentioned.

## REFERENCES

1. Assouline-Dayan Y, Chang C, Greenspan A, et al. Pathogenesis and natural history of osteonecrosis. *Semin Arthritis Rheum* 2002;32:94–124.
2. Mankin HJ. Nontraumatic necrosis of bone. *N Engl J Med* 1992;326:1473–1479.
3. Abu-Shakra M, Buskila D, Shoenfeld Y. Osteonecrosis in patients with SLE. *Clin Rev Allergy Immunol* 2003;25(1):13–24.
4. Bullough PG, TiCarlo EF. Subchondral avascular necrosis: a common cause of arthritis. *Ann Rheum Dis* 1990;49:412–420.
5. Nelson CL. Blood supply to bone and proximal femur: a synopsis. *Instr Course Lect* 1988;37:27–31.
6. Weinstein RS, Chen J, Powers CC, et al. Promotion of osteoclast survival and antagonism of bisphosphonate-induced osteoclast apoptosis by glucocorticoids. *J Clin Invest* 2002;109:1041–1048.
7. Weinstein RS, Nicholas RW, Manolagas SC. Apoptosis of osteocytes in glucocorticoid-induced osteonecrosis of the hip. *J Clin Endocrinol Metab* 2000;85:2907–2912.
8. O'Brien CA, Jia D, Plotkin LI, et al. Glucocorticoids act directly on osteoblasts and osteocytes to induce their apoptosis and reduce bone formation and strength. *Endocrinology* 2002;145(4): 1835–1841.
9. Wang Y, Li Y, Mao K, et al. Alcohol-induced adipogenesis in bone and marrow: a possible mechanism for osteonecrosis. *Clin Orthop* 2003;(410):213–224.
10. Houssiau FA, N'Zeusseu Toukap A, Depresseux G, et al. Magnetic resonance imaging-detected avascular osteonecrosis in systemic lupus erythematosus: lack of correlation with antiphospholipid antibodies. *Br J Rheumatol* 1998;37(4):448–453.
11. Tang S, Chan TM, Lui SL, et al. Risk factors for avascular bone necrosis after renal transplantation. *Transplant Proc* 2000;32: 1873–1875.
12. Allison GT, Bostrom MP, Glesby MJ. Osteonecrosis in HIV disease: epidemiology, etiologies, and clinical management. *AIDS* 2003;17(1):1–9.
13. Wenstrup RJ, Roca-Espiau M, Weinreb NJ, et al. Skeletal aspects of Gaucher's disease: a review. *Br J Radiol* 2002;75(Suppl 1):A2–A12.
14. Wanger OR, Ward WT, Herring JH. Current concepts review: Legg-Calv Perthes disease. *J Bone Joint Surg Am* 1991;73:778–788.
15. Davidson JJ, Coogan PG, Gunneson EE, et al. The asymptomatic contralateral hip in osteonecrosis of the femoral head. In: Jones JP, Urbaniak JR, eds. *Osteonecrosis: Etiology, diagnosis and treatment.* Rosemont, IL: American Academy of Orthopedic Surgery, 1997:231–246.
16. Collaborative Osteonecrosis Group. Symptomatic multi-focal osteonecrosis. *Clin Orthop* 1999;369:312–326.
17. Mont MA, Baumgarten KM, Rifai A, et al. Atraumatic osteonecrosis of the knee. *J Bone Joint Surg Am* 2000;82A:1279–1290.
18. McKee MD. Atraumatic osteonecrosis of the humeral head. *J Rheumatol* 2000;27:1582–1584.
19. Siegel LB, Alva EM. Avascular necrosis of the lumbar spine. *J Clin Rheum* 1996;250–255.
20. Watson RM, Roach NA, Dalinka MK. Avascular necrosis and bone marrow edema syndrome. *Radiol Clin North Am* 2004;42(1): 207–219.

21. Mont MA, Carbon JJ, Fairbank AC. Core decompression of non-operated versus non-operative management for osteonecrosis of the hip. *Clin Orthop* 1996;324:169–178.
22. Mont MA, Hungerford DS. Non-traumatic avascular necrosis of the femoral head. *J Bone Joint Surg Am* 1995;77A(3):459–474.
23. Association for Research on Osseous Circulation. Committee on terminology and classification. *ARCO News* 1992;4:41.
24. Stulberg BN, Bauer TW, Belhobek JH. Making core decompression work. *Clin Orthop* 1990;261:186–195.
25. Castro FP Jr, Barrack RL. Core decompression and conservative treatment for avascular necrosis of the femoral head: a meta-analysis. *Am J Orthop* 2000;29(3):187–194.
26. Lieberman JR. Core decompression for osteonecrosis of the hip. *Clin Orthop* 2004;(418):29–33.
27. Mont MA, Etiene G, Ragland BS. Outcome of non-vascularized bone grafts of the femoral head. *Clin Orthop* 2003;417:84–92.

# Calcinosis and Heterotopic Ossification

27

*Deborah Wenkert    Michael P. Whyte*

Extraskeletal mineralization [deposition of calcium (Ca) usually with phosphate,] (Pi) can be either ectopic calcification (calcinosis) or heterotopic ossification (1). Both soft tissue calcification (amorphous Ca-Pi or hydroxyapatite crystals, $Ca_{10}(PO_4)_6(OH)_2$) and ossification (true bone formation) can present as a tender erythematous mass or painless nodule or be discovered radiographically in an asymptomatic individual. Extraskeletal mineralization is most commonly classified into one of four clinical situations: (a) metastatic calcification caused by supranormal "Ca-Pi solubility product" (e.g., renal failure), (b) dystrophic calcification into diseased tissues (e.g., juvenile dermatomyositis) or into seemingly normal tissue (e.g., calcinosis cutis) despite normal serum levels of Ca and Pi, (c) traumatic (e.g., posttraumatic and neurogenic) or idiopathic heterotopic ossification (pseudomalignant myositis ossificans), and (d) genetically based heterotopic ossification (e.g., fibrodysplasia [myositis] ossificans progressiva, progressive osseous heteroplasia, Albright hereditary osteodystrophy and its variant pseudopseudohypoparathyroidism). Our chapter briefly describes several disorders among the considerable number that cause calcinosis or heterotopic ossification (Table 27.1).

## CALCINOSIS (METASTATIC AND DYSTROPHIC CALCIFICATION)

Metastatic calcification can reflect a chronically supranormal "Ca-Pi solubility product" in extracellular fluid resulting from significant hypercalcemia alone, hyperphosphatemia alone, or both elevated serum Ca and Pi concentrations

from any cause (1). Mineral precipitation occurs in adults when the Ca × Pi product exceeds 70 (mg/dl × mg/dl) (2). However, Pi supplementation during mild hypercalcemia, or vitamin-D or Ca administration during mild hyperphosphatemia, may transiently exceed this solubility product and cause mineral deposition (2). In fact, this problem can occur during hyperphosphatemia despite concomitant hypocalcemia (1).

Dystrophic calcification may involve injured tissue of any kind (1). Calcifications can occur in tumors, surgical sites (e.g., arthroplasty), burns, infections, metastases, and other forms of trauma including repetitive injury and even thumb sucking or electromyography. Granulomas can calcify in tuberculosis and histoplasmosis as well as in sarcoidosis and Wegener's granulomatosis. Dystrophic calcification can be exacerbated by elevation in Ca or Pi levels in extracellular fluid. In sarcoidosis, calcification is especially complex because increased 1,25-dihydroxyvitamin D, $1,25(OH)_2D$, production causing hypercalcemia may engender metastatic calcification. Dystrophic calcification is well-recognized in juvenile dermatomyositis (3), scleroderma (4), Calcinosis, Raynaud's phenomenon, esophageal dysfunction, sclerodactyly, telangiectasia (CREST) syndrome (4), overlap syndrome (5), and pseudoxanthoma elasticum. (6).

The local factors that predispose to calcinosis are poorly understood. Normally, various local inhibitors of mineralization (e.g., inorganic pyrophosphate, PPi), prevent ectopic calcification. Nevertheless, mineral precipitation can continue once crystal nucleation begins despite physiologic concentrations of Ca and Pi in serum (and presumably in extracellular fluid) (7).

## TABLE 27.1
### DISORDERS ASSOCIATED WITH EXTRASKELETAL CALCIFICATION OR OSSIFICATION

METASTATIC CALCIFICATION

I. Hypercalcemia
   a. Milk-alkali syndrome
   b. Hypervitaminosis D
   c. Sarcoidosis
   d. Hyperparathyroidism
   e. Renal failure

II. Hyperphosphatemia
   a. Tumoral calcinosis
   b. Hypoparathyroidism
   c. Pseudohypoparathyroidism
   d. Cell lysis following chemotherapy for leukemia
   e. Renal failure

III. Conditions of increased PPi*
   a. Familial calcium pyrophosphate dihydrate deposition
   b. Hypophosphatasia

IV. Conditions of decreased PPi*
   a. Idiopathic arterial calcification of infancy

DYSTROPHIC CALCIFICATION

I. Posttraumatic
   a. Repetitive injury (e.g., thumb sucking)
   b. Neoplasm
   c. Infectious or autoimmune disease with granuloma formation (e.g., tuberculosis, Wegener's granulomatosis, sarcoidosis)

II. Autoimmune disease
   a. Dermatomyositis (juvenile)
   b. Scleroderma
      i. Systemic
      ii. Limited or CREST*
   c. Mixed connective tissue disease
   d. Systemic lupus erythematosus
   e. Overlap syndromes

III. Calcinosis cutis

ECTOPIC OSSIFICATION

I. Myositis ossificans (posttraumatic)
   a. Burns
   b. Surgery (e.g., joint replacement)
   c. Neurologic injury
   d. Repetitive injury (e.g., adductor ossification in horseback riders, deltoid or pectoralis minor ossification in hunters)

II. Fibrodysplasia (myositis) ossificans progressiva (FOP)
III. Progressive osseous heteroplasia (POH)
IV. Osteoma cutis

*PPi, inorganic pyrophosphate; CREST, calcinosis, Raynaud's phenomenon, esophageal dysfunction, sclerodactyly, telangiectasia.

## Dystrophic Calcification

### Juvenile Dermatomyositis

Dermatomyositis is a multisystem, autoimmune disorder featuring small vessel vasculitis (8). Acute and chronic inflammation occurs predominantly in striated muscles and skin but can also affect the joints, gastrointestinal tract, lungs, and heart (9). When dermatomyositis manifests before age 18 years, it is called "juvenile dermatomyositis"

(JDMS) with an annual incidence in the United States of 3.2 cases per million (10). Peak ages of presentation in childhood are 2 to 6 years and the teenage years (10). Female predominance (10) is expressed in both the pediatric and adult forms (peak ages 50 to 60 years). Dystrophic calcification, however, is rare in the adult form.

Historically, calcinosis occurs in 10% to 50% of patients with JDMS and may be the principal cause of long-term disability. It generally manifests 1 to 3 years after diagnosis (3), yet can be the presenting complaint (11). In fact, calcinosis also follows "amyopathic JDMS" (12). In JDMS, gender and age at presentation seem unrelated to the severity of calcinosis. Early aggressive therapy, however, appears important for minimizing calcinosis and facilitating recovery (3,13). HLA-DQA1*0501 may confer disease susceptibility to JDMS. Furthermore, a polymorphism in the promoter of the gene encoding tumor necrosis factor alpha (*TNFα-308A*) has been implicated in especially severe muscle disease and calcinosis (14). Lipodystrophy is also associated with a greater prevalence of ectopic mineralization (15).

Biochemical parameters of mineral homeostasis are usually normal in the clinical laboratory, yet hypercalcemia with hypercalciuria and hyperphosphaturia may occur (16). Ectopic mineral in JDMS has a hydroxyapatite nucleus and the associated fluid contains macrophages, giant cells, eosinophils, interleukin (IL)-6, IL-1, and TNFα (17). Mechanisms for the dystrophic calcification could include release from diseased muscle of alkaline phosphatase (ALP) and Ca-binding free fatty acids or gamma-carboxylated peptides. The ALP may then hydrolyze PPi, thus decreasing local concentrations of this nucleation inhibitor. Elevated urinary levels of gamma-carboxyglutamic acid have been reported in JDMS, especially if there is calcinosis. However, warfarin administration to inhibit gamma-carboxylation has not decreased mineral deposits (18).

Four types of calcinosis occur in JDMS (19).*

1. *Calcinosis circumscripta:* Calcification occurs throughout the subcutaneous tissues but primarily in periarticular regions or areas subject to trauma (20% of cases) (Fig. 27.1). This type can interfere with joint motion or ulcerate and extrude calcific material through the skin. This complication has been called "tumoral calcinosis," but it must not be confused with idiopathic or familial tumoral calcinosis (see below).

2. *Superficial calcinosis:* Skin nodules or plaques occur most often on pressure points such as elbows, knees, extremities, and digits (33% of cases) but rarely interfere with joint function.

3. *Calcinosis universalis:* Deep, linear, sheet-like deposits occur along intramuscular fascial planes (15% of cases) and are associated with discomfort and limitation of motion.

4. *Exoskeleton calcification:* Diffuse, lacy, reticular, subcutaneous deposits encase the torso and elsewhere to form a generalized "exoskeleton" (10% of cases) and may cross joints causing significant morbidity.

*Notably, 22% of JDMS patients have mixed forms of calcinosis.

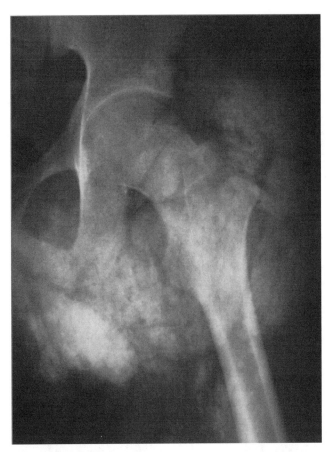

**Figure 27.1**   Juvenile dermatomyositis. The deep, soft tissues especially surrounding the left hip of this 18-year-old man show remarkable calcification that extends to the thigh and is typical of *calcinosis universalis*.

Calcinosis tends to affect skin and muscle most severely disturbed by inflammation. Reportedly, calcinosis in JDMS improves over time, yet spontaneous complete resolution is unusual (20). Numerous medical treatments have been attempted and many appear efficacious; however, there have been no controlled trials. Troublesome calcium deposits have also been removed surgically.

Antiinflammatory drugs (hydroxychloroquine, intravenous immunoglobulin, cyclosporine, infliximab) have been prescribed for recalcitrant JDMS with reports of some regression of calcinosis (21) including a report of resolution with cyclosporine. Also, beneficial responses have been attributed to diltiazem, but this drug can induce a myositis flare (21). Several case reports suggest some success from efforts to lower the blood Ca × Pi product. Included are treatment with Al(OH)$_3$ and probenecid (22). Probenecid decreases renal elimination of methotrexate however, and therefore, combined therapy must be used with increased caution. Glucocorticoid-induced osteoporosis in JDMS is often prevented by Ca and vitamin-D supplementation, but the impact on calcinosis is unclear. Bisphosphonates have been associated with diminution of calcinosis (17), and despite any added preservation or increases in bone mineral density, high-dose bisphosphonates pose unique risks to children

(23). Esophageal dysmotility complicating JDMS adds further concern for oral bisphosphonate therapy.

## Scleroderma

Calcinosis affects approximately 33% of patients with limited scleroderma (CREST) and 24% with diffuse disease (4). Typical locations include the palmar aspects of the fingers and bony prominences such as the olecranon and prepatellar bursae, ischial tuberosities, and lateral malleoli. Treatment with diltiazem, bisphosphonates, probenecid, Al(OH)$_3$, and warfarin have been attempted; however, controlled trials are wanting. Surgical intervention is often indicated when skin lesions ulcerate and risk infection or interfere with hand function. Hand surgery, however, may be hazardous because of ischemic complications (24) or delayed healing and has led to amputation.

### Metastatic Calcification

Metastatic calcification is initially amorphous Ca-Pi, but may later become hydroxyapatite (1). The location of deposits varies somewhat between hypercalcemia, hyperphosphatemia, and perhaps deficiency of inhibitors of calcification.

For metastatic calcification in hypercalcemia, deposits typically occur in the kidneys, lungs, and fundus of the stomach (1). Additionally, the media of large arteries, elastic tissue of the endocardium (especially the left atrium), conjunctiva, and periarticular soft tissues are frequently affected. Well-established causes include chronic milk-alkali syndrome, hypervitaminosis D, sarcoidosis, and hyperparathyroidism.

For metastatic calcification in hyperphosphatemia, deposits occur periarticularly and elsewhere from renal insufficiency (leading to hyperphosphatemia, hypercalcemia, or both), massive cell lysis (release of cellular Pi) because of chemotherapy for leukemia, and other metabolic disorders.

Elevated extracellular concentrations of other factors, such as oxalate, can cause calcium deposition. Hypophosphatasia [Online Mendelian Inheritance in Man (OMIM) 146300, 241500, 241510] (25) due to inactivating mutations in the gene that encodes the tissue nonspecific isoenzyme of alkaline phosphatase (TNSALP) (26) leads to PPi accumulation. PPi is incorporated into crystals accounting for the associated pseudogout, chondrocalcinosis, and PPi arthropathy. Although PPi generally inhibits hydroxyapatite crystal growth, at certain concentrations it seems to promote hydroxyapatite formation, and rarely "calcific periarthritis" complicates hypophosphatasia. Recent genetic studies of familial articular chondrocalcinosis (OMIM 118600) report mutations within the human progressive ankylosis (ANKH) gene (25). ANKH promotes extracellular movement of PPi. Hence, sequestration of PPi in this condition leads to calcium pyrophosphate dihydrate (CPPD) deposition within cartilage. Homozygous deactivating mutations of ectonucleotide pyrophosphatase/phosphodiesterase-1 (a protein that generates PPi) have been found in some patients with idiopathic arterial calcification of infancy (25). Here, decreased production of PPi leads to hydroxyapatite deposition especially of the internal elastic lamina, and death usually occurs by 6 months of age (25). Reduced extracellular PPi resulting from the genetic defect may be changing the impact of the Ca × Pi solubility product in these patients.

## Tumoral Calcinosis

Tumoral calcinosis features periarticular metastatic calcification (27). One-third of patients have the heritable disorder. Although the pathogenesis is poorly understood, there can be increased kidney tubular reabsorption of Pi causing hyperphosphatemia (28). Deranged regulation of renal 25-hydroxyvitamin D, 1α-hydroxylase activity enhances synthesis of 1,25(OH)$_2$D leading to increased dietary Ca absorption and suppressed parathyroid hormone levels.

Mineral deposition involves bursae on the extensor surfaces of major joints (Fig. 27.2). Usually, the hips (trochanteric bursae), gluteal region (ischialgluteal bursae), elbows (olecranon bursae), and shoulders are affected, although additional joints can be involved (27). Visceral calcification does not occur, yet segments of the vasculature may contain mineral deposits (28).

Typically, the calcifications in tumoral calcinosis are chronic, recurring, and painless and grow at variable rates. They may weigh 1 kg or more and are often hard, lobulated, and firmly attached to deep fascia. Swellings may begin as calcific bursitis but then grow into adjacent fascial planes. Occasionally, they infiltrate tendons and muscles. Bone scanning is a particularly useful technique for their detection.

Most clinical complications are caused by the tumor masses (e.g., compression effects). Furthermore, deposits in the skin can ulcerate and form a sinus tract draining a chalky fluid that may lead to infection. Other secondary features include low-grade fever, regional lymphadenopathy, splenomegaly, anemia, and amyloidosis. Recurrent episodes of bone inflammation have also been reported (29). This "diaphysitis" has been recognized using radiographs, computerized tomography, or magnetic resonance imaging. New bone formation occurring along the endosteal surface of diaphyses (perhaps from calcific inflammation of the marrow) (29) may be confused with osteomyelitis or a neoplasm.

Serum Ca and ALP levels are usually normal. Sedimentation rates can be elevated. Hyperphosphatemia and increased serum 1,25(OH)$_2$D levels occur in some patients (28). The phosphate transport maximum/glomerular filtration rate (TmP/GFR) may be supranormal, but renal function is otherwise unremarkable. The chalky fluid is predominantly hydroxyapatite.

The differential diagnosis for tumoral calcinosis includes periarticular metastatic calcification from hypercalcemia as a result of renal failure, milk-alkali syndrome, sarcoidosis, and vitamin-D intoxication.

Surgical removal of calcified masses may be helpful when they are painful, interfere with function, or are cosmetically unacceptable. When excision is complete, recur-

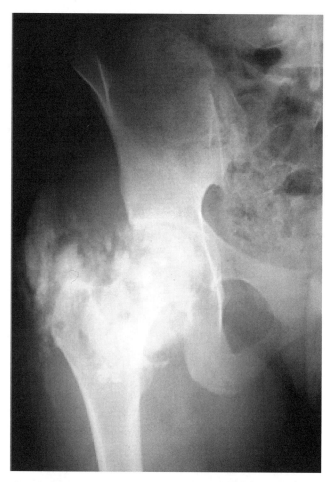

**Figure 27.2** Tumoral calcinosis. The periarticular region of the right hip of this 16-year-old girl has characteristic deep calcifications with a septated appearance consistent with tumoral calcinosis.

rence of tumors seems unlikely (30). Radiation or cortisone treatments have not been effective. Although large masses of apatite crystals might seem unlikely to dissolve, successes with dietary Pi-binding using Al(OH)$_3$ (together with dietary Ca and Pi deprivation) (31) and calcitonin have been reported.

## HETEROTOPIC OSSIFICATION

Heterotopic ossification (HO) may occur sporadically following burns, surgery (e.g., total hip replacement) (32), or neurological injury (33) and rarely is inherited. HO may present as fever, pain, swelling, erythema, or elevated serum ALP activity. The associated bone is lamellar, actively remodeled by osteoblasts and osteoclasts, has haversian systems, and sometimes contains marrow.

### Myositis Ossificans Traumatica

HO resulting from trauma is sometimes called myositis ossificans traumatica. Radiographic evidence of HO may take 3 to 4 weeks to appear. Bone scans identify lesions earlier and define matured ossification helping guide the timing of excision. Surgical treatment of HO is recommended only for significant symptoms or loss of joint motion and should be performed when the bone scan is "inactive" thereby decreasing recurrences.

Following total hip replacement, differentiation from joint infection may be difficult. Patients with previous HO, hypertrophic osteoarthritis, ankylosing spondylitis, diffuse idiopathic skeletal hyperostosis (DISH) (32), and Paget's bone disease are especially predisposed to HO. Conversely, individuals with rheumatoid arthritis are less likely to develop HO following total hip replacement (34).

High-risk patients often benefit from cyclooxygenase-2 (COX2)-inhibitors (32) and external beam radiation to prevent or minimize HO. Indomethacin, a traditional non-steroidal antiinflammatory drug (NSAID), has been extensively studied in HO but carries a high risk of bleeding in patients receiving anticoagulation. COX2-inhibitors are begun within 1 or 2 days after surgery and continued for 1 to 2 weeks (32). For external beam radiation prophylaxis, a single-dose regimen is given either preoperatively within 24 hours or postoperatively within 3 days (35) and seems to be effective.

## Neurogenic Heterotopic Ossification

Neurogenic HO can follow any significant trauma to the central nervous system (e.g., near drowning, hemorrhage, hydrocephaly, spinal cord injury, tumors). Ectopic bone develops distant to the injury and has a predilection for appearing near joints. The prevalence is 10% to 20% for significant head trauma and 20% to 30% for significant spinal cord injury (33). Ossification from spinal cord injury develops 3 to 12 weeks after trauma and is most often found (in descending prevalence) in hips, knees, shoulders, elbows, and feet. Bone scans help detect HO after spinal cord injury. NSAIDs and/or bisphosphonates may be useful for prophylaxis (32).

## Pseudomalignant Heterotopic Ossification

Myositis ossificans occurring without antecedent trauma or a genetic basis is also called pseudomalignant heterotopic ossification (36). Seventy-five percent of affected individuals are younger than age 30 years, with peak prevalence at age 11 to 20 years (37). Equal numbers of males and females are affected (38). Localized pain is followed by an erythematous, warm, enlarging soft tissue mass typically growing for 8 weeks (36). The sedimentation rate is elevated as it expands. This circumscribed, rapidly proliferating, mesenchymal lesion contains nonneoplastic bone and cartilage (38). It develops in muscle adjacent to, but separated from, bone (near a hip, metacarpals, or shoulder) and reaches 1 to 6 cm in diameter (36). Unlike other forms of HO, pseudomalignant heterotopic ossification reportedly can be excised with minimal risk of recurrence even if not "mature" (36).

## Heritable Heterotopic Ossification

Ectopic ossification occurs as the major feature of fibrodysplasia (myositis) ossificans progressiva (FOP) (OMIM 135100) and progressive osseous heteroplasia (POH) (OMIM 166350) and complicates Albright hereditary osteodystrophy (AHO) (OMIM 103580) or pseudohypoparathyroidism, type IA.

Maternally inherited, inactivating mutations in the *GNAS1* gene encoding the stimulating alpha subunit of G proteins ($G_s\alpha$) cause AHO. AHO is characterized by defects in skeletal development including growth, modeling, and remodeling and resistance to several hormones with short stature, round faces, obesity, brachydactyly, and subcutaneous ossification (25). Paternally inherited, deactivating *GNAS1* mutations lead to POH, characterized by cutaneous calcifications in infancy that later spread to become debilitating bone deposition in deep muscle, fat, and fascia, yet typically without endocrinopathy (25).

## Fibrodysplasia Ossificans Progressiva

FOP is increasingly attributed to a connective tissue defect (fibrodysplasia ossificans progressiva) as opposed to muscle abnormality (myositis ossificans progressiva). Reports of mutations in the gene encoding noggin have not been verified (25). HO is typically present by five years of age, first involving the region of neck, spine, and shoulder girdle (39). Hallux valgus deformity (a congenital malformation of the great toe) is a critical characteristic and important clue for diagnosis (Fig. 27.3).

Current treatment involves injury prevention (avoiding intramuscular and dental injections), use of a helmet, walker, or cane to avoid trauma from falls, and antiinflammatory agents. Experimental therapies are being evaluated (40) (http://www.ifopa.org).

In 2004, two genes were implicated in autosomal recessive forms of tumoral calcinosis (41,42). Linkage analysis

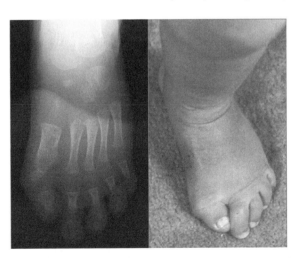

**Figure 27.3** Fibrodysplasia ossificans progressiva. Radiographic and clinical depiction of a hallux valgus deformity in a child, a critical clue for diagnosis of fibrodysplasia ossificans progressiva.

followed by candidate gene sequencing revealed deactivating mutations in *GALNT3* (a glycosyltransferase which initiates mucin-type O-glycosylation) in two kindreds (41). A preliminary report, based on candidate gene sequencing, uncovered homozygous mutation of the FGF-23 gene affecting protein processing and resulting in increased renal phosphate reclamation (42).

# REFERENCES

1. Favus MJ, Whyte MP. Extraskeletal (ectopic) calcification and ossification. In Favus M. ed. Primer on metabolic bone diseases and disorders of mineral metabolism. New York: American Society for Bone and Mineral Research, 2003:427–437.
2. Harrison HE, Harrison HC. *Disorders of calcium and phosphate metabolism in childhood and adolescence.* Philadelphia: WB Saunders, 1979:291–304.
3. Pachman LM, Hayford JR, Chung A, et al. Juvenile dermatomyositis at diagnosis: clinical characteristics of 79 children. *J Rheumatol* 1998;25:1198–1204.
4. Medsger TA. Natural history of systemic sclerosis and the assessment of disease activity, severity, functional status, and psychologic well-being. *Rheum Dis Clin North Am* 2003;29:1–15.
5. Chan AT, Wordsworth BP, McNally J. Overlap connective tissue disease, pulmonary fibrosis, and extensive subcutaneous calcification. *Ann Rheum Dis* 2003;62(7):690–691.
6. Buka R, Wei H, Sapadin A, et al. Pseudoxanthoma elasticum and calcinosis cutis. *J Am Acad Dermatol* 2000;43:312–315.
7. Fawthrop FW, Russell RGG. Ectopic calcification and ossification. In: Nordin BEC, Need AG, Morris HA, eds. *Metabolic bone and stone disease*, 3rd ed. Edinburgh, UK: Churchill Livingstone, 1993:325–338.
8. Pachman L. Juvenile dermatomyositis: immunogenetics, pathophysiology, and disease expression. *Rheum Dis Clin North Am* 2002;28:579–602.
9. Spiera R, Kagen L. Extramuscular manifestations in idiopathic inflammatory myopathies. *Curr Opin Rheumatol* 1998;10:556–561.
10. Mendez EP, Lipton R, Ramsey-Goldman R, et al. US incidence of juvenile dermatomyositis, 1995–1998: Results from the National Institute of Arthritis and Musculoskeletal and Skin Diseases Registry. *Arthritis Rheum* 2003;29:300–305.
11. Wananukul S, Pongprasit P, Wattanakrai P. Calcinosis cutis presenting years before other clinical manifestations of juvenile dermatomyositis: report of two cases. *Australas J Derm* 1997;38:202–205.
12. Plamondon S, Dent PB. Juvenile amyopathic dermatomyositis: results of a case finding descriptive survey. *J Rheumatol* 2000;27:2031–2034.
13. Fisler RE, Liang MG, Fuhlbrigge RC, et al. Aggressive management of juvenile dermatomyositis results in improved outcome and decreased incidence of calcinosis. *J Am Acad Dermatol* 2002;47:505–511.
14. Pachman LM, Liotta-Davis MR, Hong DK, et al. TNFα-308A Allele in juvenile dermatomyositis. *Arthritis Rheum* 2000;43:2368–2377.
15. Rider L, Ruiz-Hidalgo M, Labora J, et al. Lipodystrophy in juvenile dermatomyositis is associated with calcinosis, but not with adipocyte differentiation factor DLK levels (abstract). *Arthritis Rheum* 2001;44:S264.
16. Perez MD, Abrams SA, Koenning G, et al. Mineral metabolism in children with dermatomyositis. *J Rheumatol* 1994;21:2364–2369.
17. Mukamel M, Horev G, Mimouni M. New insight into calcinosis of juvenile dermatomyositis: a study of composition and treatment. *J Pediatr* 2001;138:763–766.
18. Moore SE, Jump AA, Smiley JD. Effect of warfarin sodium therapy on excretion of 4-carboxy-l-glutamic acid in scleroderma, dermatomyositis, and myositis ossificans progressiva. *Arthritis Rheum* 1986;29:344–351.
19. Bowyer SL, Blane CE, Sullivan DB, Cassidy JT. Childhood dermatomyositis: factors predicting functional outcome and development of dystrophic calcification. *J Pediatr* 1983;103:882–888.
20. Ramanan AV, Feldman BM. Clinical outcomes in juvenile dermatomyositis. *Curr Opin Rheumatol* 2002;14:658–662.
21. Rider LG. Calcinosis in juvenile dermatomyositis: pathogenesis and current therapies. *Pediatric Rheumatology* on-line journal 2003;(2), www.pedrhemonlinejournal.org/April/calinosis.html.
22. Eddy MC, Leelawattana R, McAlister WH, Whyte MP. Calcinosis universalis complicating juvenile dermatomyositis: resolution during probenecid therapy. *J Clin Endocrinol Metab* 1997;82: 3536–3542.
23. Whyte MP, Wenkert D, Clements KL, et al. Bisphosphonate-induced osteopetrosis. *N Engl J Med* 2003;349:455–461.
24. Hussmann, J, Russell, RC, Kucan JO, et al. Soft-tissue calcifications: differential diagnosis and therapeutic approaches. *Ann Plast Surg* 1995; 34:138–147.
25. McKusick VA. *Mendelian inheritance in man: a catalog of human genes and genetic disorders.* 12th ed. Baltimore: Johns Hopkins University Press, 1998 *and Online mendelian inheritance in man, OMIM.* Baltimore, MD: McKusick-Nathans Institute for Genetic Medicine, Johns Hopkins University and Bethesda, MD: National Center for Biotechnology Information, National Library of Medicine, 2000.
26. Mumm S, Jones J, Finnegan P, et al. Denaturing gradient gel electrophoresis analysis of the tissue non-specific alkaline phosphatase isoenzyme gene in hypophosphatasia. Mol Genet Metabo 2002;75:143–153.
27. Martinez S. Tumoral calcinosis: 12 years later. *Semin Musculoskelet Radiol* 2002;6:331–339.
28. Slavin RE, Wen J, Kumar D, Evans EB. Familial tumoral calcinosis. A clinical, histopathologic, and ultrastructural study with an analysis of its calcifying process and pathogenesis. *Am J Surg Pathol* 1993;17:788–802.
29. Martinez S, Vogler JB, Harrelson JM, Lyles KW. Imaging of tumoral calcinosis: new observations. *Radiology* 1990;174:215–222.
30. McGuinness FE. Hyperphosphataemic tumoral calcinosis in Bedouin Arabs—clinical and radiological features. *Clin Radiol* 1995;50:259–264.
31. Gregosiewicz A, Warda E. Tumoral calcinosis: successful medical treatment. *J Bone Joint Surg Am* 1989;71A:1244–1249.
32. Romano CL, Duci D, Romano D, et al. Celecoxib versus indomethacin in the prevention of heterotopic ossification after total hip arthroplasty. *J Arthroplasty* 2004;19:14–18.
33. van Kuijk AA, Geurts ACH, van Kuppevelt HJM. Neurogenic heterotopic ossification in spinal cord injury. *Spinal Cord* 2002;40:313–326.
34. Eggli S, Woo A. Risk factors for heterotopic ossification in total hip arthroplasty. *Arch Orthop Trauma Surg* 2001 Oct;121: 531–535.
35. Padgett DE, Holley KG, Cummings M, et al. The efficacy of 500 CentiGray radiation in the prevention of heterotopic ossification after total hip arthroplasty: a prospective, randomized, pilot study. *J Arthroplasty* 2003;18:677–686.
36. Ogilvie-Harris DJ, et al. Pseudomalignant myositis ossificans: heterotopic new-bone formation without a history of trauma. *J Bone Joint Surg* 1980:62:1274–1284.
37. Jouve JL, Cottalorda J, Bollini G, et al. Myositis ossificans: report of seven cases in children. *J Pediatr Orthop B* 1997;6:33–41.
38. Heinrich SD, Zembo MM, MacEwen GD. Pseudomalignant myositis ossificans. *J Pediatr Orthop* 1989;12:599–602.
39. Cohen RB, et al. The natural history of heterotopic ossification in patients who have fibrodysplasia ossificans progressiva. *J Bone Miner Res* 1993; 75-A:215–219.
40. *Clinical proceedings of the Third International Symposium on Fibrodysplasia Ossificans Progressiva.* July 2001. www.ifopa.org/treatment.pdf
41. Topaz O, Shurman DL, Bergman R, et al. Mutations in *GALNT3*, encoding a protein involved in O-linked glycosylation, cause familial tumoral calcinosis. *Nature Genet* 2004;36:579–581.
42. Araya K, Fukumoto S, Backenroth R, et al. A mutation in FGF-23 gene enhances the processing of FGF-23 protein and causes tumoral calcinosis (abstract). *J Bone Miner Res* 2004; 19 (Suppl 1): s41.

# Index

Note: Page numbers followed by f indicate figures; those followed by t indicate tables.

## A

Acquisitions, in magnetic resonance imaging, 60
Adipogenesis, glucocorticoids in, 107–108
Adynamic bone, bisphosphonates for, 142
Aggrecan(s)
  structure of, 29–30
  turnover of, 29–30
Aggrecan-based markers, of cartilage turnover, 30–31, 30t, 31f
Albright hereditary osteodystrophy, 201
Alendronate. See also Bisphosphonates
  clinical trials of, 143, 143t, 144–145, 144t
  efficacy of, 143, 143t, 144–145, 144t
  for glucocorticoid-induced osteoporosis, 112–114, 113f, 116
  with calcium supplements, 112
  for Paget's disease, 178–179
  with parathyroid hormone, 165–167
  for primary hyperparathyroidism, 189
  with raloxifene, 152
  side effects of, 146
Alexander technique, 132
Alfacalcidiol, with glucocorticoids, 112, 112f, 114
αν β3 integrin, 172
American College of Rheumatology (ACR), bone densitometry guidelines of, 41
Analgesia, 132
  calcitonin in, 139–140
  for complex regional pain syndrome, 139–140
Anastrozole, bone loss due to, 121
Andersson lesions, 88
Androgen(s), 154–159
  endogenous
    deficiency of, male osteoporosis and, 155
    skeletal effects of, 154–155, 155t
  pharmacologic
    with estrogen, 155–156
    immunosuppressive effects of, 157–158
    for male osteoporosis, 155, 156t
    for postmenopausal osteoporosis, 155–156, 157t
    for rheumatoid arthritis, 156–159, 158t
  side effects of, 156

Androgen receptors, 154
Angiogenic factors
  in rheumatoid arthritis, 12
  in spondyloarthropathies, 12
Ankylosing spondylitis
  Andersson lesions in, 88
  angiogenesis in, 12
  bisphosphonates for, 147
  bone formation in, 88–89
  bone loss in, 11–12, 87–89
  magnetic resonance imaging in, 63–64
  Romanus lesions in, 88
Anticoagulants, for systemic lupus erythematosus, bone loss due to, 81
Anticonvulsants, bone loss due to, 81, 120
Antiinflammatory agents
  for juvenile dermatomyositis, 199
  for myositis ossificans traumatica, 201
Anti-RANK ligand antibody, 172
Antiresorptive agents. See also Osteoporosis therapy
  in glucocorticoid therapy, 103
Antirheumatic drugs, clinical trials of, 125–129, 126f–128f
Anxiety, in osteoporosis, 67–68
Aromatase, 154
Aromatase deficiency, 154
Aromatase inhibitors, bone loss due to, 121
Arthritis
  degenerative. See Osteoarthritis
  inflammatory bowel disease–related, bone loss in, 11–12
  psoriatic. See Psoriatic arthritis
  reactive, bone loss in, 11–12
  rheumatoid. See Rheumatoid arthritis
Arthroplasty, for osteonecrosis, 195
Autoimmunity, estrogens and, 135

## B

B cells, in osteoclastogenesis, 16
Biochemical markers
  of bone turnover, 25–28, 26f, 26t, 28f, 28t
    clinical utility of, 27–28, 28f, 28t, 29f
    in psoriatic arthritis, 89
    in systemic lupus erythematosus, 81–82
    variability in, 28
  of cartilage turnover, 28–33

Biopsy, in osteomalacia, 183
Birth control pills, in systemic lupus erythematosus, 136
Bisphosphonates, 141–147. See also Osteoporosis therapy
  absorption of, 142
  for ankylosing spondylitis, 147
  chemical structure of, 142f
  for children, 146–147
  clinical trials of, 143–145, 143t, 144t
  deposition of, 141
  development of, 141
  efficacy of, 143t
  focal bone erosions and, 17
  for geriatric patients, 147
  for glucocorticoid-induced osteoporosis, 50, 51t, 52, 112–114, 113f, 116, 168
  indications for, 143
  intravenous, 146
    for osteogenesis imperfecta, 146–147
    side effects of, 146
  for juvenile dermatomyositis, 199
  mechanism of action of, 26, 141–143
  metabolism of, 142
  nitrogen, 141, 142t
  nonnitrogen, 141, 142t
  for osteoarthritis, 147
  for osteogenesis imperfecta, 146–147
  overview of, 141
  for Paget's disease, 178–179
  with parathyroid hormone, 147, 165–167
  in pregnancy, 147
  for primary hyperparathyroidism, 189
  renal excretion of, 142
  response to, biochemical markers of, 27–28, 285t
  for rheumatoid arthritis, 147
  with selective estrogen receptor modulators, 152
  for systemic lupus erythematosus, 83–84
Bone. See also under Skeletal
  adynamic, bisphosphonates for, 142
  cancellous (spongy), 3, 4f
  core decompression of, for osteonecrosis, 195
  cortical (compact), 3, 4f
  glucocorticoid effects on, 105–109
  properties of, 3

Bone (*continued*)
structure and function of, 3–6, 4f, 5f
subchondral trabecular, in osteoarthritis, 94
Bone biopsy, in osteomalacia, 183
Bone densitometry
in ankylosing spondylitis, 87–88
in children, 37, 38, 40–41
in complex regional pain syndrome, 140
in degenerative spinal disease, 38
in diagnosis, 45–46
in disease monitoring, 37, 46–47, 50–52
DXA, 35–37, 40–41
in children, 40–41
indications for, 40, 41
vs. quantitative computer tomography, 37–38
in fracture risk assessment, 38–40, 45–46, 47, 47f, 50–52
in glucocorticoid-induced bone loss, 49–52, 50, 50f
historical perspective on, 35–36
indications for, 40, 41
interpretive report for, 42
measurement sites in, 41
in obese patients, 37–38
patient selection for, 40–41
peripheral, 45–47
in fracture risk assessment, 45, 47, 47f
indications for, 45–47
limitations of, 45–47
quantitative computer tomography in, 38, 41, 45–47
quality improvement for, 42
quantitative computer tomographic, 35–36, 37–40
central, vs. peripheral QCT, 41
in children, 40–41
in glucocorticoid-induced osteoporosis, 51–52
indications for, 40, 41
measurement sites in, 41
peripheral, 38, 45–47
indications for, 41, 45–47
radiation dose in, 38, 38t
3D, 38, 39f
vs. DXA, 37–38
quantitative ultrasonographic, in glucocorticoid-induced osteoporosis, 51
radiation dose in, 38, 38t
reference databases for, 36–37, 46
reimbursement for, 41
reporting results of, 42
in scoliosis, 38
in systemic lupus erythematosus, 81
in therapeutic monitoring, 25–26, 27–28, 28f, 28t, 46–47
T scores in, 37
in central vs. peripheral testing, 45–47, 46f
for children, 40–41
fracture risk and, 47
in scoliosis, 38, 39t

in vertebral body compression, 38, 39t
Z scores in, 37
for children, 40–41
Bone erosions. *See* Focal bone erosions
Bone formation, 5–6, 5f
in ankylosing spondylitis, 11–12, 88–89
glucocorticoid effects on, 107–108, 107t, 108–109
Bone grafts, for osteonecrosis, 195
Bone growth, glucocorticoid effects on, 102–103, 108
Bone loss, 8–13. *See also* Focal bone erosions; Joint space narrowing; Osteopenia; Osteoporosis
in ankylosing spondylitis, 87–89
drug-induced
anticonvulsants in, 81, 120
aromatase inhibitors in, 121
calmodulin-calcineurin phosphatase inhibitors in, 121
depot medroxyprogesterone acetate in, 121
glucocorticoids in. *See* Glucocorticoid-induced osteoporosis
heparin in, 81, 120
luteinizing hormone–releasing hormone agonists in, 121
methotrexate in, 76, 121
thyroid hormone in, 120–121
in hyperparathyroidism, 187–188, 187f, 188f
inflammatory cytokines and, 8–13, 75
interleukins, 17–18, 18f, 19t
in juvenile idiopathic arthritis, 19
measurement of. *See* Bone densitometry
in osteoarthritis, 91–95
pathophysiology of, in rheumatic disorders, 8–13
in psoriatic arthritis, 11–12, 89
radiological measurement of
magnetic resonance imaging in, 59–65. *See also* Magnetic resonance imaging (MRI)
radiographic scoring systems for, 54–57, 55t
in rheumatoid arthritis, 9–11, 73–76
androgens for, 156–159, 158t
glucocorticoid-induced, 10, 49–52, 75–76, 99–100, 105–106
osteoclasts in, 16–18
pathogenesis of, 15–20, 74–76
risk assessment for, biochemical markers in, 27, 27f
severity of, 37
in systemic lupus erythematosus, 12, 79–85
tumor necrosis factor-α in, 17–18, 18f, 19t
Bone mass
measurement of. *See* Bone densitometry in osteoarthritis
of hip, 91–92, 92f
of knee, 92–93

Bone Mass Measurement Act, 41
Bone matrix
androgen effects on, 154
glucocorticoid effects on, 106–107
Bone metabolism, immune system in, 4, 4f, 9, 9t, 11, 16–19, 18f, 19t, 75. *See also* RANK/RANKL/OPG system
Bone mineral content
in complex regional pain syndrome, 140
vs. bone mineral density, 41
Bone mineral density (BMD)
in ankylosing spondylitis, 87–88
biochemical markers of, 25–28, 26t
bone size and, 40
in children, 41
classification of, 37
in diagnosis, 45–46
in disease monitoring, 46–47
fracture risk and, 38–40, 45–46, 47, 47f
in glucocorticoid-induced osteoporosis, 49–52
in low bone mass, 37
measurement of, 35–52. *See also* Bone densitometry
monitoring of, 37
in osteoarthritis, 91–95
in osteopenia, 37
in osteoporosis, 37
in primary hyperaparthyroidism, 91–95, 187–188, 187f
in scoliosis, 38, 39f, 39t
in systemic lupus erythematosus, 79, 81–82
in therapeutic monitoring, 25–26, 27–28, 28f, 28t, 46–47
in vertebral body compression, 38, 39f, 39t
vs. bone mineral content, 41
Bone remodeling, 3–6, 4f, 5f, 8, 26f
biochemical markers of, 25–28, 26f, 26t, 28f, 28t
clinical utility of, 27–28, 28f, 28t, 29f
in psoriatic arthritis, 89
in systemic lupus erythematosus, 81–82
variability in, 28
bisphosphonate effects on, 141–143
bone strength and, 26f
glucocorticoid effects on, 105–106, 106t
in hyperparathyroidism, 106
inflammatory cytokines in, 9
in osteoarthritis, 94, 94f
osteocytes in, 6
in osteoporosis, 6
rate of
biochemical markers of, 26–28, 26t
fracture risk and, 6, 26
in rheumatoid arthritis, 9–11
sites of, 142
in spondyloarthropathy, 11–12
Bone remodeling units, 142
Bone resorption, 4, 5f

bisphosphonate suppression of, 141–143
osteoprotegerin in, 9
RANKL in, 4, 4f, 9, 9t
regulation of, 8–9, 9t
Bone scan
in osteomalacia, 183, 183f
in osteonecrosis, 193
Bone strength, bone turnover and, 26f
Bone turnover. See Bone remodeling
Breast cancer, raloxifene for, 152

**C**

Calciferol, 183. See also Vitamin D, supplemental
Calcification
extraskeletal, 197–200, 198t
metastatic, 197, 199–200
Calcinosis, 197–200
in juvenile dermatomyositis, 198–199, 199f
in scleroderma, 199
tumoral, 200, 200f
Calcinosis circumscripta, 198
Calcinosis universalis, 198, 199f
Calcitonin, 138–140. See also Osteoporosis therapy
analgesic effects of, 139–140
clinical studies of, 138–140
in combination therapy, 139
for complex regional pain syndrome, 139–140
dosage of, 139
for glucocorticoid-induced osteoporosis, 114, 139
for Paget's disease, 139, 179–180
response to, biochemical markers of, 27–28, 285t
routes of administration for, 139
side effects of, 139
for systemic lupus erythematosus, 84
Calcitriol, with glucocorticoids, 112, 112f
Calcium metabolism
parathyroid hormone and, 161–162, 185
teriparatide and, 163
Calcium pyrophosphate deposition disease, hyperparathyroidism and, 185, 186
Calcium supplements
in glucocorticoid therapy, 111–112, 112f, 114
in systemic lupus erythematosus, 83
Calculi, renal, in hyperparathyroidism, 185
Calmodulin-calcineurin phosphatase inhibitors, bone loss due to, 121
Cancellous bone, 3, 4f
Cancer
breast, raloxifene for, 152
hypercalcemia in, bisphosphonates for, 146
osteomalacia in, 184
Carbamazepine, bone loss due to, 81, 120
Cardiovascular disease, raloxifene for, 152
Cartilage, glucocorticoid effects on, 109
Cartilage matrix proteins, 30f, 30t, 31–33

Cartilage oligomeric protein (COMP), 30f, 30t, 31–33
Cartilage proteoglycan aggrecan core protein, 30–31, 30f, 30t
Cartilage turnover, 28–33
biochemical markers of, 29–33, 30f, 30t, 32f
clinical utility of, 31–33, 32f
in therapeutic monitoring, 32–33, 32f
types of, 29–31, 30f, 30t
Cathepsin K, 172
C/EBP proteins, glucocorticoids and, 107
Children. See also under Juvenile
bone densitometry in, 37, 38, 40–41
dermatomyositis in, 198–199, 199f
glucocorticoids in, 102–103, 108, 109
osteonecrosis in, 192
Cholecalciferol, 183. See also Vitamin D, supplemental
Chondrocalcinosis, familial articular, 199–200
Chondroitin sulfate, in aggrecan, 30
Chondroitin sulfate epitopes, as cartilage degradation marker, 30–31, 30f, 30t
Cinacalcet, for primary hyperparathyroidism, 189
Clodronate, 146. See also Bisphosphonates
Clomifene, 150–153. See also Selective estrogen receptor modulators (SERMs)
Codfish vertebrae, 183
Collagen
type I, glucocorticoid effects on, 106–107
type II, in cartilage turnover, 30t, 31, 31f
type III propeptides, in cartilage turnover, 30f, 30t, 31–33
Collagenases, glucocorticoid effects on, 106–107, 107
Collagen peptides, in bone turnover, 26–28
Compact bone, 3, 4f
Complex regional pain syndrome, calcitonin for, 139–140
Computer tomography
in bone densitometry. See Quantitative computer tomography (QCT)
in osteonecrosis, 193
Core decompression of bone, for osteonecrosis, 195
Cortical bone, 3, 4f
Corticosteroids. See Glucocorticoid(s)
Cortisol, glucocorticoids and, 107, 108
Crescent sign, in osteonecrosis, 192, 194f
C-telopeptide (CTx)
in bone turnover, 27
in osteoarthritis, 94
as cartilage degradation marker, 30f, 30t, 31, 32, 32f
C-terminal procollagen peptide, as cartilage degradation marker, 30f, 30t, 31, 32
Cyclophosphamide, bone loss due to, 81

Cyclosporine, bone loss due to, 81, 121
Cytokines
in bone loss, 8–13, 75
in bone remodeling, 9
in osteoclastogenesis, 17–18, 18f, 19t
in rheumatoid arthritis, 11, 15, 75
in spondyloarthropathies, 12
in systemic lupus erythematosus, 80

**D**

Databases, reference, for bone densitometry, 36–37, 46
Degenerative arthritis. See Osteoarthritis
Degenerative spinal disease, bone mineral density measurement in, 38
Dehydroepiandrosterone (DHEA)
endogenous
immunosuppressive effects of, 157–158
skeletal effects of, 154–155, 155t, 156
pharmacologic
for glucocorticoid-induced osteoporosis prevention, 84
for osteoporosis, 156
for rheumatoid arthritis, 156–159, 158t
for systemic lupus erythematosus, 157–158
Densitometry. See Bone densitometry
Depot medroxyprogesterone acetate, bone loss due to, 121
Depression, in osteoporosis, 67–68
Dermatomyositis, juvenile, 198–199, 199f
Diet, osteoporosis and, 68
Disease-modifying antirheumatic drugs, clinical trials of, 125–129, 126f–128f
Disodium etridonate. See Etidronate
Diuretics, thiazide, for glucocorticoid-induced osteoporosis, 84
Drug-induced bone loss. See Bone loss, drug-induced
Dual energy photon absorptiometry (DPA), 35–36. See also Bone densitometry
Dual-energy X-ray absorptiometry (DXA), 35–37. See also Bone densitometry
in children, 40–41
indications for, 40, 41
measurement sites in, 41
radiation dose in, 38, 38t
vs. quantitative computer tomography, 37–38
Dystrophic calcification, 197–199

**E**

Education, patient, in disease management, 68
Elderly, bisphosphonates for, 147
Emotional impact, of osteoporosis, 67–68
Ergocalciferol, with glucocorticoids, 112, 112f
Estradiol. See Estrogen therapy
Estrogen
endogenous
autoimmunity and, 135

Estrogen (*continued*)
  deficiency of, glucocorticoid-
      induced, 106
  in systemic lupus erythematosus,
      135–136
  pharmacologic. *See* Estrogen therapy
Estrogen receptors, selective estrogen
      receptor modulators and, 150,
      151f. *See also* Selective estrogen
      receptor modulators (SERMs)
Estrogen therapy. *See also* Hormone
      replacement therapy
  with androgens, 155–156
  with bisphosphonates, 143
  declining use of, 134
  for osteoarthritis, 136
  with parathyroid hormone, 167
  for primary hyperparathyroidism, 189
  for rheumatoid arthritis, 136
Etidronate, 143t, 144, 144t. *See also*
      Bisphosphonates
  for glucocorticoid-induced osteoporo-
      sis, 112–114, 113f
  for Paget's disease, 179
Exercise
  inadequate, bone loss and, 75
  in osteoarthritis, 131–132
  in osteoporosis, 68, 80, 131–132
  protective effects of, 68, 80
  in rheumatoid arthritis, 131–132
  in systemic lupus erythematosus, 80
Exercises, for back pain, 132
Exoskeleton calcification, 198–199
Extraskeletal calcification, 197–200, 198t
Extraskeletal mineralization, 197–202,
      198t
Extraskeletal ossification, 197, 198f,
      200–202, 200f

**F**
Falls
  fear of, 67–68
  fractures from. *See* Fractures
  prevention of, 131–132
Familial articular chondrocalcinosis,
      199–200
Fast low-angle shot (FLASH) sequences,
      60
Fast spin-echo imaging, 60
Fear of falling, in osteoporosis, 67–68
Feet. *See* Foot
Femoral head/neck. *See* Hip
Fibroblast growth factor (FGF)
  androgen effects on, 154–155, 155t
  in osteoclastogenesis, 17–18, 18f, 19t
Fibroblasts, in bone resorption, 17
Fibrodysplasia ossificans progressiva,
      201–202, 201f
FLASH sequences, 60
Focal bone erosions. *See also* Bone loss;
      Radiographic progression
  in ankylosing spondylitis, 88
  in juvenile idiopathic arthritis, 19
  prevention of, 126–129, 126f–128f
  progression of, 125–126
      as outcome measurement, 64
  in psoriatic arthritis, 19, 89

  in rheumatoid arthritis, 16–18, 18f
      magnetic resonance imaging of,
          60–64, 61, 62f, 62t
      radiographic scoring of, 54–57, 55t
  scoring systems for
      magnetic resonance imaging,
          60–64, 61, 62f, 62t
      radiographic, 54–57, 55t
Foot
  magnetic resonance imaging of, 63
  radiography of, 54–57, 55t
Forearm
  in bone densitometry, 41, 45–46. *See
      also* Bone densitometry
  fractures of. *See* Fractures
Fractures
  in ankylosing spondylitis, 88, 88f
  back pain in, 132
  bone remodeling rate and, 6
  in children, 103
  exercise and rehabilitation for,
      131–132
  in glucocorticoid-induced osteoporo-
      sis, 50, 50f, 100–103, 101f, 102f
  in hyperparathyroidism, 187–188
  management of, 132
  in osteoarthritis, 93–94
  in osteoporosis, 6
  pain management for, 132
  physical inactivity and, 75
  prevention of, 131–132
      androgens for, 155–159, 155t–158t
      bisphosphonates for, 141–147,
          143–145, 143t, 144t
      calcitonin for, 138–140
      factors in, 143
      hormone replacement therapy for,
          134–135
      mechanisms of, 142
      parathyroid hormone for, 161–168
      selective estrogen receptor modula-
          tors for, 150–153, 151–153
      teriparatide for, 161–168
      threshold effect in, 142
  in psoriatic arthritis, 89
  psychological impact of, 67–68
  quality of life and, 67–69
  in rheumatoid arthritis, 74–76, 156
      glucocorticoid-related, 100–103,
          101f, 102f
  risk of
      biochemical markers for, 27, 27f
      bone mineral density and, 38–40,
          45–46, 47, 47f, 50–52
      T scores and, 37
  in systemic lupus erythematosus,
      80–85
FUSE-binding protein, glucocorticoids
      and, 107

**G**
Gastrointestinal toxicity, of bisphospho-
      nates, 146
Gaucher's disease, osteonecrosis in, 192
Genant's scoring method, 55t, 56
Geriatric patients, bisphosphonates for,
      147

Glucocorticoid(s)
  in adipogenesis, 107–108
  calcium supplements with, 111–112,
      112f, 114
  in children, 102–103, 108, 109
  chronic therapy with, definition of,
      111
  effects of
      on bone, 102–103, 105–109. *See
          also* Glucocorticoid-induced
          osteoporosis
      on cartilage, 109
      on skeletal growth, 102–103, 108,
          109
  enzymatic regulation of, 108
  vitamin D supplements with, 111–112,
      112f, 183–184
Glucocorticoid-induced hypogonadism,
      106
Glucocorticoid-induced osteonecrosis,
      191, 192. *See also* Osteonecrosis
Glucocorticoid-induced osteoporosis,
      99–103. *See also* Osteoporosis
  bone densitometry in, 49–52, 51t
  bone formation in, 107–109
  bone loss in, 10, 49–52, 75–76,
      105–106, 106t
      pattern and timing of, 99–100
  bone matrix in, 106–107
  bone resorption in, 105–106, 106t
  in children, 103
  dose effects in, 99
  epidemiology of, 99–103
  fractures in, 50, 50f, 100–103, 101f, 102f
  growth factors in, 108
  in juvenile dermatomyositis, 199
  lifestyle changes for, 50
  osteoblasts in, 107–109
  osteoclasts in, 105–106
  pathophysiology of, 105–109, 106t
  prevention and treatment of, 50, 51t,
      52, 103, 111–117. *See also*
          Osteoporosis therapy
      bisphosphonates in, 50, 51t, 52,
          112–114, 113f, 116, 168
      calcitonin in, 114, 139
      calcium in, 50, 52, 111–112, 112f
      cost effectiveness of, 116
      dehydroepiandrosterone in, 84
      estrogen in, 114, 115, 115f
      indications for, 50, 52
      parathyroid hormone in, 115, 168
      practice pattern variations in,
          115–116
      quality improvement in, 116
      selective estrogen receptor modula-
          tors in, 115
      teriparatide in, 115, 168
      testosterone in, 114
      thiazide diuretics in, 84, 115
      vitamin D in, 111–112, 112f
  in rheumatoid arthritis, 10, 49–50,
      75–76
  in systemic lupus erythematosus,
      80–81
Glycosaminoglycans, in aggrecan, 30, 30f
Gout, hyperparathyroidism and, 185, 186

GP-39/YKL-40, as cartilage degradation marker, 30f, 30t, 31–33
Gradient echo sequences, 60
Gradient recalled acquisition in steady state (GRASS) sequences, 60
Growth factors
    androgen effects on, 154–155, 155t
    glucocorticoid effects on, 108
Growth inhibition, glucocorticoid-induced, 102–103, 108, 109

**H**

Hallux valgus deformity, in fibrodysplasia ossificans progressiva, 201f, 202
Hand
    magnetic resonance imaging of, 54–57, 55t, 63
    radiography of, 54–57, 55t
Health insurance, for bone densitometry, 41
Heparin, bone loss from, 81, 120
Heterotopic ossification, 200–202, 201f
Hip
    in bone densitometry, 41. See also Bone densitometry
    fractures of. See Fractures
    osteoarthritis of, 91–92, 92f. See also Osteoarthritis
        estrogen for, 136
    osteonecrosis of, 192, 194f. See also Osteonecrosis
Home safety hazards, 131–132
Hormone replacement therapy, 134–136. See also Estrogen therapy; Osteoporosis therapy
    clinical studies of, 134–135
    declining use of, 134
    efficacy of, 134–135
    for fracture prevention, 134–135
    in glucocorticoid-induced osteoporosis, 114–115
    response to, biochemical markers of, 27–28, 285t
    for rheumatoid arthritis, 136
    in systemic lupus erythematosus, 83, 84
Human immunodeficiency virus infection, osteonecrosis in, 192
Hyaluronan, in aggrecan, 31
Hyaluronic acid, as cartilage degradation marker, 30f, 30t, 31
Hydroxychloroquine, for systemic lupus erythematosus, bone loss due to, 84
11β-Hydroxysteroid dehydrogenase, in glucocorticoid regulation, 108
Hydroxyvitamin D, in osteomalacia, 181, 182t
Hypercalcemia
    of malignancy, bisphosphonates for, 146
    metastatic calcification in, 199
    in primary hyperparathyroidism, 185, 188
    teriparatide-related, 163
Hyperparathyroidism
    bone remodeling in, 106

    primary, 185–189
        asymptomatic, 185, 187
        bone loss in, 187–188, 187f, 188f
        calcium pyrophosphate deposition disease and, 186
        clinical manifestations of, 185–186
        diagnosis of, 188–189, 189f
        gout and, 185, 186
        laboratory findings in, 185
        pseudogout and, 185, 186
        treatment of, 189
    secondary, in osteomalacia, 181, 182f, 183
Hyperphosphatemia, metastatic calcification in, 199
Hyperthyroidism, bone loss in, 121
Hyperuricemia, hyperparathyroidism and, 185, 186
Hypocalcemia, pseudogout and, 186
Hypogonadism
    glucocorticoid-induced, 106
    male osteoporosis and, 155, 156t, 163
Hypophosphatasia, 184
    metastatic calcification in, 199–200

**I**

Ibandronate, 143t, 144t, 146. See also Bisphosphonates
    for glucocorticoid-induced osteoporosis, 113–114
Idiopathic arterial calcification of infancy, 200
IL-1. See Interleukins
Immune system
    androgen effects on, 156
    in bone loss, 8–13, 75
    in bone metabolism, 4, 4f, 9, 9t, 11, 16–19, 18f, 19t, 75
    RANK/RANKL/OPG system and, 16, 75. See also RANK/RANKL/OPG system
    in rheumatoid arthritis, 11, 16–19, 18f, 19t, 75
Immunosuppressive therapy, for systemic lupus erythematosus, bone loss from, 81
Inactivity. See also Exercise
    bone loss and, 75
    in systemic lupus erythematosus, 80
Inflammatory bowel disease–related arthritis, bone loss in, 11–12
Inflammatory cytokines
    in bone loss, 8–13, 75
    in bone remodeling, 9
    in osteoclastogenesis, 17–18, 18f, 19t
    in rheumatoid arthritis, 11, 15, 75
    in spondyloarthropathies, 12
    in systemic lupus erythematosus, 80
Infliximab, for psoriatic arthritis, 89
Insulin-like growth factor (IGF)
    androgen effects on, 155, 155t
    glucocorticoid effects on, 108
Insurance coverage, for bone densitometry, 41
Interferon-γ, in osteoclastogenesis, 17–18, 18f, 19t
Interleukins

    androgen effects on, 155, 155t
    in bone loss, 17–18, 18f, 19t
    in osteoclastogenesis, 17–18, 18f, 19t
International Society for Clinical Densitometry, patient selection guidelines of, 40

**J**

Joint space narrowing. See also Bone loss; Radiographic progression
    in osteonecrosis, 192, 192f, 194f
    progression of, 125–126
    radiologic assessment of
        magnetic resonance imaging in, 61–65, 62f
        radiographic scoring systems in, 54–57, 55t
Juvenile dermatomyositis, 198–199, 199f
Juvenile idiopathic arthritis, focal bone erosions in, 19
Juvenile rheumatoid arthritis
    bone loss in, 12
    glucocorticoids for, 102–103
        bone loss/fractures and, 103
        growth effects of, 102–103

**K**

Kaye's scoring method, 55t, 56
Kellgren's scoring method, 54, 55t
Keratan sulfate, as cartilage degradation marker, 30–31, 30f, 30t
Kidney stones, in hyperparathyroidism, 185
Knee, osteoarthritis of, 92–93. See also Osteoarthritis
    estrogen for, 136
Kyphosis, 132

**L**

Larsen score, 54–56, 55t, 125
    modifications of, 55t, 56
Legg-Calvé-Perthes disease, 192
Letrozole, bone loss due to, 121
Looser's zones, 182–183, 182f
Low bone mass, definition of, 37
Lupus. See Systemic lupus erythematosus
Luteinizing hormone–releasing hormone agonists, bone loss due to, 121
Lymphocytes
    in bone loss, 16
    in osteoclastogenesis, 16

**M**

Macrophage–colony-stimulating factor (M-CSF), in osteoclastogenesis, 17–18, 18f, 19t
Macrophages, in bone resorption, 17
Magnetic resonance imaging (MRI), 59–65
    in osteoarthritis, 64–65
    in osteonecrosis, 193–194
    physical basis of, 59–60
    in rheumatoid arthritis, 60–64
        bony damage on, 60–63, 61f, 62f, 62t
        cartilage damage on, 61
        scanners for, 60

Magnetic resonance imaging (*continued*)
 scoring systems for, 61–64, 62t
 sequences in, 60
 signal acquisitions in, 60
 in spondyloarthropathies, 63–64
 T1/T2 relaxation time in, 60
 vs. conventional radiography, 63
Magnetic resonance scanners, 60
Male osteoporosis, 154–155, 156t, 163.
  *See also* Osteoporosis
Markers. *See* Biochemical markers
Matrix metalloproteinases (MMPs), in
  rheumatoid arthritis, 15
Matrix vesicles, 5–6
Medroxyprogesterone acetate, bone loss
  due to, 121
Men, osteoporosis in, 154–155, 156t,
  163. *See also* Osteoporosis
Menopause, bone loss after. *See also*
  Osteoporosis
 in rheumatoid arthritis, 10
Metastatic calcification, 197, 199–200
Methotrexate, bone loss due to, 76, 121
 in systemic lupus erythematosus, 81
Milkman's syndrome, 182
MRI. *See* Magnetic resonance imaging
  (MRI)
Myositis ossificans
 neurogenic, 201
 nontraumatic, 201
 traumatic, 201
Myositis ossificans progressiva, 201

**N**
Nasal calcitonin. *See* Calcitonin
National Health and Nutrition
  Educational Survey III (NHANES
  III), 37, 46
Neurogenic heterotopic ossification, 201
NF-κB, receptor for. *See*
  RANK/RANKL/OPG system
Notch genes, glucocorticoids and, 108
N-telopeptides (NTx), in bone turnover,
  27, 27f
 in osteoarthritis, 94, 94f
Nutrition counseling, for osteoporosis, 68

**O**
Obese patients, bone densitometry in,
  37–38
OPG. *See* Osteoprotegerin (OPG)
Oral contraceptives, in systemic lupus erythematosus, 136
Ossification, extraskeletal, 197, 198f,
  200–202, 200f
Osteitis fibrosa cystica, 185
Osteoarthritis
 biochemical markers in
  clinical utility of, 31–33, 32f
  in disease progression, 31–32, 32f
  in therapeutic monitoring, 32–33
  types of, 29–31, 30f, 30t
 bisphosphonates for, 147
 bone mass in, 91–95
 bone turnover in, 94, 94f
 cartilage defects in, magnetic resonance imaging of, 64–65

cartilage turnover in, biochemical
  markers of, 29–33, 30f, 30t, 32f
 estrogen for, 136
 exercise in, 131–132
 fractures in, 93–94
 of hip, 91–92, 92f
 of knee, 92–93
 radiologic assessment of
  magnetic resonance imaging in,
   64–65
  radiographic scoring in, 54–57, 55t
 rehabilitation in, 132
 subchondral trabecular bone in, 94
Osteoblasts, 5–6, 5f
 androgen effects on, 154, 155t
 characteristics of, 5, 5f
 fate of, 5–6
 functions of, 5–6
 glucocorticoid effects on, 107–109,
  107t
 origin of, 5
 precursors of, 5
Osteocalcin, in bone turnover, 26
 in osteoarthritis, 94
Osteochondritis dessicans, 191. *See also*
  Osteonecrosis
Osteochondrosis, 191. *See also*
  Osteonecrosis
Osteoclast(s), 4, 4f, 5f
 androgen effects on, 155
 in bone loss, in rheumatoid arthritis,
  16–18
 formation of, 15–16
 glucocorticoid effects on, 105–106,
  106t
 precursors of, 15–16
Osteoclast inhibitory factor. *See*
  Osteoprotegerin (OPG)
Osteoclastogenesis
 androgen effects on, 155
 glucocorticoid effects on, 105–106,
  106t
 inflammatory cytokines in, 16–18,
  18f, 19t, 75
 physiology of, 15–16, 75
 RANK/RANKL/OPG system in, 15–16,
  18f, 75, 170–171
Osteocytes, 6
 function of, 6
Osteogenesis, in ankylosing spondylitis,
  88–89
Osteogenesis imperfecta, intravenous
  pamidronate for, 146–147
Osteomalacia, 3, 181–184
 biopsy in, 183
 clinical manifestations of, 181
 diagnosis of, 181–183
 etiology of, 181, 182t
 radiologic findings in, 182–183, 182f,
  183f
 treatment of, 183–184
 tumor-induced, 184
Osteonecrosis, 191–195
 clinical manifestations of, 192
 diagnosis of, 192–194
 epidemiology of, 191
 etiology of, 191–192, 193t

 glucocorticoid-induced, 191, 192
 pathogenesis of, 191–192
 radiologic findings in, 192–194, 192f,
  194f
 staging of, 194, 194t
 terminology of, 191
 treatment of, 194–195
Osteopenia. *See also* Bone loss
 bone mineral density in, 37
 in osteomalacia, 182–183, 182f
Osteoporosis, 3. *See also* Bone loss
 in ankylosing spondylitis, 87–89
 biochemical markers in, 25–28
  clinical utility of, 27–28, 28f, 28t
  types of, 25–27, 26f, 26t
  variability in, 28
 bone mineral density in, 37
  biochemical markers of, 25–28
  in diagnosis, 49–50
  in disease monitoring, 50
  measurement of. *See* Bone densitometry
 bone remodeling in, 6
 calcitonin for, 138–140
 estrogen for, 134–136
 exercise in, 131–132
 fear of falling in, 67–68
 fractures in. *See* Fractures
 glucocorticoid-induced. *See*
  Glucocorticoid-induced osteoporosis
 lifestyle changes in, 50, 68
 male, 154–155, 156t, 163
 pathophysiology of, 155–156
 prevention and treatment of. *See*
  Osteoporosis therapy
 in psoriatic arthritis, 89
 psychological impact of, 67–68
 quality of life in, 67–69
 rehabilitation in, 132
 in rheumatoid arthritis, 9–11, 49–52,
  73–76. *See also* Rheumatoid arthritis, bone loss in
 risk assessment for, biochemical markers in, 27, 27f
 severity of, 37
 social impact of, 68
 in systemic lupus erythematosus,
  79–85. *See also* Systemic lupus erythematosus, osteoporosis in
Osteoporosis Assessment Questionnaire
  (OPAQ), 68–69
Osteoporosis therapy
 androgens in, 154–159, 156t, 157t
 bisphosphonates in, 141–147
 for glucocorticoid-induced osteoporosis,
  50, 51t, 52, 103, 111–117. *See also*
  Glucocorticoid-induced osteoporosis, prevention and treatment of
 for male osteoporosis, 154–155, 156t,
  163
 mechanism of action of, 26
 monitoring of, 25–26, 27–28, 28f, 28t
  bone mineral density in, 26,
   27–28, 28f, 28t, 29f, 46–47
  peripheral bone densitometry in,
   45–46

osteoprotegerin in, 171–172
for postmenopausal osteoporosis,
   141–146, 155–156, 157t, 162–163
recombinant parathyroid hormone
   for, 161–168
selective estrogen receptor modulators
   in, 150–153
teriparatide in, 161–168
Osteoprotegerin (OPG), 8–9, 9t, 75,
   170–172. *See also*
   RANK/RANKL/OPG system
   in bone homeostasis, 171
   glucocorticoids and, 106
   in immune response, 16
   in osteoclastogenesis, 16, 170–171,
      171f
   in psoriatic arthritis, 19
   in rheumatoid arthritis, 11, 16–19,
      19t, 75
   therapeutic uses of, 171–172
Osteosarcoma, in rats, teriparatide and,
   163
Osteotomy, for osteonecrosis, 195
Outcome measures
   focal bone erosion progression as, 64
   quality of life as, 68–69
Ovarian dysfunction, in systemic lupus
   erythematosus, 80, 81

**P**

Paget's disease of bone, 177–180
   calcitonin for, 139
   diagnosis of, 178
   epidemiology of, 177
   pamidronate for, 146
   signs and symptoms of, 177–178,
      178t
   tiludronate for, 145
   treatment of, 178–180
Pain management, 132
   calcitonin in, 139–140
   for complex regional pain syndrome,
      139–140
Pamidronate, 146. *See also*
   Bisphosphonates
   for ankylosing spondylitis, 147
   bone loss due to, 121
   for glucocorticoid-induced osteoporo-
      sis, 113
   for Paget's disease, 146, 179
   for psoriatic arthritis, 89
   for rheumatoid arthritis, 147
Parathyroidectomy
   hyperparathyroidism after, 186. *See
      also* Hyperparathyroidism, primary
   for primary hyperparathyroidism,
      188–189, 189t
Parathyroid hormone (PTH)
   endogenous
      bone loss and, 187–188
      elevated. *See also*
         Hyperparathyroidism
      differential diagnosis of, 188
      skeletal effects of, 161–162,
         187–188, 187f, 188f
   pharmacologic, 161–168
      adverse effects of, 163, 189

anabolic potential of, 164–165,
   187, 189
with bisphosphonates, 147,
   166–168
clinical studies of, 162–163
efficacy of, 162–163, 189
with estrogen, 167
for glucocorticoid-induced osteoporosis, 84, 106, 115, 115f, 168
mechanism of action of, 161–162
for primary hyperparathyroidism,
   188, 189
recombinant human, 161, 164
in sequential/combination therapy,
   165–167
skeletal effects of, 164–165, 188,
   189
for systemic lupus erythematosus,
   84
Parathyroid hormone–related peptide
   (PTHrP), in osteoclastogenesis,
   17–18, 18f, 19t, 106
Pathologic fractures. *See* Fractures
Patient education, in disease management, 68
Pediatric patients. *See also under* Juvenile
   bone densitometry in, 37, 38, 40–41
   dermatomyositis in, 198–199, 199f
   glucocorticoids in, 102–103, 108, 109
   osteonecrosis in, 192
Peripheral bone densitometry. *See* Bone
   densitometry, peripheral
Peripheral quantitative computer tomography (pQCT), 38. *See also*
   Quantitative computer tomography
   (QCT)
   indications for, 41, 45–47
   vs. central QCT, 41
Peroxisome proliferator activated receptor
   γ2 (PPARγ2), 172
   glucocorticoids in, 107
Phenobarbital, bone loss due to, 81, 120
Phenytoin, bone loss due to, 81, 120
Physical activity
   inadequate, bone loss and, 75
   in osteoarthritis, 131–132
   in osteoporosis, 68, 80, 131–132
   protective effects of, 68, 80
   in rheumatoid arthritis, 131–132
   in systemic lupus erythematosus, 80
Pilates exercises, 132
Plicamycin, for Paget's disease, 180
Pool therapy, 132
Posterioanterior spine, in bone densitom-
   etry, 41
Postmenopausal osteoporosis. *See*
   Osteoporosis
Posttraumatic heterotopic ossification, 201
PPARγ2, 172
   glucocorticoids in, 107
Predisone/prednisolone-induced bone
   loss. *See* Glucocorticoid-induced
   osteoporosis
Pregnancy, bisphosphonates in, 147
Prevention, definition of, 126–128
Prevent Recurrence of Osteoporotic
   Fracture (PROOF) study, 138–140

Primary hyperparathyroidism. *See*
   Hyperparathyroidism, primary
Procollagen peptides
   in bone turnover, 26
   in cartilage turnover, 30f, 30t, 31, 32
Progestin. *See* Hormone replacement
   therapy
Progressive osseous heteroplasia, 201
Pro-inflammatory cytokines. *See*
   Cytokines
PROOF study, 138–140
Prostaglandin E2, in osteoclastogenesis,
   16–18, 18f
Pseudoarthrosis, in ankylosing spondyli-
   tis, 88, 88f
Pseudofractures, in osteomalacia,
   182–183, 182f
Pseudogout, hyperparathyroidism and,
   185, 186
Pseudohyperparathyroidism, ectopic ossification in, 201
Pseudomalignant heterotopic ossification,
   201
Psoriatic arthritis
   bone loss in, 11–12, 89
   focal bone erosions in, 19
   fractures in, 89
   radiographic scoring systems for,
      54–57, 55t
Psychological impact, of osteoporosis,
   67–68
Pyridinoline crosslinks, in bone turnover,
   26

**Q**

Quality of life, in osteoporosis, 67–69
Quality of Life Questionnaire of the
   European Foundation for
   Osteoporosis (QUALEFFO), 68–69
Quantitative computer tomography
   (QCT), 35–36, 37–40. *See also*
   Bone densitometry
   central vs. peripheral, 41
   in children, 40–41
   in glucocorticoid-induced osteoporo-
      sis, 51
   indications for, 40, 41
   measurement sites in, 41
   peripheral, 38, 45–47
      indications for, 41, 45–47
      vs. central QCT, 41
   radiation dose in, 38, 38t
   3D, 38, 39f
   vs. DXA, 37–38
Quantitative ultrasound. *See also* Bone
   densitometry
   in bone density measurement, in glu-
      cocorticoid-induced osteoporosis,
      51

**R**

Radiation dose, in bone densitometry, 38,
   38t
Radiographic assessment, 53–58. *See also
   specific disorders and modalities*
   abnormalities detected on, 54
   film interpretation in, 128

Radiographic assessment (*continued*)
  scoring systems for, 54–57, 55t,
    125–126, 126f–128f
    advantages and disadvantages of, 55t
    assessing progression with, 57
    data analysis and reporting for, 57
    detailed, 56
    global, 54–56
    interobserver reliability of, 57
    observer number in, 57
    selection of, 55t, 56–57
    types of, 54–56, 55t
    vs. magnetic resonance imaging, 63
Radiographic progression, 125–129. *See
    also* Focal bone erosions; Joint
    space narrowing
  components of, 125–126
  in control populations, 128
  estimated yearly, 127f, 128
  meta-analyses on, 128–129
  pharmacologic inhibition of,
    125–129, 126f–128f
  quantification of, 126
  scoring systems for, 55t, 56, 125–126,
    126, 126f–128f
  treatment effects on, 128–129
Radionuclide bone scan
  in osteomalacia, 183, 183f
  in osteonecrosis, 193
Raloxifene, 150, 151–152. *See also*
    Selective estrogen receptor modula-
    tors (SERMs)
  with bisphosphonates, 143, 152
  clinical trials of, 151–152
  duration of therapy with, 152
  efficacy of, 151–152
  indications for, 151–152
  nonskeletal effects of, 152
  with parathyroid hormone, 166–167
  for primary hyperparathyroidism, 189
  side effects of, 152
  in systemic lupus erythematosus, 84
RAMRIS scoring system, 62–63
RANK/RANKL/OPG system, 4, 4f, 9, 9t,
    75
  in bone homeostasis, 171
  glucocorticoids and, 106
  in immune response, 16, 75
  in osteoclastogenesis, 16–17, 18f, 75,
    170–171, 171f
  in psoriatic arthritis, 19, 89
  in rheumatoid arthritis, 11, 16–19,
    18f, 19t, 75
Ratingen score, 55t, 56
Reactive arthritis, bone loss in, 11–12
Receptor activator for NF-κB. *See*
    RANK/RANKL/OPG system
Recombinant human parathyroid hor-
    mone, 161, 164. *See also*
    Parathyroid hormone (PTH), phar-
    macologic
5-alpha-Reductase, 154
Reference databases, for bone densitome-
    try, 36–37, 46
Reflex sympathetic dystrophy, 139–140
Rehabilitation, exercise programs in,
    131–132

Renal calculi, in hyperparathyroidism,
    185
Renal osteodystrophy, bisphosphonates
    for, 142
Rheumatic disorders, bone loss in, 8–13.
    *See also* Bone loss; Osteoporosis
Rheumatoid arthritis
  androgens for, 156–159, 158t
  angiogenesis in, 12
  biochemical markers in, 28–33
    clinical utility of, 31–33, 32f
    in disease progression, 31–32, 32f
    in therapeutic monitoring, 32–33
    types of, 29–31, 30f, 30t
  bisphosphonates for, 147
  bone loss in, 9–11, 73–76
    androgens for, 156–159, 158t
    glucocorticoid-induced, 10, 49–50,
      49–52, 75–76
    magnetic resonance imaging of,
      60–64
    osteoclasts and, 16–18, 18f
    pathogenesis of, 15–20, 74–76,
      156–158
    radiographic scoring for, 54–57,
      55t
  bone mass in
    determinants of, 10
    osteoclasts in, 16–18
  bone remodeling in, 9–11
  cartilage turnover in, biochemical
    markers of, 29–33, 30f, 30t, 32f
  dehydroepiandrosterone for, 156–159,
    158t
  estrogen for, 136
  exercise in, 131–132
  focal bone erosions in, 16–18, 18f
    magnetic resonance imaging of,
      60–64, 61, 62f, 62t
    osteoclasts and, 16–18, 18f
    radiographic scoring of, 54–57, 55t
  fractures in, 74–76, 156
    glucocorticoid-related, 100–103,
      101f, 102f
  glucocorticoids for
    bone loss and, 10, 49–50, 75–76,
      99–103. *See also* Glucocorticoid-
      induced osteoporosis
    fractures and, 100–103, 101f, 102f
  joint space narrowing in
    magnetic resonance imaging of, 61,
      62f, 62t
    radiographic scoring systems for,
      54–57, 56t
  lymphocytes in, 16–17
  osteoclastogenesis in, 16–18, 18f
  radiologic assessment in
    magnetic resonance imaging in,
      59–64, 61f, 62f, 62t. *See also*
      Magnetic resonance imaging
      (MRI)
    radiographic scoring in, 54–57, 55t
  RANK/RANKL/OPG system in, 11,
    16–19, 18f, 19t, 75
  rehabilitation in, 132
Rickets, 3, 181–184. *See also* Osteomalacia
Risedronate. *See also* Bisphosphonates

  for geriatric patients, 147
  for glucocorticoid-induced osteoporo-
    sis, 113–114, 113f
  for osteoarthritis, 147
  for Paget's disease, 179
Rolfing, 132
Romanus lesions, 88

**S**
Safety precautions, 131–132
Scanners, magnetic resonance, 60
Scleroderma, 199
Scoliosis
  bone densitometry in, 38
  bone mineral density in, 38, 39f, 39t
  T scores in, 38, 39t
Scoring systems
  quality of life, for osteoporosis, 68–69
  radiologic
    magnetic resonance imaging,
      61–64, 62t
    radiographic, 54–57, 55t, 125–126,
      126f. *See also* Radiographic
      assessment, scoring systems for
Selective estrogen receptor modulators
    (SERMs), 150–153. *See also*
    Osteoporosis therapy
  with bisphosphonates, 152
  clinical trials of, 151–152
  efficacy of, 151–152
  in glucocorticoid-induced osteoporo-
    sis, 115, 151–152
  indications for, 151–152
  mechanism of action of, 150
  response to, biochemical markers of,
    27–28, 285t
  in systemic lupus erythematosus, 83,
    151–152
Sharp's scoring method, 55t, 56, 126,
    126f
  modifications of, 55t, 56
Short erosion scale, 55t, 56
Short tau inversion recovery (STIR)
    sequences, 60
Signal acquisitions, in magnetic reso-
    nance imaging, 60
Simple erosion narrowing score, 55t, 56
Single energy photon absorptiometry
    (SPA), 35–36. *See also* Bone densit-
    ometry
Single energy x-ray absorptiometry (SXA),
    36. *See also* Bone densitometry
Skeletal alkaline phosphatase, in osteo-
    porosis, 27, 27f
Skeletal growth
  androgen effects on, 154–155, 155t
  glucocorticoid effects on, 102–103, 108
Social impact, of osteoporosis, 68
Spinal disease, degenerative, bone miner-
    al density measurement in, 38
Spinal fractures. *See* Vertebral compres-
    sion fractures
Spine, in bone densitometry, 41. *See also*
    Bone densitometry
Spoiled gradient recalled acquisition in
    steady state (GRASS) sequences, 60
Spondyloarthropathies

angiogenesis in, 12
bone loss in, 11–12, 87–89
magnetic resonance imaging in, 63–64. *See also* Magnetic resonance imaging (MRI)
Spongy bone, 3, 4f
Src tyrosine kinase, 172
Steinbrocker index, 54, 55t
Steroids. *See* Glucocorticoid(s)
STIR sequences, 60
Subchondral trabecular bone, in osteoarthritis, 94
Sulfasalazine, bone loss and, 76
Systemic lupus erythematosus
  bone loss in, 12
  bone mineral density in, 79
  osteonecrosis in, 191
  osteoporosis in, 12, 80–85
    dehydroepiandrosterone for, 157–158
    epidemiology of, 79
    estrogen for, 135–136
    evaluation of, 81–82, 82f
    fractures in, 79–80i
    glucocorticoid-induced, 80–81
    prevention of, 82–84, 82f
    progression of, 79–80
    risk factors for, 80–81
    treatment of, 82–84, 82f
    treatment-related, 80–81
  ovarian dysfunction in, 80, 81

**T**

T1/T2 weighted spin-echo sequences, 59–65
Tacrolimus, bone loss due to, 121
Tai chi, 132
Tamoxifen, 150–151, 150–153. *See also* Selective estrogen receptor modulators (SERMs)
  in systemic lupus erythematosus, 84
T cells, in osteoclastogenesis, 16
Telopeptides
  in bone turnover, 27
    in osteoarthritis, 94, 94f
    in cartilage turnover, 30f, 30t, 31, 32
Teratogenicity, of teriparatide, 163
Teriparatide, 161–168. *See also* Parathyroid hormone (PTH), pharmacologic
  adverse effects of, 163
  clinical studies of, 162–163
  efficacy of, 162–163
  for glucocorticoid-induced osteoporosis, 115, 115f, 168
  indications for, 165
  for male osteoporosis, 163
  osteosarcoma and, 163
  for postmenopausal osteoporosis, 162–163
  in sequential/combination therapy, 165–166
  skeletal effects of, 164–165
Testosterone. *See also* Androgen(s)
  immunosuppressive effects of, 157–158

pharmacologic
  with estrogen, 155–156
  indications for, 155
  for male osteoporosis, 155, 156t
  for postmenopausal osteoporosis, 155–156, 157t
  for rheumatoid arthritis, 156–159, 158t
  safety of, 155
  skeletal effects of, 154–155, 155t
Tetracycline-labeled bone biopsy, in osteomalacia, 183
TGF-β. *See* Transforming growth factor (TGF-β)
Therapeutic monitoring, 25–26, 27–28, 28f, 28t, 46–47
Thiazide diuretics, for glucocorticoid-induced osteoporosis, 84, 115
Thyroid hormone, bone loss due to, 120–121
Tiludronate, 145. *See also* Bisphosphonates
  for Paget's disease, 179
TNF-α. *See* Tumor necrosis factor-α
Toremifene, 150–153. *See also* Selective estrogen receptor modulators (SERMs)
  in systemic lupus erythematosus, 84
Transforming growth factor (TGF-β), in osteoclastogenesis, 17–18, 18f, 19t
Traumatic heterotopic ossification, 201
T scores
  in central vs. peripheral densitometry, 45–47, 46f
  for children, 40–41
  fracture risk and, 47
  in scoliosis, 38, 39t
  in vertebral body compression, 38, 39t
Tumoral calcinosis, 200, 200f
Tumor-induced osteomalacia, 184
Tumor necrosis factor-α (TNF-α)
  in bone loss, 17–18, 18f, 19t
    in ankylosing spondylitis, 87
    in osteoclastogenesis, 17–18, 18f, 19t
Type I collagen, glucocorticoid effects on, 106–107
Type II collagen, in cartilage turnover, 30t, 31, 31f
Type III collagen amino (N) propeptides, as cartilage degradation markers, 30f, 30t, 31–33

**U**

Ultrasound, quantitative. *See also* Bone densitometry
  in bone density measurement, in glucocorticoid-induced osteoporosis, 51
Urate, elevated serum, hyperparathyroidism and, 186

**V**

Valproic acid, bone loss due to, 81, 120
Van der Heijde's scoring method, 55t, 56
Vascular endothelial growth factor (VEGF)
  in osteoclastogenesis, 17–18, 18f, 19t

in rheumatoid arthritis, 12
in spondyloarthropathies, 12
Vertebrae
  in bone densitometry, 41. *See also* Bone densitometry
  codfish, 183
  lesions of, in osteomalacia, 182–183, 182f
Vertebral body compression
  bone mineral density and, 38, 39f, 39t
  T scores in, 38, 39t
Vertebral compression fractures. *See also* Fractures
  in ankylosing spondylitis, 11–12
  back pain in, 132
  exercises for, 132
  glucocorticoid-related, 50, 50f
  in hyperparathyroidism, 187–188
  management of, 132
  risk of, bone mineral density and, 38–40
  silent, 132
Vinculin, glucocorticoids and, 107
Vitamin D, supplemental
  in glucocorticoid therapy, 111–112, 112f
  guidelines for, 183–184
  in osteomalacia, 183–184
  in systemic lupus erythematosus, 83
Vitamin D deficiency
  in osteomalacia, 181, 182t
  prevention and treatment of, 183–184
  in systemic lupus erythematosus, 80
Vitamin D resistance, in glucocorticoid-induced osteoporosis, 105–106

**W**

Walking programs, 132
Water therapy, 132

**X**

X-ray films. *See* Radiographic assessment

**Y**

YKL-40, as cartilage degradation marker, 30f, 30t, 31–33
Yoga, 132

**Z**

Zolendronate, 146. *See also* Bisphosphonates
  bone loss due to, 121
  for glucocorticoid-induced osteoporosis, 113
  for hypercalcemia of malignancy, 146
Z scores, 37
  for children, 40